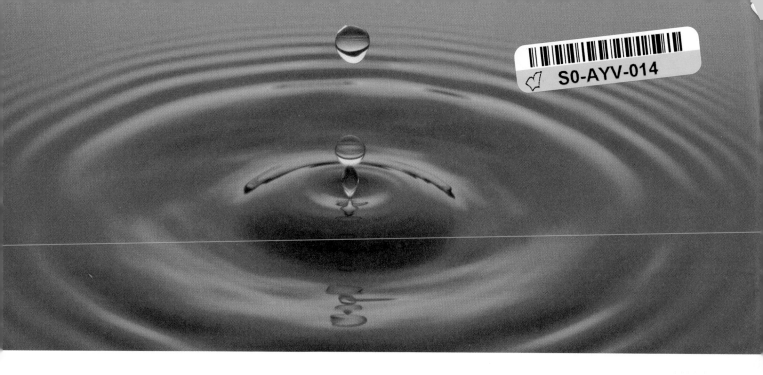

Natural Spa and Hydrotherapy
Theory and Practice

ANN L. MIHINA, LMT
Massage School Director, Providence Institute, Tucson, AZ

SANDRA K. ANDERSON, BA, LMT, NCTMB
Tucson Touch Therapies, Tucson, AZ

Pearson

Boston   Columbus   Indianapolis   New York   San Francisco   Upper Saddle River
Amsterdam   Cape Town   Dubai   London   Madrid   Milan   Munich   Paris   Montreal   Toronto
Delhi   Mexico City   Sao Paulo   Sydney   Hong Kong   Seoul   Singapore   Taipei   Tokyo

Library of Congress Cataloging-in-Publication Data

Mihina, Ann L.
  Natural spa and hydrotherapy : theory and practice / Ann L. Mihina,
Sandra K. Anderson. — 1st ed.
    p. ; cm.
Includes bibliographical references and index.
ISBN-13: 978-0-13-174471-4
ISBN-10: 0-13-174471-2
1. Hydrotherapy. 2. Health resorts. I. Anderson, Sandra Kauffman. II. Title.
  [DNLM: 1. Hydrotherapy. 2. Health Resorts. WB 520 M636n 2010]
  RM811.M54 2010
  615.8'53—dc22
                                                              2008053882

Publisher: Julie Levin Alexander
Publisher's Assistant: Regina Bruno
Executive Editor: Mark Cohen
Associate Editor: Melissa Kerian
Assistant Editor: Nicole Ragonese
Senior Media Editor: Amy Peltier
Development Editor: Stephanie Kelly, Triple SSS Media Development
Managing Production Editor: Patrick Walsh
Production Liaison: Yagnesh Jani
Production Editor: Bruce Hobart, Pine Tree Composition, Inc.
Manufacturing Manager: Ilene Sanford
Manufacturing Buyer: Pat Brown
Senior Art Director: Maria Guglielmo-Walsh
Photographer: Haskell Photography
Interior/Cover Designer: Ilze Lemesis
Director of Marketing: Karen Allman
Executive Marketing Manager: Katrin Beacom
Marketing Specialist: Michael Sirinides
Marketing Assistant: Judy Noh
Media Project Manager: Lorena Cerisano
Manager, Rights and Permissions: Zina Arabia
Manager, Visual Research: Beth Brenzel
Manager, Cover Visual Research & Permissions: Karen Sanatar
Image Permission Coordinator: Vicki Menanteaux
Composition: Pine Tree Composition, Inc.
Printer/Binder: Courier Companies, Inc.
Cover Printer: Lehigh-Phoenix
Cover Photos: Amy Haskell

Credits and acknowledgments borrowed from other sources and reproduced, with permission, in this textbook appear on the appropriate pages within text.

Pearson® is a registered trademark of Pearson plc

Pearson Education, Ltd., London
Pearson Education Singapore, Pte. Ltd.
Pearson Education, Canada, Inc.
Pearson Education—Japan
Pearson Education Australia PTY, Limited

Pearson Education North Asia Ltd., Hong Kong
Pearson Educación de Mexico, S.A. de C.V.
Pearson Education Malaysia, Pte. Ltd.
Pearson Education, Upper Saddle River, New Jersey

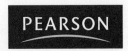

10 9 8 7 6 5 4 3 2 1
ISBN-13: 978-0-13-174471-4
ISBN-10: 0-13-174471-2

Dedication

This book is dedicated to my entire loving family. With special thanks to

Grandma Ding—she inspired and encouraged my passion for bodywork and natural healing

My mother, Marian, and my father, Ralph—they taught me love and compassion for others

My beautiful sisters, Mary, Barbara, Nancy, and my late sister, Joan—their wisdom, love, and encouragement have always been there when I've needed it

In loving memory of my late husband, Michael—he taught me what true strength is

My children who are, and always will be, the very center of my life—Christopher, Katie and Matt, Mike and Karen, and my most adorable granddaughters, Zoe Rose and Lily Bean

—Ann L. Mihina

This book is dedicated to my family and friends

David Kent Anderson—my husband, my wellspring of inspiration

My friends Annie Gordon, Carol Davis, Garnet Adair, Jeanie Hayes, and Annette Desmarais—they keep me laughing and keep me grounded

—Sandra K. Anderson

Things should be made as simple as possible, but not any simpler.

—Albert Einstein

Contents

It is a wholesome and necessary thing for us to turn again to the earth and in the contemplation of her beauties to know of wonder and humility.—Rachel Carson, American marine biologist, nature writer, and author of *Silent Spring*

Preface

In recent years, the spa industry has experienced unprecedented growth. Going to spas has become a mainstream activity, with a focus on health as well as beauty. The number of consumer visits to spas has steadily increased, and consumers have also become more knowledgeable about treatment options. They are demanding the most current treatments, the best-quality products, and the most skillful treatment performance. Additionally, some consumers, instead of going to a spa, look to massage therapists and bodyworkers in private practice for spa and hydrotherapy treatments for stress reduction and health maintenance.

Today's culture focuses on "green," or natural, trends. People are concerned about having as minimal an impact on the environment as possible, and the spa and massage and bodywork professions are no exception. Spa guests and bodywork clients want to know what is in the products being applied to their bodies and how these products are made. They are choosing natural or green substances over chemically processed preparations, and they are choosing natural therapies in addition to allopathic methods for health and healing.

All of these developments have resulted in a need for highly educated practitioners of spa and hydrotherapy treatments. Practitioners not only need to know about the treatments themselves—what substances to use; what equipment is needed; how to perform them; and their benefits, indications, contraindications, and cautions—they also need to know how to assist guests and clients in choosing the best treatments, how to answer questions knowledgeably, and how to convey the natural basis of spa and hydrotherapy treatments to contemporary consumers.

Natural Spa and Hydrotherapy: Theory and Practice does just that. This text can be used for spa training as well as for skill enhancement for individual therapists. It will assist instructors and students of massage and bodywork as well as practitioners in spa settings and private practice who have the desire to increase their knowledge and understanding of, and competency in, natural spa and hydrotherapy.

Further, students sometimes are not prepared for the work environment of the spa and may have unrealistic expectations. To help students become more informed, *Natural Spa and Hydrotherapy: Theory and Practice* discusses what it means to work in a spa in a clear and direct manner.

The text is easy to read and offers numerous pedagogical features that support learning and information retention and increase interest in the subject matter. Readers are encouraged to make the information their own through various activities and are supported in integrating the subject matter into their own experience. Since most spa and massage and bodywork practitioners learn by doing, there are basic treatment protocols to follow as well as suggestions for readers to design their own personal, unique methods.

FROM CONCEPT TO REALITY

Many years ago, both Ann L. Mihina's and Sandra K. Anderson's primary massage education included a course in hydrotherapy. Although they had attended the same school but at different times, both had found the hydrotherapy course to be tremendously rewarding. It was fascinating, tactile, historic, and useful all at the same time. Sandra could not believe how such simple methods could effect positive change in the body so easily; Ann realized that many of the methods were similar to the ones her German grandmother, Grandma Ding, had shown her. There was no required text for this course. Instead, a series of instruction sheets were used, sheets that had been handed down from instructor to instructor.

As time went on, both Sandra and Ann became bodywork educators as well as private practitioners. Since they taught at the same school, they were colleagues who were not only friends, but who also had a great deal of respect for each other. With her background in biology, Sandra focused on the sciences—anatomy, physiology, kinesiology, and pathology. She also developed an interest and received training in shiatsu and Thai massage and taught courses in shiatsu theory and technique. As an instructor, then Anatomy and Physiology department head, then director of education, Sandra not only taught, she also developed curricula, wrote lesson plans, designed practical and written tests, and oversaw faculty.

Ann instructed massage technique classes and, over time, became the hydrotherapy instructor. A pivotal point in her career occurred when she became a Certified Kneipp and Hydrotherapy Spa Therapist. This helped her understand how the traditional methods of hydrotherapy have a modern context and how it would be possible to make these "old methods" meaningful for new practitioners. Ann branched into spa work and developed entry-level as well as continuing education courses in spa techniques, aromatherapy, and hot and cold stones.

During this time, Ann had greatly improved and consolidated course information, but the material was still in handout form; there was not yet a definitive text on spa and hydrotherapy techniques. There were a few books available, and although they were valuable for historical information and "tried and true" hydrotherapy treatments, they had been published quite a while ago and did not contain up-to-date information. In order to be as timely as possible, Ann had to conduct continual searches for spa and hydrotherapy information, which was a time-consuming and sometimes frustrating process.

Meanwhile, Sandra (with her husband) opened a center that offered continuing education courses for massage therapists and other bodyworkers. Ann's spa, hydrotherapy, and hot and cold stone courses were featured and proved immensely popular. Sandra conducted continuing education courses in Asian bodywork techniques and also had the opportunity to co-author (with Susan Salvo) the first edition of *Pathology for Massage Therapists* and to author *The Practice of Shiatsu*. Because of her writing experience, she was asked by Pearson if she could write a text on spa techniques.

Sandra immediately asked Ann to be a co-author. Both realized what a tremendous impact this text could have—namely, people who perform spa and hydrotherapy treatments could now be considered educated professionals.

Ann and Sandra both agreed that the text should not only be about spa but should also include hydrotherapy, and it should cover not only spa settings but also have information for private practitioners who want to augment their treatment menus with spa and hydrotherapy. The authors also determined that there needed to be a blending of science and technique, historical and present-day information, current trends and time-proven methodologies. With these ideas in mind, Ann and Sandra got to work, and the result is *Natural Spa and Hydrotherapy: Theory and Practice*.

ORGANIZATION

The eight chapters of *Natural Spa and Hydrotherapy: Theory and Practice* present core material necessary for massage and bodywork students, spa practitioners, and practitioners in private practice to successfully learn and integrate spa and hydrotherapy information and techniques. The selection of information is based on current trends in the spa and bodywork professions, competency requirements from the Commission on Massage Therapy Accreditation (COMTA), and requirements for National Certification in Therapeutic Massage and Bodywork (NCTMB).

The text starts with the history of spa and hydrotherapy, the science behind spa and hydrotherapy, and crucial components of spa practice. Hydrotherapy is discussed in its own chapter. Other types of spa treatments, based on natural therapeutics—exfoliations, pelotherapy, thalassotherapy, and aromatherapy—are covered in individual chapters. Within each chapter is a brief history of the natural therapeutic to give readers a context on how it formed and developed through the ages and how the therapeutics can be used in various treatment protocols, including rationale, benefits, indications, contraindications, cautions, equipment and supplies, preparation, procedure, after-treatment care, and hygiene. Appendices on poultices and Ayurveda, as well as resources, answers to multiple choice questions from each chapter, references, and a glossary have been included to round out important and necessary information.

Chapter 1, "History of Spa and Hydrotherapy," is centered on the idea that spa is not a new concept even though it may seem to be, and, by the same token, hydrotherapy is not just "folk medicine" even though it may seem to be. The progression of spa and bodywork throughout the ages is discussed, as well as the scientific advances and contributions of prominent figures. Different types of treatments are introduced as well as descriptions of different types of spas.

Chapter 2, "The Science Behind Spa and Hydrotherapy," is included because an understanding of how the body works, and how spa and hydrotherapy treatments affect the body, lends validity to the spa, massage, and bodywork professions. Basic chemistry, the flow of body fluids, the systems of the body, and thermoregulation are covered, as well as the physiological impact of spa and hydrotherapy treatments on the body.

Chapter 3, "Elements of Practice," gives basic, realistic information necessary for a successful practice, whether in a spa or private office setting. Clear communication with clients, what it means to work in a spa, universal precautions, hygiene and sanitation, indications, contraindications, methods to help clients choose the best treatments, and considerations for incorporating spa and hydrotherapy treatments into a bodywork practice are all included.

Chapter 4, "Hydrotherapy," encompasses the realm of treatments that have water as their basis. The properties of water; effects and variables of hydrotherapy; benefits; indications; contraindications; and considerations for hot, cold, and alternating (hot and cold) applications are all discussed. Basic hydrotherapy treatment procedures are outlined. The benefits of baths and showers at certain temperatures are covered as well as inhalation treatments, steam baths, and saunas. The chapter finishes with descriptions of Watsu®, Aquatic Massage, and Water Dance.

Chapter 5, "Exfoliation," explains what exfoliation is and discusses the benefits it has on the body. Both manual and chemical, also known as enzyme or dissolving, exfoliations are covered. Treatment protocols for full body and quick-prep dry brushing, manual exfoliations using natural substances, including salt and sugar glows, and how to perform enzyme exfoliations using natural substances are discussed.

Chapter 6, "Pelotherapy," distinguishes among the different types of pelotherapy and explains the therapeutic properties of muds, clays, peats, earth salts, paraffin, and geothermal therapy. Treatment protocols for mud or peat body wraps; mud, peat, or clay masks; earth salt glows; paraffin applications; and hot and cold stone therapy are included.

Chapter 7, "Thalassotherapy," discusses the various elements of thalassotherapy—seawater, seaweed, sea mud, and sea salt. Treatment protocols for seaweed, other algae, or sea mud body wraps and masks, as well as sea salt glow, are included.

Chapter 8, "Aromatherapy and Herbs," explains what essential oils are, how they are extracted, and how they affect the body. Included are precautions for working with essential oils, how to tell if an essential oil is pure, and how to store essential oils. There is discussion of the characteristics, uses, and cautions of ten foundational essential oils practitioners can purchase as a "starter set," as well as ten additional essential oils practitioners may want to purchase. Ways to use essential oils in a spa or private practice are outlined. The effects of common herbs on the body, how to make and use an herbal infusion, and treatment protocols for herbal wraps complete the chapter.

Appendix 1, "Poultices," explains what poultices are, gives a brief history of their use, and explains the link between these "folk remedies" and modern-day body wraps. Various types of poultices, their benefits and cautions for use, and how to apply them to the body are described.

Appendix 2, "Ayurveda," explains what Ayurveda is, gives a brief history of its development and principles, and outlines some basic Ayurvedic treatment procedures.

Appendix 3, "Resources," gives readers a comprehensive list of resources for further study and information. Topics include Equipment and Supplies, Spa Location Search Sites, Business and Marketing, Associations, Treatment Clinics, Schools and Programs of Study, Publications, and Research.

Appendix 4, "Answers to Multiple Choice Questions," has the answers to the Study Questions at the end of each chapter.

Appendix 5, "References," is a compilation of all the references used in writing this text.

FEATURES

Each chapter has a number of pedagogical features designed to help readers generate interest in the material, retain information, and integrate the knowledge into their own experience. What follows is a list of the features and how readers can use them as sign posts as they negotiate each chapter:

Chapter Learning Objectives

Each chapter-opening page contains measurable objectives for the reader. Each objective allows the reader to identify the key goals and what information should be studied thoroughly. Readers can use these as a checklist for recall of important information. Student readers can use the objectives in preparation for exams.

Key Terms

When key terms are initially introduced and defined within the text, they are boldfaced to highlight their importance. Readers can watch for these bolded key terms, knowing that they point to useful information.

Treatment Boxes

To ensure clarity of information, all the treatment protocols are set apart in individual boxes within the text. Within the treatment box are Rationale, Indications, Contraindications, Equipment and Supplies, Preparation, Procedure, After the Treatment, and Hygiene. Readers can be assured that the information they need for any given procedure is contained in one place and that they will not have to hunt through the text.

Clinical Alert Boxes

Clinical Alert boxes contain essential cautionary information readers need as they prepare for and perform treatments.

Did You Know?

Did You Know margin notes appear throughout each chapter and contain information designed to add more interest to a particular subject matter.

To Get You Started

To Get You Started boxes are found throughout Chapters 4 through 8 and contain recipes for various treatment substances and applications that readers can try. The recipes are designed to stimulate creativity and can be used by readers as tools for designing their own treatment menus.

Chapter Summaries

Summaries at the end of each chapter provide an overview of major topics and information discussed. Readers can use these as quick references and for quick searches of the material presented in the chapter.

Activities

Activities at the end of each chapter contain questions designed to stimulate readers' retention of the material presented in the chapter. Readers are also encouraged to receive treatments presented in the chapters, perform assessments of these treatments, and formulate the improvements they would make. Other activities are designed to support readers in thinking about the material presented in the chapter in new and different ways.

Study Questions

The study questions are in the traditional multiple-choice format. Readers can use these as a method to retain the information presented in the chapter. Student readers can use these to prepare for exams.

Case Samples

Case samples are found at the end of Chapters 4 through 8. They are drawn from real-life experiences and are de-signed to be situations readers are likely to encounter. Critical-thinking skills are enhanced when readers decide which questions the client should be asked; determine which treatment would be best for the client; and delineate the rationale, equipment and supplies, indications, contraindications, preparation, after-treatment care, and hygiene for the treatment.

Instructor Resources

The instructor's manual for *Natural Spa and Hydrotherapy: Theory and Practice* includes learning objectives, key terms, content outlines, teaching tips, classroom activities, classroom discussion questions, and worksheets designed to stimulate student creativity and critical thinking skills for each chapter. Suggestions on how instructors can create practical examinations for the techniques presented throughout the text are also included. Additionally, there is a test bank with multiple choice, fill-in-the-blank, true/false, and short answer questions that instructors can use in constructing written classroom examinations. PowerPoint slides for each chapter round out the supplements package, helping instructors to prepare for class by providing presentation notes and figures from the book.

About the Authors

Ann L. Mihina, LMT, Certified Kneipp Hydrotherapy and Spa Therapist, graduated in 1994 from the Desert Institute of the Healing Arts in Tucson, AZ, with certification in massage therapy. Ann has written curriculum for and taught foundation courses in massage therapy, hydrotherapy, aromatherapy, and spa techniques at the Desert Institute of the Healing Arts (now Cortiva Institute–Tucson) and the Providence Institute in Tucson, AZ, for more than ten years. Additionally, she presents continuing education workshops in hydrotherapy and spa treatments that she has developed, such as her Desert Spa series, Lotions and Potions I and II, Hot and Cold Stone Massage, and her Thermodynamic series. She is a consultant and maintains a private practice in massage, hydrotherapy and spa treatments, and hot and cold stone therapy and is currently the Massage School Director at the Providence Institute in Tucson, AZ.

Sandra K. Anderson, BA, LMT, NCTMB, graduated with a BA in biology from Ithaca College in Ithaca, NY. She went on to graduate from the Desert Institute of the Healing Arts in 1991 with certification in massage therapy, in 1999 with certification in zen shiatsu, and in 2002 with certification in Thai massage. She taught classes at the Desert Institute of the Healing Arts (now Cortiva Institute–Tucson) in Tucson, AZ, for twelve years in anatomy, physiology, kinesiology, pathology, and shiatsu theory techniques, and she supervised massage and shiatsu student clinics and was head of the Anatomy and Physiology Department for five years. From 2006 to 2007, Sandra was the director of education at Cortiva Institute–Tucson During her time as instructor, department head, and director of education, she developed curriculum for all program courses, which included designing course outlines, syllabi, learning objectives, and lesson plans. She also taught instructor training programs that included workshops on teaching classes on classroom management; test writing; and developing course outlines, syllabi, learning objectives, and lesson plans. Sandra observed instructors during class, gave feedback to strengthen teaching skills; and identified possible new instructors.

Additionally, Sandra is co-author of the first edition of *Pathology for Massage Therapists* and author of *The Practice of Shiatsu*. She is on the board of the Arizona chapter of the American Massage Therapy Association, was a member of the National Certification Board for Therapeutic Massage and Bodywork's Examination Committee from 1999 to 2006, and was chair of the Examination Committee from 2001 to 2006.

Currently, Sandra is focusing on writing and maintaining her practice at Tucson Touch Therapies in Tucson, AZ, a private massage practice she and her husband, David, own. Tucson Touch Therapies has eleven treatment rooms and thirty independent contractors who perform integrated massage therapies, Asian bodywork therapies, and energy therapies. More information can be found at www.tucsontouchtherapies.com.

Acknowledgments

- A special thank you to Amy Haskell—a phenomenal photographer with a true artist's eye
- Stephanie Kelly—for her invaluable collaboration, stores of information, and extraordinary attention to detail
- Michaela Johnson—for her amazing editing and ability to get right to the point
- Todd Edwards, Jenny Mendoza, Dave Nelson, Jillian Balda, Katie Mihina, Jan Neubauer, Jacque Pierce, Dana Mohaupt, Megan Dickinson, David Adix, Donna Goodheart, Keith and Mindy McDaniel, Jeff and Pam Haskell—models who graciously gave their time
- Dave Nelson—whose professionalism and hard work are inspiring
- David Adix—who radiates love and keeps us laughing
- Megan Dickinson, Yvonne Esker, Jesseca Maglothin, and all the tireless teaching assistants and colleagues who always made the job a lot less work and a lot more fun
- Patricia Warne, Gloria Gomez, Judy Moses, Patti McNulty, Mary Nelson—colleagues who share the passion
- All of our fellow instructors—we've only been as good as our sustaining network
- All of our students through the years—they have taught us more than they'll ever know
- Jenny and Noah Providence—for their patience, support, and encouragement
- Jeff and Pam Haskell—for the use of their beautiful home and lush desert property
- Keith and Mindy McDaniel—for the use of their Watsu® and aquatic massage facilities
- Tom Borland—for the use of Touch of Tranquility
- Margaret Avery Moon—for her friendship, support, and dedication to the massage and bodywork profession
- Diane Trieste—for her expertise and knowledge of the spa industry
- German and Sissi Schleinkofer, Kneipp Schule, Bad Worshofen, Bavaria—they taught Ann's first formal Kneipp workshop and continue to bring the magic of Kneipp to the United States
- Dr. Jonathon Paul de Vierville—he inspired Ann's passion for the history of spa and hydrotherapy treatments and helped forge the integration of spa and hydrotherapy with massage and bodywork
- Tucson Touch Therapies—all the wonderful practitioners and staff make going to work a joy for Sandra
- Sue Kauffman—Sandra's beautiful, intelligent and very capable sister as well as friend
- Mark Cohen and Melissa Kerian—for giving us this opportunity, and for their support and guidance
- Dwight Yoakam—whose music provided a backdrop when Sandra needed to get crucial writing done
- We'd also like to acknowledge each other for shared teamwork, encouragement, and workload (and for remaining friends!) through the long process of writing this book.

When you drink the water, remember the spring.
—Chinese proverb

Reviewer List

Chantel Anstine
Rasmussen College
Brooklyn Park, Minnesota

Anne Berwick, BSc
Coordinator, Spa and Advanced Bodywork Studies
Boulder College of Massage Therapy
Boulder, Colorado

Bernice Bicknase, BS, AAS
Program Chair, Therapeutic Massage
Ivy Tech Community College
Fort Wayne, Indiana

Shelli Davis-Redford, BS, MTI, LMT
Director of Education
Texas Massage Institute
Haltom City, Texas

Maggie Fenimore, LMT, RA
Instructor, Aromatherapy
St. Charles School of Massage Therapy
St. Charles, Missouri

Beverly Giroud, LMT
Instructor, Massage Therapy
The Desert Institute of Healing Arts
Tucson, Arizona

Lisa Jakober, NCMT, BS
Corporate Director of Education
National Massage Therapy Institute
Philadelphia, Pennsylvania

Marjorie Johnson, CMT
Faculty, Massage Therapy
Cortiva Institute – Colorado
Broomfield, Colorado

Tiffany Leigh
California Institute of Healing Arts
Golden River, California

Kelli Lene, NCTMB
Department Head, Massage Therapy
Community Care College
Tulsa, Oklahoma

Sherry Parker, AS
National Director of Skin Care Education
Florida College of Natural Health
Pompano Beach, Florida

Beth Rinard, BSc, LMT
Instructor, Massage Therapy
American Institute of Alternative Medicine
Columbus, Ohio

Judy Scheller, MT
Licensed Skincare Specialist, Spa Consultant/Educator
Somerset School of Massage Therapy
Wall Township, New Jersey

Joanna Sechuck, BS
Executive Director
Academy of Massage Therapy
Hackensack, New Jersey

Emily Sibley, BS, LMT
Instructor, Hydrotherapy
Downeast School of Massage
Waldoboro, Maine

Deborah Taylor, BS, LMT
Instructor, Massage Therapy
East West College
Portland, Oregon

Florent Villenueve, BA
Eastern Regional Director
ICT Schools
Toronto, Ontario, Canada

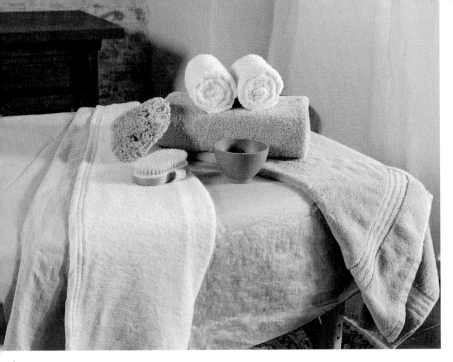

History of Spa and Hydrotherapy

1

LEARNING OBJECTIVES

After studying this chapter, the reader will have the information to

1. Describe components of the spa experience.
2. Trace the early history of spa.
3. Explain the contributions of the Greeks and Romans to spa.
4. Describe the factors involved in the decline of hydrotherapy during the Middle Ages.
5. Delineate the scientific advances and contributions of prominent figures in the hydrotherapy field.
6. Discuss the reasons why spa has developed into its current forms.
7. Explain the differences among the major categories of spas.

Tis True: the noblest of the elements is water.
—Poet Pindar, from the "Olympian Odes," 476 BC
(inscription over the old pump house in Bath, England)

KEY TERMS

Ayurveda	Frigid	Nutrition	Sento
Banya	Hammam	Onsen	Spa
Compress	Hydrotherapy	Phytotherapy	Spa experience
Day spas	Hygiene	Regulative therapy	Sweat lodge
Destination spas	Kinesiotherapy	Resort/hotel spas	Tepid
Exfoliation	Medical spas	Ryokan	
Fomentation	Mineral spring spas	Sauna	

WHAT IS SPA?

With the remarkable number of services and treatments available to consumers seeking health and wellness, a clear definition of **spa** and the **spa experience** is somewhat elusive. Spas range from simple to complex. A spa venue could be a hair salon or massage therapy office that offers a few select treatments all the way to destination spas that offer multiple-day stays that offer every amenity imaginable, including strategies for major lifestyle changes. However, what they have in common is the offering of health and wellness services to consumers.

These health and wellness services are part of the spa experience. Depending on the type of spa, these services can include bodywork such as massage therapy, shiatsu, and Thai massage; body treatments such as facials, wraps, and salt glows; exercise and fitness routines; programs for **nutrition**, weight loss, smoking cessation, and detoxification; spiritual renewal classes such as yoga, meditation, and labyrinth walking; and cosmetic treatments for skin rejuvenation, liposuction, and plastic surgery. The atmosphere is also an important part of the spa experience. The décor, ambient aromas, printed information, and staff appearance are just a few of the factors that make up the atmosphere.

No matter how great the menu of services or tasteful the surroundings, without well-trained and professional staff, a spa experience can be disappointing. From the people who answer the phone, schedule appointments, and greet clients to those who perform treatments and consultations, all the way to the spa managers, how spa staff members present themselves is crucial. Their professionalism and communication skills and how they perform the actual treatments or consultations all set the tone for the spa experience the client will have. Because spas face many challenges today that stem either directly or indirectly from issues involving communication and professionalism, a special section in Chapter 3 is devoted to these areas.

Today, spas and spa treatments are flourishing, and they are flourishing for the same reasons that natural healing methods have always done so in the human experience: they provide a sense of well-being—a chance to renew, refresh, and reintegrate the body, mind, and spirit. There is no doubt that consumers are interested in what spas have to offer. According to the International Spa Association (www.experienceispa.com), there were more than 130 million visits to spas in the United States in 2005, representing almost $10 billion of revenue.

As there are many options available to spa consumers, there are also many opportunities for employment within the spa industry. Dieticians, yoga practitioners, fitness experts, estheticians, cosmetologists, and bodyworkers are just few examples. Not everyone, though, who has an interest in spa and natural therapies wants to work in a spa setting. There are massage therapists and bodyworkers who want to learn treatments to augment their menu of services but do not consider their practices spas. This text is designed to illustrate methods and techniques that can be used for spa training as well as for skill enhancement for individual therapists.

EARLY HISTORY OF SPA

The actual origin of the word *spa* is not known. A popular theory is that it may be an acronym for the Latin phrases *sanitas per agua* or *salud per agua*—health or healing via water. The letters "S-P-A" were sometimes seen as graffiti on the walls of ancient Roman baths. Another theory is that it may come from the village of Spa, located high in the Ardennes Mountains of eastern Belgium. The village is known to have been a well-liked stopover for Roman soldiers on the march in the time of the Roman Empire. The town's mineral springs became so well known for their curative powers that the word *spa* may have become synonymous in the English language for a place where one is restored and refreshed (Croutier, 1992).

Water

Water is the original natural medicine. The earliest spas were mineral springs, and the earliest healing remedies were based on natural substances. Early civilizations, including the Babylonians, Hebrews, Persians, Indians, Chinese, Egyptians, Greeks, and Romans, have recorded the healing properties of water. Some of these records, as well as archeological discoveries, are the basis of modern hydrotherapy and spas. Archeological digs have uncovered structures for bathing in many of these early civilizations.

The use of water in the treatment of various mental and physical disorders came to be known as **hydrotherapy**—from the Greek *hydro,* which means "water" and *therapies,* which means "treatment." The first hydrotherapy treatments developed in indigenous cultures after the discovery that drinking and bathing in certain waters cured particular ailments. Over time, rituals were created around the use of water for healing, and water became more than just a component for physical health—it took on an almost mystical and spiritual aspect. These rituals for mind-body-spirit connection and wellness became extremely important for some cultures and are still practiced today. For example, in orthodox and conservative

Judaism, a mikvah is a ritual bath designed for achieving purity. Christian religions have long used baptism, which is essentially a ritual bath, to admit recipients to the Christian community. For other cultures, bathing may no longer have a spiritual aspect, but it is hard to deny that a long, hot shower or an afternoon spent swimming still remain potentially uplifting.

The water sources used for health and ritual were, and are, many and varied. Freshwater streams, pools, and lakes were all attractive to early communities as plentiful sources of water. Coastal populations discovered how fortifying bathing in the ocean can be (from both the relaxation of floating in the water and the nourishment of certain vitamins and minerals), and communities living near hot springs bathed in those waters (Barron, 2003; Sinclair, 2008; Williams, 2007).

Origins of Organized Hydrotherapy and Spas

Greece

By the fifth century BC, Greeks believed in the healing properties of water and recognized a correlation between personal **hygiene** and health. Initially, they used only cold baths, but later incorporated the use of hot water, steam baths, sponges, oils rinses, and a metal instrument for scraping residue left from water treatments off the body (the first record of **exfoliation,** which is the removal of the surface layers of dead skin cells) (Barron, 2003; Sinclair, 2008).

In the Greek pantheon, Asclepios, the son of Apollo, became revered as the Greek god of healing and medicine. He used water in all its forms—solid, liquid, and vapor—to heal his patients. One of his five daughters, Hygeia, was the goddess of health and sanitation. Whereas Asclepios was linked most closely with healing, Hygeia was connected with disease prevention and wellness. Her name is the origin of the word *hygiene,* which denotes cleanliness and practices contributing to health.

Hippocrates (see ▶Figure 1.1) (circa 460–370 BC), the "Father of Modern Medicine," was thought by many of his time to be Asclepios' descendant. He prescribed water to treat common conditions such as fever, gout, ulcers, hemorrhages, and rheumatism. He ascribed to a regimen of hydrotherapy, exercise, herbs, and nutrition. Because of water's calming effect, he used it to treat the mentally

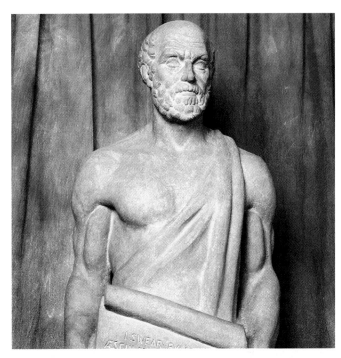

▶ **Figure 1.1** Hippocrates, the "Father of Modern Medicine," documented the phenomenon of using water at various temperatures to create a healing response. *(Brian Warling/International Museum of Surgical Science, Chicago, IL)*

disturbed. Most important, however, Hippocrates documented the phenomenon of using water at various temperatures to create a healing response.

In 347 BC, Aristotle, a student of Plato, opened the first Western university in Athens. Hygiene was part of the curriculum. Also around this time, the Greeks introduced water treatments to the Roman Empire. Greek healing methods included massage, exercise, and hydrotherapy, particularly hot and cold baths, **compresses** (soft cotton cloths soaked in hot or cold water and applied to the body), and **fomentations** (special types of hot compresses). The Romans even adopted Asclepius' philosophies of health and changed his name to the Latin Aesculapius. Of all these modes for health, the Romans seemed to be particularly captivated by baths.

Romans

At first, the Roman baths were designed on a small scale and used only cold water. These *balnea* were private baths or neighborhood baths and were employed for cleansing after physical exercise. When the Emperor Augustus (63 BC to AD 14) was cured of illness by cold baths, bathing became very popular. The Roman physicians Galen (circa AD 200) and Celsus (circa AD 175) incorporated baths as an integral part of their remedies. As the balnea became more popular, public baths, or *thermae,* were built on a

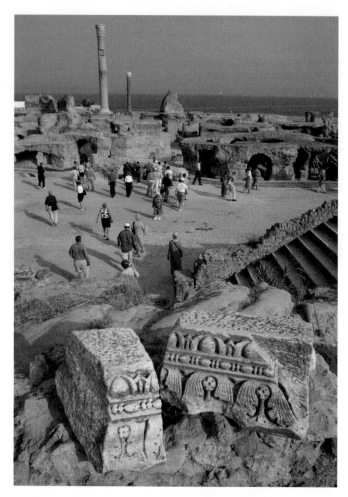

▶ **Figure 1.2** The Romans constructed baths throughout the empire, wherever a conquest was made, including at Carthage, Tunisia. *(Dave Bartruff/DanitaDelimont.com)*

massive scale. These included the Baths of Titus (AD 81), Baths of Domitian (AD 95), Trajan's Baths (circa AD 100), the Baths of Caracalla (AD 217), and the thermae of Diocletian (Diocletian ruled the Roman Empire from AD 284–305), which had a capacity for 6,000 bathers. Roman baths were also built whenever and wherever the Romans made conquests (see ▶Figure 1.2), and the imperial bathing institution was replicated in its basic form throughout the Roman Empire. Ruins of these baths are found all over Europe, the British Isles, northern Africa, and the Near East.

Magnificent public baths became centers for health, wellness, and social interaction. A typical public bath could accommodate about 10,000 bathers daily, with separate facilities for men and women. Although the baths were initially meant for the wealthy, over time public baths became available to working people. Romans would go daily to bathe, steam, receive massage, relax, and listen to po-

etry, often after their workday (see ▶Figure 1.3 for a diagram of Roman bathing facilities). A large, central courtyard was the exercise area; it was surrounded by a shady portico that led into the bathing rooms. Bathers would either swim in the large outdoor pool or apply oil to themselves and participate in physical exercise. After exercise, since soap had not been invented yet, the bathers would have the dirt and oil scraped off with a curved metal instrument called a *strigil*.

The bathers then had several rooms from which to choose. The *tepidarium* was the warm room and had heated walls and floors, but sometimes no pool of water. The *caldarium* was the hot bath. There was a large tub or small pool with very hot water and a waist-high fountain called a *labrum* with cool water to splash on the head and neck. Roman engineers had an ingenious system, called the *hypocaust,* to heat the baths. Pillars raised the floor off the ground and spaces were left inside the walls in which hot air from the furnace could circulate. The furnaces contained wood-fed fires and made the floors scorching hot, which necessitated the wearing of thick sandals. Rooms requiring the most heat were placed closest to the furnace. The cold room was the *frigidarium,* which had a cold pool. Other rooms offered moist steam, dry heat like a sauna, and massage with perfumed oils. The order in which a bather visited the rooms would vary. Generally, however, the *tepidarium* and *caldarium* were used first, and the *frigidarium* last.

After bathing, patrons could stroll in gardens, visit a library, watch performances by entertainers, listen to a literary piece, or get a snack from food vendors.

It is easy to see the origin of terms used today to describe different temperatures. **Tepid** means moderately warm or lukewarm; **frigid** means intensely cold; a *cauldron* is a large kettle or boiler, and the word comes from the Latin *caldarius,* which means "used for hot water" (Barron, 2003; Sinclair, 2008).

Finland and Russia

Sometime during Europe's Middle Ages, Finnish **saunas** and Russian **banyas** came into existence. Both of these are for hot vapor baths and evolved from portable **sweat lodges** used by nomadic tribes that became the Finns and Russians. The sweat lodges were similar to those used by Native American tribes. The saunas and banyas were small wooden rooms or huts with benches. Water was thrown on hot stones to create clouds of steam vapor that induced bathers to sweat. To increase circulation, bathers rubbed and whipped themselves and one another with birch twigs. The treatment ended with a cold plunge into icy water or snow. Saunas

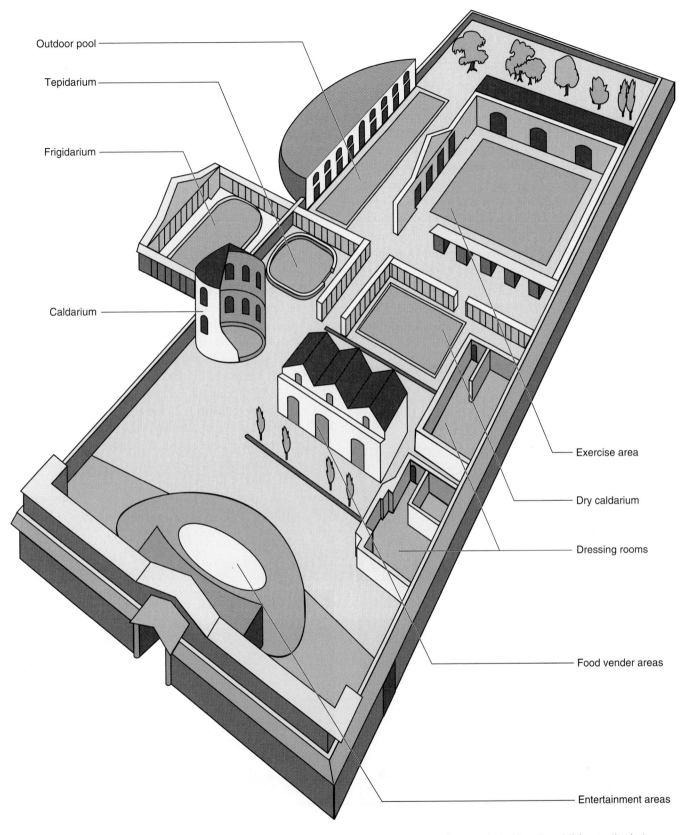

Outdoor pool

Tepidarium

Frigidarium

Caldarium

Exercise area

Dry caldarium

Dressing rooms

Food vender areas

Entertainment areas

▶ **Figure 1.3** Roman bathing facilities became centers for health and wellness, as well as socialization. In addition to the hot, warm, cool, and cold rooms, bathers might find pools for swimming, an exercise area, and food vendors. *(Stephen Conlin © Dorling Kindersley)*

became spiritual places as well for health and relaxation. They became places of ritual for milestones in a person's life—marriage, birth of a baby, and as places where the dead were laid out prior to funerals. (Barron, 2003).

The Middle East

In the Middle East and Byzantium, people adopted the Roman bathing traditions. Hebrews took frequent baths as required by their religion. Lacking baths or running water at home, Turkish baths or **hammams** (also spelled hamams) (see ▶Figure 1.4), were built and evolved into places to cleanse body and soul and to socialize and gossip. Bathing practices at a hammam closely resembled those of the Romans. First, bathers relaxed in a warm room that had a constant flow of dry, hot air. This caused the bathers to perspire profusely. They could then move on to an even hotter room to perspire even more. After that, they splashed themselves with cold water and then washed themselves completely in a warm room before

receiving a massage. The massage was followed by sitting in a cooling room and relaxing for a period of time.

Everyone gathered at hammams. Ritual celebrations of birth, marriage, and transition to the next life took place there. The bathing process at hammams became popular and spread throughout Europe; it became known as taking a Turkish bath. Turkish baths continue to be enjoyed today, and some of the historic Turkish baths have even survived to the present day. In Istanbul, the Cagaloglu and the Cemberlitas Hammam were constructed in the 1500s and are still fully functioning (Williams, 2007).

Japan

Japan is primarily a mountainous and volcanic country. The benefit of being situated on top of one of the most thermally active areas in the world is the thousands of natural hot springs scattered across the country. Hot-spring bathing first became popular in Japan more than 1,000 years ago. Originally, it was limited to aristocrats, but when it was discovered how effective the springs were in healing battle wounds, warlords began using them. This continued throughout the Warring States period (1477–1568). During the Edo period (1603–1867), peace and stability were instituted, and the custom of bathing in hot springs was adopted by everyone, from monarchs to farmers. **Onsens** (see ▶Figure 1.5) are natural, mineral-rich hot springs where, to this day, people go to soak away aches and pains or just relax. Onsens can be found as simple open-air pools near rivers, on mountaintops, as part of beautiful traditional inns (**ryokans**), or within modern buildings in the heart of Japan's cities.

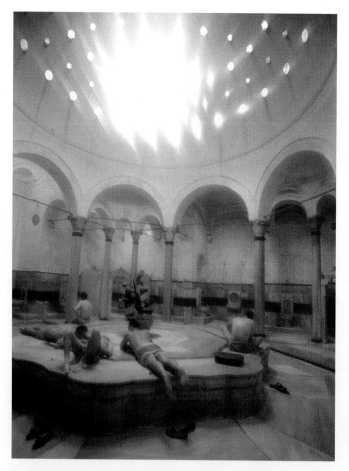

▶ **Figure 1.4** Turkish hammams were public places for cleansing body and soul and socializing. This facility in Turkey was constructed in the sixteenth century and is still in use today. *(D E Cox/Getty Images Inc.—Stone Allstock)*

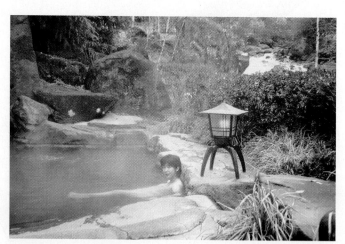

▶ **Figure 1.5** Natural, mineral-rich hot springs, such as this onsen, can be found throughout Japan because of the prevalence of thermal activity on the island nation. *(Dallas and John Heaton/Stock Connection)*

If a village was not located near hot springs, a **sento**, or public bath, was built. Sentos date back to the eighth century and are still used to this day. The main difference between an onsen and a sento is that onsens use only hot mineral water, and sentos may use other types of water. Since onsens and sentos were public venues, washing and rinsing were required before people entered the bath. In present-day Japanese culture, the bath is still used primarily for soaking; people cleanse their bodies before entering the bath. Most Japanese families have their own deep soaking tub (*o-furo,* see ▶Figure 1.6) where they find relief from the stress of the day; as part of their culture, they cleanse before they enter the tub (Neff, 1999).

The Americas

The medicine of various Native American tribes has been used for move than 10,000 years. Hot springs are found throughout the Americas, and Native Americans who lived near them have used them from early times to the present day. Other Native American nations use sweat lodges. These are huts, lodges, caverns, or other small buildings that are heated by steam from water poured on hot stones for ritual and/or therapeutic sweating. Originally, the lodges of the people of the Northeast were made of willow poles covered with birch bark or animal skins; on the plains, they were covered with buffalo skins. Native Amer-

icans of the Southwest dug out earth mounds for their sweats. When the Spaniards came to Mexico, they observed what they called *temezcalli.* In the Aztec language of Nahuatl, *teme* meant "to bathe," and *calli* is the word for "house." In arctic regions, the Inuit people performed sweats in their igloos.

Sweat lodges today may be built of traditional materials or modern items, such as tarps (see ▶Figure 1.7). Inside the sweat lodge, the patient, the healer, and any helpers pray, sing, and perhaps drum to purify the spirits. At the same time, water is poured onto red-hot stones to create large amounts of sweat-producing steam. The sweating that is stimulated purges and cleanses the body of disease (Barron, 2003; Nikola, 1997; Sinclair, 2008).

DECLINE OF HYDROTHERAPY

As the Roman Empire fell into decay, many of the Roman traditions fell into disuse. Baths gradually were no longer used for health and socializing. The fall of the Roman Empire, about AD 450, marked the beginning of the Middle

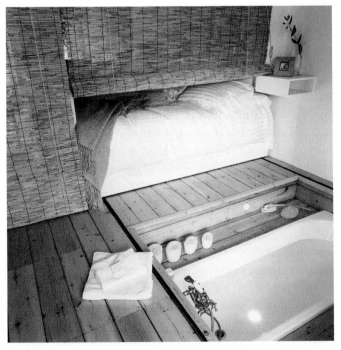

▶ **Figure 1.6** In today's Japanese culture, many homes have an o-furo, or deep soaking tub. It is common for Japanese people to cleanse their bodies before entering the tub. *(Jake Fitzjones © Dorling Kindersley)*

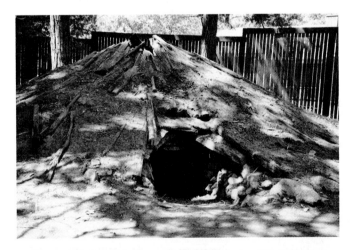

▶ **Figure 1.7** Sweat lodges, such as this one made of timber and earth, are common in Native American nations. They may be constructed of a variety of materials but all serve the same purpose—ritual or therapeutic sweating. *(EMG Education Management Group)*

Ages, which lasted for about 1,000 years. During this time, there were many wars and migrations and much social disorganization. As villages, towns, and cities grew larger, there was no infrastructure built for waste management or to ensure a clean water supply. Wastes from humans and animals intermingled with water needed for drinking and washing.

Christianity and Islam

With the rise in Christianity, more emphasis was placed on spiritual and heavenly matters than on earthly matters, including the body. Bathing was viewed as unhealthy and self-indulgent and was thus forbidden. In practical terms, it was also a risky venture since water was not clean. Perfumes and cosmetics were developed to mask body odors and the lack of good hygiene. Wines, beer, and ale were drunk instead of water. Knowledge that was considered pagan, earthly, or non-Christian was outlawed, and many texts containing such information were destroyed. Practitioners of ancient healing methods were called heretics and not allowed to practice openly.

Medical care came under the authority of priests, who did not believe in the ancient healing methods that used water. Only the medical school at Salerno, Italy, taught the Hippocratic treatments and the use of cold water. The knowledge of hydrotherapy was almost lost entirely. Fortunately, monks in certain monasteries throughout Europe dedicated themselves to collecting, studying, and replicating classic Greek and Roman texts. Additionally, Middle Eastern physicians kept alive the tradition of water therapies and bathing. In fact, during the Middle Ages of Europe, Islamic countries became the centers of classical Western scientific thought. Because of this, the knowledge of Aristotle, Hippocrates, Celsus, Galen, and others survives to this day.

Ibn Sina (see ▶Figure 1.8), also known as Avicenna (AD 973–1037), was a Persian physician who practiced throughout Arabia. He based his practice on the teachings of Galen and did further research and experimentation in medicine. His chief work, *Canon Medicinae,* served as the most important textbook for physicians in Western society until the Renaissance (Barron, 2003, Buckle, 2007; Sinclair, 2008; Tisserand, 1985).

RESURGENCE OF HYDROTHERAPY

Toward the end of the medieval era, two historical figures played roles in the resurgence of hydrotherapy in Western culture. One was St. Thomas Aquinas (1225–1274), who

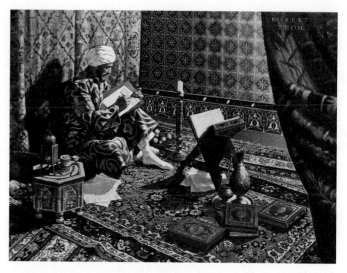

▶ **Figure 1.8** Ibn Sina, a follower of the teachings of Galen, wrote *Canon Medicinae,* which served as the most important textbook for physicians in Western society until the Renaissance. *(Courtesy of Parke, Davis & Co. Used with permission.)*

was both a scholar and a member of the Dominican order and one of the most influential Christian philosophers. His study and interpretations of the works of Aristotle countered the Catholic Church's tendency to reject Greek philosophy and led, eventually, to a new acceptance of Aristotle's philosophies, including the virtues of cleanliness.

The other historical figure is Henry VIII (1491–1547). During his time, people still visited hot springs for health reasons, although there were strict regulations on their use because of unsanitary conditions and lack of moral decency. In fact, many warm springs were still connected with pagan rituals during this time (for being part of the Roman custom of bathing), so they were renamed as holy wells where saints of the Catholic Church had performed miracles. They became pilgrimage sites, where pilgrims could be cured of ills by drinking or bathing in the water. Henry VIII closed most of the wells because the pilgrimages seemed to be superstitious and pagan in nature, resembling too closely the methods used to worship Roman gods. These wells were also sometimes gathering sites for political dissidents, so the English government chose to limit the number of people traveling to wells outside England and to encourage the use of public baths, which had been forbidden for a long time. England's Privy Council encouraged bathing at several places, notably Bath in the west, Buxton and Harrogate in the north, and a spring located in central England whose location has been lost.

Innovations in Science and Medicine

Thus, in the sixteenth century, as part of the Renaissance, there was a renewed interest in medicine and in bathing for health. Besides the springs in England, there were more than 200 other springs in Germany, Italy, Belgium, Switzerland, and France that became popular. Advances in methods to analyze chemicals allowed physicians to uncover the composition of mineral springs to determine how they heal the body. The invention of the thermometer is generally credited to Galileo in 1592. Daniel Gabriel Fahrenheit (1686–1736) was a German physicist who also made scientific instruments. He invented the alcohol thermometer in 1709 and the mercury thermometer in 1714. He also developed the Fahrenheit temperature scale, which is still in use in the United States. The creation of a reliable thermometer was a major step forward for hydrotherapy.

Prominent Persons

Prominent people also started questioning the then currently accepted practices of Western medicine, which paved the way for modern uses of hydrotherapy. In England, Dr. Thomas Sydenham (1624–1689) challenged common medical practices, especially blood letting. He did not believe in an authoritarian medical system; instead, he based his practice and teaching on independent reasoning. He is considered one of the most important revivers of the views of Hippocrates and regularly used ancient applications, such as the use of water, to treat common ailments.

Sir John Floyer (1649–1734) was an English physician who was a passionate advocate of hydrotherapy. In 1697, he wrote *An Enquiry into the Right Use and Abuses of Hot, Cold and Temperate Baths in England,* which was later released as *The History of Cold Bathing.* At the time, it was extremely controversial within the medical community. It did, however, influence Dr. Johann Sigmund Hahn (1696–1773), who is credited with instituting the principles of modern hydrotherapy in Germany.

John Wesley (1703–1791) was the founder of the Methodist Church. He recognized the correlation between bathing and health and coined the saying, "Cleanliness is next to Godliness." In 1747, he wrote *Primitive Physick,* which asserted that cold baths could cure certain afflictions. This book, in fact, brought social awareness to cold bathing and was a profound influence in the popularization of hydrotherapy.

Along with an interest in cold-water bathing was an increasing interest in the benefits of bathing in seawater. Dr. Richard Russell of Lewes published his *Dissertation on the Use of Sea Water* in 1752, and it encouraged people to visit the seaside to improve their health. Seawater cures became very popular in France and Sweden as well (de Vierville, 2000).

BIRTH OF MODERN SPA AND HYDROTHERAPY

Prominent Persons

A number of people are responsible for bringing ancient hydrotherapy techniques to prominence today. One of the most important is Vincent Preissnitz (1799–1851). Early in the nineteenth century as a young Austrian peasant boy, Preissnitz mangled his fingers in a farm accident. He had noticed that the cold-water folk remedies used on farm animals were extremely effective. By applying repeated cold-water applications, he was able to restore the use of his fingers. Shortly thereafter, he was on a hill, loading hay into a cart when the horses bolted and the heavy cart rolled over his body, crushing him. The doctors in his village told him he would be crippled for life. He decided to use the same cold-water therapies that had healed his mangled fingers. After putting his ribs back in place, he used cold compresses to relieve his pain; drank large amounts of water; and wrapped himself in cold, wet sheets. To his amazement, he recovered fully. In 1829, he established a clinic in Graefenberg and performed the Priessnitz cure: a regimen of wrapping the body with wet sheets, cold baths, fresh air, healthy diet, and physical exercise. When people heard the news of his miraculous cure, they came from far and wide to his small village of Grafenberg to experience his healing water therapies. Being analytical, he experimented and developed new techniques involving water. He also carefully organized and documented his treatments and so was instrumental in bringing the world's attention to hydrotherapy. Unhappy physicians in the area took Preissnitz to court. However, he won his case and the leading physician of the empire, Baron Turkheim, came to observe and learn his techniques. From then on, Preissnitz was protected by the crown. His clinic, now called a spa, is still in operation today.

In nearby Bavaria, Sebastian Kneipp (1821–1897) (see ►Figure 1.9), the son of a weaver, dreamt of going into the priesthood, but he suffered from tuberculosis and did not have the stamina to attend the seminary. He read Dr. Hahn's book and came across a pamphlet describing Preissnitz's successful cold water therapies. Kneipp decided to use the treatments to challenge his system and strengthen his vitality. He began by taking daily plunges into the icy Danube River; over a period of time, he was completely restored to health and was able to complete his study for the priesthood.

Father Kneipp dedicated his life to treating his parishioners and all others who came to him, including the royalty of Europe and the pope of his time. He developed

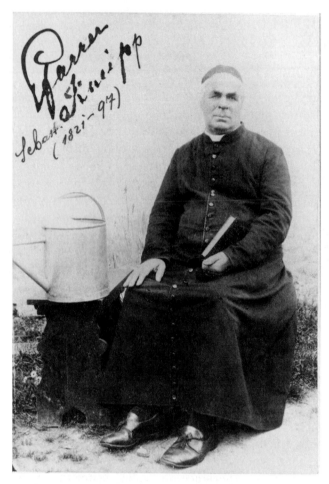

▶ **Figure 1.9** Father Sebastian Kneipp followed the teachings of Hahn and Preissnitz to overcome his tuberculosis, which allowed him to complete his training at the seminary. *(Courtesy of Kneipp-Werke)*

cold-water treading and walking on early morning cool dew to strengthen the body, wet sheet packs, and alternating compresses. A wet nightshirt dipped in salt water or hayflower (a term for wild plants that grow in hayfields; they are used to improve circulation and aid in the relief of colds and flu) became a procedure used for many childhood illnesses (Frohlich, 1997). He is known today as the "Father of Hydrotherapy." Kneipp wrote *Meine Wasser Kur* (*My Water Cure),* which was published in 1866. *Kur* actually means a course of treatments; it describes his course of water treatments, and how they are based on five fundamental principles:

1. **Hydrotherapy**—thermal and mechanical water applications and baths
2. **Kinesiotherapy**—movement, exercise, and massage
3. **Phytotherapy**—natural herbal remedies, teas, oils, and juices
4. **Nutrition**—a well-balanced diet

5. **Regulative Therapy**—mental, emotional, and spiritual balance in one's life (Kneipp, 1956).

Father Kneipp's approach to healing was truly holistic, encouraging balance and harmony between work and relaxation, and among the body, mind and spirit. He especially emphasized that people need to be active participants in achieving and maintaining their health. The Kneipp Institute exists today in the town of Bad Worshofen, Bavaria. Bavaria has more than 200 spas (Kur Houses) offering Kneipp hydrotherapy. The Kneipp system is practiced predominantly at European Spas and some American spas as well (Bruggerman, 1982).

Benedict Lust (1872–1945) was born in Germany and came to the United States in 1892 to seek his fortune. Unfortunately, he contracted a severe case of tuberculosis and returned to Germany. He went to Father Kneipp who was able to help him heal. In 1896, he returned to the United States and, with Father Kneipp's blessing, distributed information on the water cure. Lust had an eclectic approach to healing; he combined the Kneipp cure with other modalities he had learned from other European physicians who focused on natural cures. In 1900, members of a committee of Kneipp practitioners, including Lust, decided to expand their practice to include homeopathy, psychology, and bony manipulation and thus formed the foundation of Naturopathic Medicine, as it is known today.

Dr. John Bastyr (1912–1995), known as the "Father of Naturopathic Medicine," was born in New Prague, MN. He was greatly influenced both by his mother, who was an herbalist and student of Father Kniepp, and his father, who was trained as a pharmacist. This combination gave him a unique blend of science and naturopathic remedies. Dr. Bastyr was always looking for the connections among mind, body, and spirit in the pursuit of health and wellness. His modalities included hydrotherapy, homeopathy, botanical medicine, nutrition, and chiropractics. In 1956, he established the National College of Naturopathic Medicine in Seattle, WA. The college moved to Portland, Oreson, in 1978, the same year Bastyr College was founded in Seattle.

Ellen G. White (1827–1915) (see ▶Figure 1.10) was one of the founders of Seventh Day Adventism. She was also a noted health reformer. She had a vision that focused on the importance and benefits of nature's remedies: pure water, clean air, sunshine, healthy diet, and exercise. Ellen and her husband James opened the Health Reform Institute in Battle Creek, MI, where hydrotherapy was practiced. The Institute had some success but needed a full-time medical director.

The Whites helped finance John Harvey Kellogg's (1852–1943) medical education at Bellevue Medical Col-

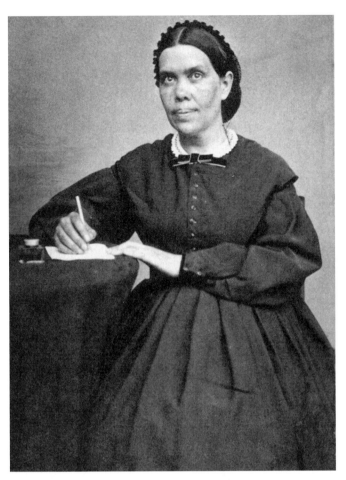

> **Figure 1.10** The noted health reformer Ellen G. White opened the Health Reform Institute with her husband, where they could practice hydrotherapy. *(Courtesy of Ellen G. White Estate Inc.)*

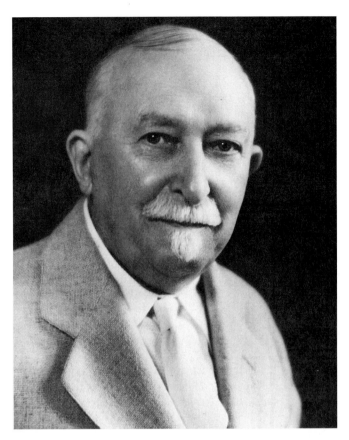

> **Figure 1.11** Dr. John Harvey Kellogg became the medical superintendent of Ellen and James White's Health Reform Institute, which Dr. Kellogg renamed the Battle Creek Sanitarium. *(Corbis/Bettmann)*

lege in New York City. When he graduated in 1875, Dr. Kellogg (see ▶Figure 1.11) returned to Battle Creek and became the medical superintendent of the Health Reform Institute. Dr. Kellogg also studied at the Vienna Medical School with Dr. William Winternitz, who was known for his research into the scientific aspects of hydrotherapy. Benedict Lust was also an influence in Dr. Kellogg's education. Dr. Kellogg coined the term *sanitarium* and changed the name of the Institute to the Battle Creek Sanitarium. He developed the "Battle Creek Idea" that good health and fitness were the result of good diet, exercise, correct posture, fresh air, and proper rest. The rich and famous traveled to Battle Creek and stayed for several weeks to restore their bodies to health. In 1901, Dr. Kellogg wrote *Rational Hydrotherapy, Vols. 1 & 2,* a thorough reference to the scientific aspects of hydrotherapy. It is still an authoritative text on hydrotherapy (Barron, 2003; Kellogg, 1903; Nikola, 1997; Sinclair, 2008; Williams, 2007).

Hydrotherapy and Spa Today

Finland and Russia remained relatively untouched by the Catholic Church's ban on bathing because of their geographic distance from central Europe (Barron, 2003). Saunas, therefore, did not decrease in popularity until industrialization and urbanization relegated them to folk medicine. World War II contributed to their resurgence. With the war, food and entertainment were scarce. To alleviate their dreary life, people once again turned to saunas. The military especially found them helpful and healthful for the troops. With innovations in safe heating methods, and aggressive marketing, saunas have once again become popular.

Three types of saunas are used in Finland today. Saunas with electric heaters are popular because of convenience. Traditional saunas with wood-burning heaters are used more in rural areas. The third type is the *savusauna* or smoke sauna (see ▶Figure 1.12). It has a large wood-burning heater with 200- to 300-pound rocks and no stove pipe. The smoke is allowed to remain in the sauna while the sauna is heating up to the desired temperature.

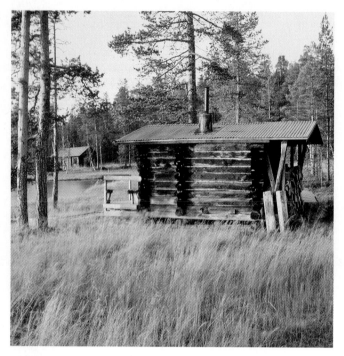

▶ **Figure 1.12** Saunas, such as this traditional wood-burning model, are still common in Finland today, along with those that use electricity. *(Mark de Fraeye/Photo Researchers, Inc.)*

The smoke is released through a small vent before the sauna is used (Roy, 2004).

Throughout the end of the nineteenth century and into the twentieth century, mineral-spring spas were popular in both Europe and the United States. Those who could afford to travel to them did so and could spend weeks at a time "taking the waters." The European spas were already well known. People regularly stayed at spas in Evian-les-Bains, France; Tuscany, Italy; Budapest, Hungary; Bavaria and Baden-Baden, Germany; and Bath, England. Many of these spas are still in use today, such as Gellert Spa in Budapest, Hungary (see ▶Figure 1.13).

In the United States, spas became fashionable centers for relaxation starting around the 1850s. Saratoga Springs, NY and Warm Springs, AR are two examples of places to which people would travel. During both world wars, wounded veterans were sent to spas for treatment of their injuries. The warmth of the water was soothing to muscles, and the high mineral content of the water allowed bathers buoyancy and a sensation of floating that they could not experience with their limited movement. After Franklin Delano Roosevelt contracted polio, he

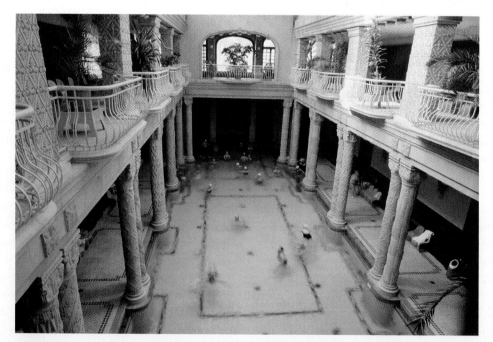

▶ **Figure 1.13** Mineral springs spas, such as this one, Gellert Spa in Budapest, Hungary, became popular in the early twentieth century and are still in use today. *(Chad Ehlers/Stock Connection)*

went to Warm Springs on a regular basis to alleviate his symptoms.

However, starting in the 1930s, interest in going to spas declined in the United States. As more people were able to buy cars, more vacation areas around the country were developed. There was less interest in traveling to just one place, such as a spa, for several weeks, and more interest in making shorter trips to many more places, such as national parks. During this time, additional Western scientific healing methods, including diagnostic tools, medications, and surgery, were being discovered and developed. The natural approach to healing was discarded for the scientific approach. Traditional methods were considered folk medicine; spas were considered relics of the past. This continued for some time as more and more advances in medicine were made, such as the discovery of penicillin, the development of blood transfusions, the creation of the polio vaccine on up to the wide array of complex procedures and medications that are available today.

There is no doubt that Western science and medicine have saved thousands of lives. However, even as modern technology and practices have become generally accepted and sought after, there have always been threads of interest in natural health techniques. Traditional methods have been kept alive and handed down through generations. In the 1960s, a movement began for simpler ways of life that were closer to nature. Along with food grown organically and ways to center oneself such as yoga and meditation, mineral spas were appealing to naturalists and health enthusiasts.

Also during this time, programs to help people lose weight began developing; these programs included a regimen of rigorous exercise and low-calorie food. As more and more people were making use of these programs, retreats were built for those who wanted to lose weight in seclusion, and be pampered while they did so. Classes for relaxation and self-development, such as meditation, were added, as well as treatments for beauty, such as facials.

In the late 1970s and 1980s, fitness began to be a priority for many people. Hotels and resorts determined that in order to remain competitive, they needed to provide workout facilities in addition to pools for swimming. Some went further and added saunas and salons for hair styling, skin care, and nail care. This was the start of the amenity spas, and it was a natural progression to evolve from offering beauty treatments to offering bodywork.

Offerings at destination spas were also expanded. There began to be a focus on wellness and health maintenance and an integrated approach to connecting the mind, body, and spirit. In addition to healthy food, exercise, relaxation, and stress-relief techniques, bodywork therapies became available to spa goers. Old-fashioned treatments, which had not gone out of style in European spas, were rediscovered. Hydrotherapy in the form of Vichy showers (special showers with multiple nozzles used for rinsing spa substances off clients) whirlpool baths, mineral baths, hot tubs, and cold plunges were added to spa menus. Substances known to ancient populations were researched; seaweed and muds appeared in the form of wraps and facials. Scrubs using salts, sugar, and other abrasives were developed. Other ancient healing traditions were incorporated, such as aromatherapy and the traditional medicine of India, **Ayurveda** (see Appendix 2 for more information). Because of an increase in interest in optimal fitness and vitality, and because of an increase in disposable income, these new treatments met with success (Crebbin-Bailey, Harcup, and Harrington, 2005; Sinclair, 2008; Williams, 2007).

To better understand the development of spa and hydrotherapy throughout history, see ▶Figure 1.14 for a time line of events.

Types of Spas

According to International SPA Association 2007 statistics, there are more than 14,000 spas in the United States. This means there are many options from which consumers can choose when deciding which treatments will meet their needs. Additionally, there are many businesses, including bodywork offices and salons, that may not consider themselves spas but do offer spa and other natural healing therapies. Most spas fit under at least one of five major categories of spas; ▶Box 1.1 lists and describes these categories.

Today, health and well-being may be the reason for a visit to a spa. Or it may be to relax and be pampered. Perhaps it is for a day of beauty, to try something new, or to reconnect with nature. No matter what the reason, it is undeniable that the spa industry and spa techniques have hit on just the right blend of old and new philosophies and skills. It is true that the spa experience is different for everyone, and it is also true that there is something for everyone in the spa experience.

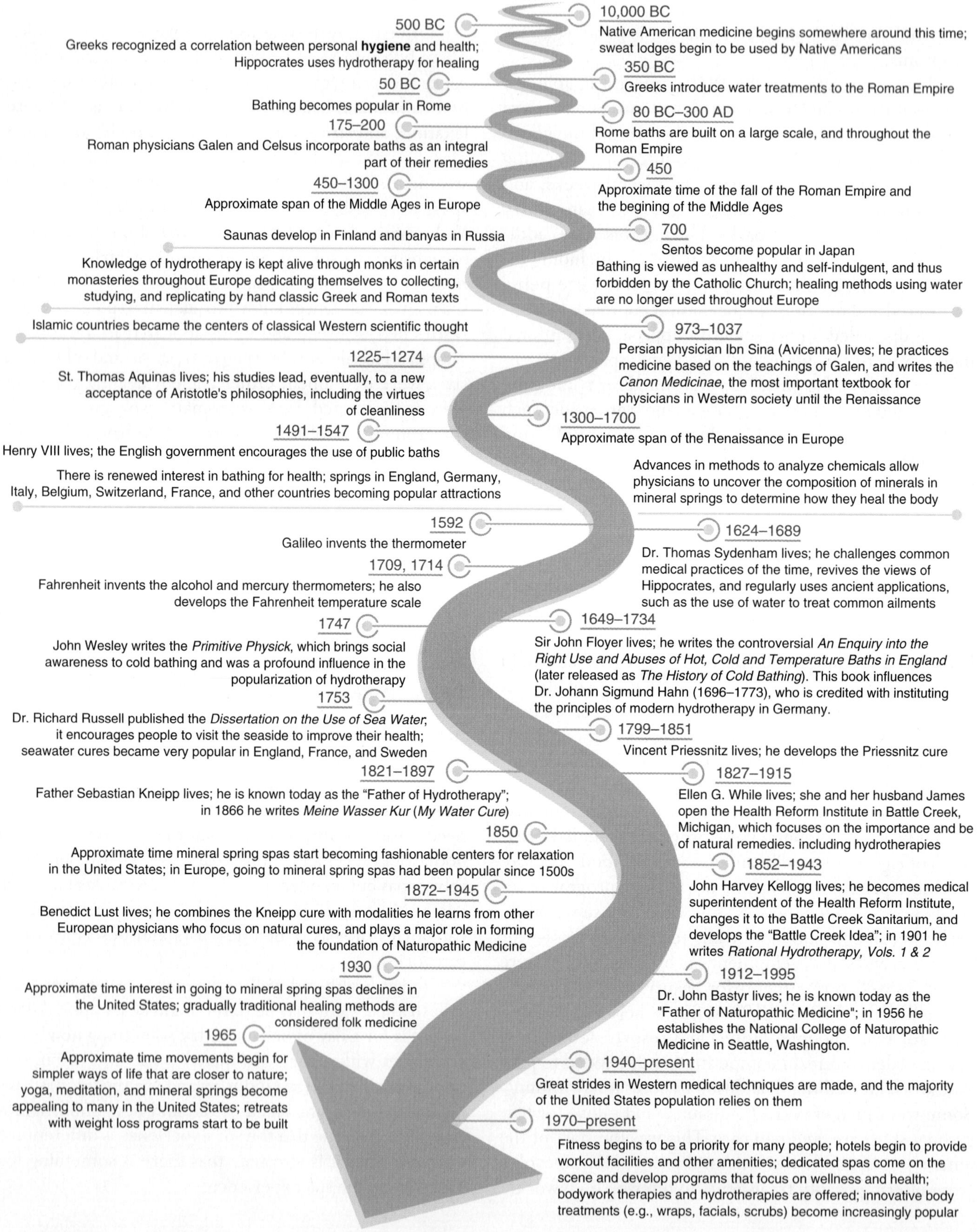

500 BC
Greeks recognized a correlation between personal **hygiene** and health; Hippocrates uses hydrotherapy for healing

10,000 BC
Native American medicine begins somewhere around this time; sweat lodges begin to be used by Native Americans

350 BC
Greeks introduce water treatments to the Roman Empire

50 BC
Bathing becomes popular in Rome

175–200
Roman physicians Galen and Celsus incorporate baths as an integral part of their remedies

80 BC–300 AD
Rome baths are built on a large scale, and throughout the Roman Empire

450
Approximate time of the fall of the Roman Empire and the begining of the Middle Ages

450–1300
Approximate span of the Middle Ages in Europe

Saunas develop in Finland and banyas in Russia

700
Sentos become popular in Japan
Bathing is viewed as unhealthy and self-indulgent, and thus forbidden by the Catholic Church; healing methods using water are no longer used throughout Europe

Knowledge of hydrotherapy is kept alive through monks in certain monasteries throughout Europe dedicating themselves to collecting, studying, and replicating by hand classic Greek and Roman texts

Islamic countries became the centers of classical Western scientific thought

973–1037
Persian physician Ibn Sina (Avicenna) lives; he practices medicine based on the teachings of Galen, and writes the *Canon Medicinae*, the most important textbook for physicians in Western society until the Renaissance

1225–1274
St. Thomas Aquinas lives; his studies lead, eventually, to a new acceptance of Aristotle's philosophies, including the virtues of cleanliness

1300–1700
Approximate span of the Renaissance in Europe

1491–1547
Henry VIII lives; the English government encourages the use of public baths

There is renewed interest in bathing for health; springs in England, Germany, Italy, Belgium, Switzerland, France, and other countries becoming popular attractions

Advances in methods to analyze chemicals allow physicians to uncover the composition of minerals in mineral springs to determine how they heal the body

1592
Galileo invents the thermometer

1624–1689
Dr. Thomas Sydenham lives; he challenges common medical practices of the time, revives the views of Hippocrates, and regularly uses ancient applications, such as the use of water to treat common ailments

1709, 1714
Fahrenheit invents the alcohol and mercury thermometers; he also develops the Fahrenheit temperature scale

1649–1734
Sir John Floyer lives; he writes the controversial *An Enquiry into the Right Use and Abuses of Hot, Cold and Temperature Baths in England* (later released as *The History of Cold Bathing*). This book influences Dr. Johann Sigmund Hahn (1696–1773), who is credited with instituting the principles of modern hydrotherapy in Germany.

1747
John Wesley writes the *Primitive Physick*, which brings social awareness to cold bathing and was a profound influence in the popularization of hydrotherapy

1799–1851
Vincent Priessnitz lives; he develops the Priessnitz cure

1753
Dr. Richard Russell published the *Dissertation on the Use of Sea Water*; it encourages people to visit the seaside to improve their health; seawater cures became very popular in England, France, and Sweden

1827–1915
Ellen G. While lives; she and her husband James open the Health Reform Institute in Battle Creek, Michigan, which focuses on the importance and be of natural remedies. including hydrotherapies

1821–1897
Father Sebastian Kneipp lives; he is known today as the "Father of Hydrotherapy"; in 1866 he writes *Meine Wasser Kur* (*My Water Cure*)

1850
Approximate time mineral spring spas start becoming fashionable centers for relaxation in the United States; in Europe, going to mineral spring spas had been popular since 1500s

1852–1943
John Harvey Kellogg lives; he becomes medical superintendent of the Health Reform Institute, changes it to the Battle Creek Sanitarium, and develops the "Battle Creek Idea"; in 1901 he writes *Rational Hydrotherapy, Vols. 1 & 2*

1872–1945
Benedict Lust lives; he combines the Kneipp cure with modalities he learns from other European physicians who focus on natural cures, and plays a major role in forming the foundation of Naturopathic Medicine

1912–1995
Dr. John Bastyr lives; he is known today as the "Father of Naturopathic Medicine"; in 1956 he establishes the National College of Naturopathic Medicine in Seattle, Washington.

1930
Approximate time interest in going to mineral spring spas declines in the United States; gradually traditional healing methods are considered folk medicine

1940–present
Great strides in Western medical techniques are made, and the majority of the United States population relies on them

1965
Approximate time movements begin for simpler ways of life that are closer to nature; yoga, meditation, and mineral springs become appealing to many in the United States; retreats with weight loss programs start to be built

1970–present
Fitness begins to be a priority for many people; hotels begin to provide workout facilities and other amenities; dedicated spas come on the scene and develop programs that focus on wellness and health; bodywork therapies and hydrotherapies are offered; innovative body treatments (e.g., wraps, facials, scrubs) become increasingly popular

▶ **Figure 1.14** The development of spa and hydrotherapy treatments can be traced as far back as 10,000 BC. A number of cultures, geographic areas, and religious groups have contributed to the growth and transformation of these treatments to make them what they are today.

Medical Spas and **Medispas**

- These are also known as medspas.

- They focus on integrating mind-body-spirit connection with medical procedures.

- Staff includes full-time, licensed health-care professionals (physicians, nurses, nurse practitioners) who manage and oversee programs and facilities.

- Treatments can include Botox injections; chemical and laser skin treatments; liposuction; breast augmentation; plastic surgery; dentistry; naturopathic medicine; and traditional Asian medicine methods, such as herbal remedies and acupuncture, and Ayurveda.

- Medical spas draw from European spa wellness approaches: focus on lifestyle changes for wellness and preventative health care (weight loss, nutritional counseling, smoking cessation, strength and flexibility training programs may be offered along with methods to manage specific medical conditions such as heart disease, high cholesterol, and respiratory conditions).

- Complementary treatments contributing to mind-body-spirit connection include bodywork, hypnotherapy, meditation, aromatherapy, yoga, and spa therapies (wraps, salt glows, etc.).

- Guests at medical and medispas are given thorough medical examinations; health histories are discussed.

- Individualized treatment plans are designed for guests and progress is closely monitored.

- Some medical spas are for day use only; some have on-site accommodations for multiple-day stays.

Examples of medical spas

Cooper Spa in Dallas, TX

www.cooperaerobics.com

Greenbrier Spa in White Sulfur Springs, WV

www.greenbrier.com

Canyon Ranch in Tucson, AZ

www.canyonranch.com

Destination Spas

- These are locations that guests travel to for multiple-day stays.

- Focal point of programs is enhancement of health and well-being.

- Programs individualized for each guest assist in detoxifying, smoking cessation, increasing strength and flexibility, eating better, incorporating stress reduction techniques.

- Guests' progress is closely monitored by health care professionals.

- Complementary treatments and activities that help guests integrate their body, mind, spirit include bodywork and spa therapies, yoga, hiking, labyrinth walking, and meditation.

- Some medical spas also considered destination spas.

Examples of destination spas

Miraval in Tucson, AZ

www.miravalresort.com

Chopra Centers in California, New York, and Colorado

www.chopra.com

Resort/Hotel Spas

- Spas in settings such as hotels and cruise ships offer guests choices for relaxation, stress relief, and beauty enhancement.

- Bodywork, wraps, facials, aromatherapy, and body polishes are some treatments provided by professional practitioners.

- Spa cuisine consisting of healthy, light fare may also be available.

Examples of resort/hotel spas

The Breakers Palm Beach in Palm Beach, FL

www.thebreakers.com

Mirbeau Inn and Spa in Skaneateles, NY

www.mirbeau.com

Princess Cruise Lines

www.princess.com

Mineral Spring Spas

- These are based around a source of mineral or hot spring water that is used for its healing properties.

- Some use seawater in addition to or instead of mineral springs.

- There are pools for guests to enjoy.

- Some offer bodywork and spa therapies.

- Spas may be for day use only, although some have accommodations for multiple-day stays.

Examples of mineral spring spas

The Springs Resort in Pagosa Springs, CO

www.pagosahotsprings.com

The Fairmont Banff Springs in Banff, Alberta, Canada

www.fairmont.com/banffsprings

Gideon Putnam Resort and Spa in Saratoga Springs, NY

www.gideonputnam.com

Day Spas

- There is no concrete definition of what a day spa is; generally it is a location to which guests travel to spend part or all of a day.

- There are many different types; menus of services vary depending on individual spa.

- Examples include hair and nail treatments, bodywork and spa therapies, esthetic treatments, yoga classes, and weight loss consultations.

Examples of day spas

Crowne Point Historic Inn and Spa in Provincetown, MA

www.crownepointe.com

Spa Space in Chicago, IL

www.spaspace.com

Seattle Art of Wellness in Seattle, WA

www.seattleartofwellness.com

Note: Most spas fit under at least one of five major categories.

(Spa listings courtesy of www.spafinder.com)

Summary

The earliest spas were mineral springs, and the earliest healing remedies were based on natural substances. The modern spa experience has its origins in these. There have been periods in history when spas and natural remedies were quite fashionable, and times when they have fallen out of favor. A number of significant scientific advances, and the work of leaders in the field of traditional healing methods, have formed the foundation of modern spa therapies. Additionally, an interest in connecting with nature, fitness, and overall health and wellness has helped form the integrative approach to body, mind, and spirit that is another aspect of the spa experience. People are visiting spas and requesting spa therapies in record numbers. Today, it is a billion-dollar industry.

Activities

1. What does the "spa experience" mean to you? What factors would make going to a spa a good experience for you?

   _____

   _____

   _____

   _____

2. Give five examples of how spa and hydrotherapy treatments have been developed and used by various cultures throughout history.

   _____

   _____

   _____

   _____

3. Who do you think has had the most significant impact on spa and hydrotherapy? Why did you choose this person?

   _____

   _____

   _____

   _____

   _____

   _____

   _____

4. Choose five of the spas listed in the section "Types of Spas." View their websites, and then list three components you found attractive about the spa and three components you did not like about the spa.

	What you like	What you did not like
Spa 1	_____	_____
	_____	_____
	_____	_____
Spa 2	_____	_____
	_____	_____
	_____	_____
Spa 3	_____	_____
	_____	_____
	_____	_____
Spa 4	_____	_____
	_____	_____
	_____	_____

Spa 5 _____   _____

_____   _____

_____   _____

Study Questions

1. What is the term for the use of water for various disorders?
   a. hydrotherapy
   b. exfoliation
   c. hygiene
   d. sauna

2. What is the name of natural hot springs people use in Japan?
   a. hammam
   b. caldarium
   c. onsen
   d. sweat lodge

3. Which ancient figure is considered the "Father of Modern Medicine"?
   a. Galen
   b. Hippocrates
   c. Asclepios
   d. Augustus

4. Who is credited with bringing water cures to modern prominence?
   a. Dr. John Harvey Kellogg
   b. Dr. John Bastyr
   c. Father Sebastian Kneipp
   d. Vincent Preissnitz

5. During the bathing process in ancient Rome, what was the warm room called?
   a. labrum
   b. caldarium
   c. tepidarium
   d. frigidarium

6. Who wrote the most important textbook for physicians in Western society until the Renaissance?
   a. Ibn Sina
   b. Galen
   c. Bastyr
   d. Ellen G. White

7. Which of the following contribute to a "spa experience"?
   a. bodywork services
   b. professionalism of staff
   c. décor
   d. all of the above

8. Which of the following are credited with recognizing a correlation between personal cleanliness and health by the fifth century BC?
   a. Chinese
   b. Babylonians
   c. Greeks
   d. Romans

9. Which of the following rooms in an ancient Roman bath gave rise to a word meaning very cold?
   a. tepidarium
   b. frigidarium
   c. caldarium
   d. labrum

10. What is another term for Turkish bath?
    a. sauna
    b. onsen
    c. hamman
    d. banya

11. St. Thomas Aquinas helped the acceptance hydrotherapy toward the end of the Middle Ages because he
    a. played a role in the acceptance of Aristotle's philosophies, including the virtues of cleanliness
    b. established foundational work in the study of naturopathy
    c. closed small mineral spring wells and encouraged the use of public baths
    d. invented the thermometer

12. Who developed the "Battle Creek Idea" that good health and fitness depended on good diet, exercise, fresh air, and proper rest?
    a. Dr. John Bastyr
    b. Dr. John Harvey Kellogg
    c. Benedict Lust
    d. Father Sebastian Kneipp

13. Which type of spa is most likely to have physicians and nurses on staff?
    a. day spa
    b. resort spa
    c. medispa
    d. mineral spring spa

14. Which of the following is least likely to have overnight accommodations for guests?
    a. medispa
    b. day spa
    c. destination spa
    d. resort spa

15. Which of the following occupations can be found in a spa?
    a. athletic trainer
    b. facialist
    c. massage therapist
    d. all of the above

16. Who is considered the "Father of Hydrotherapy"?
    a. Vincent Priessnitz
    b. Father Sebastian Kneipp
    c. Hippocrates
    d. Ibn Sina

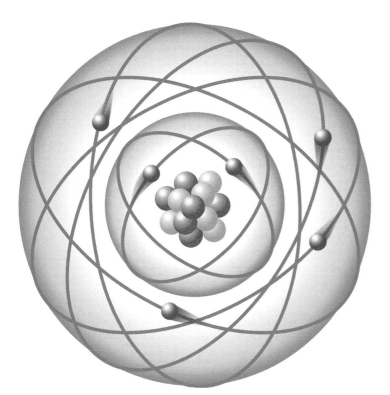

(Robin Hunter © Dorling Kindersley)

Water is life's matter and matrix, mother, and medium. There is no life without water.
—Albert Szent-Gyorgyi, Hungarian biochemist and winner of the Nobel Prize in Medicine

LEARNING OBJECTIVES

After studying this chapter, the reader will have the information to

1. Explain what the water of the body and the water of the ocean have in common.

2. Explain basic chemistry concepts.

3. Describe the ebb and flow of fluids in the body.

4. Briefly describe the structures and functions of each of the systems of the body.

5. Explain the importance of knowledge of the integumentary, cardiovascular, nervous and lymphatic, and immune systems to spa and hydrotherapy.

6. Delineate the factors involved in thermoregulation.

KEY TERMS

Acid	Dehydration	Ionic bond	Radiation
Acidosis	Dermis	Ions	Rehydration
Alkalosis	Electrolytes	Metabolic rate	Sebaceous (oil) gland
Anion	Electrons	Metabolism	Shell temperature
Atoms	Element	Mineral	Solutes
Base (alkali)	Epidermis	Molecules	Solution
Cation	Evaporation	Neutrons	Solvent
Chemical bond	Fluid balance	Nucleus	Subcutaneous layer
Conduction	Homeostasis	Osmosis	Sudoriferous (sweat) glands
Convection	Hydration	Pathogen	Thermoregulation
Core temperature	Hypodermis	pH scale	Vasoconstrict
Covalent bond	Hypotension	Protons	Vasodilate

THE CONNECTION BETWEEN SCIENCE AND SPA AND HYDROTHERAPY

To understand how spa therapies and hydrotherapy work, it is essential to have an understanding of how the human body functions. These therapies are not merely applied to clients' bodies; the therapies interact with human tissue. Practitioners need to be able to recommend specific treatments for their clients' needs. It is also the practitioner's responsibility to know which treatments would not be useful to particular clients and would, perhaps, even be harmful to them. Knowing the basic physiology of the body and how treatments affect organs and systems gives practitioners the tools they need to make these decisions.

Homeostasis is the term for the relative consistency in the body's internal environment. Homeostasis is not a fixed state. Instead, many regulatory processes monitor conditions in the body and then respond in particular ways to keep the internal environment within normal limits. When the body is in homeostasis, metabolic processes are working as they were intended.

Disorders and diseases occur when the body is not able to return to homeostasis by itself. Intervention from outside the body is necessary. Depending on the disorder or disease, people can choose from numerous treatments to alleviate their symptoms and address the cause. These include Western allopathic methods, naturopathy, Eastern traditional medicine, Ayurvedic medicine, bodywork, hydrotherapy, and, of course, many others.

WATER

Water is abundant, versatile, naturally available, inexpensive, and easy to use. Since hydrotherapy is defined as the use of water in the treatment of various mental and physical disorders, perhaps it can be considered a natural medicine. Water has properties that are important to hydrotherapy's effectiveness. It is the best and most effective solvent known. (In a **solution**, the **solvent** is the liquid that dissolves substances called **solutes**. So, *solutes + solvent = solution*.) Because of its versatility, there are many different ways to use water in treatments designed to address and alleviate certain conditions.

Ways Water Is Used in Treatments

Water as a solid is used for:

▶ ice packs
▶ ice massage

Water as a liquid is used for:

▶ baths
▶ showers
▶ hot tubs
▶ cold plunges
▶ whirlpools
▶ compresses
▶ fomentations
▶ contrast applications
▶ body wraps

Water as a vapor is used for:

▶ inhalation treatments
▶ steam baths

Additionally, substances within water, such as those found in mineral springs and seawater, or used with water can enhance vitality and healing. Muds, clays, peat, seaweed, salt, essential oils, herbs, and ginger are some substances that can be used to supplement water therapies. Even treatments that use little or no water, such as paraffin, dry brushing, and certain other exfoliation methods, can be used with water-based treatments, such as body wraps, and add to their therapeutic properties. So there are quite a few treatments from which to choose and quite a few combinations of treatments that can be performed. The beauty of spa and hydrotherapy treatments is this variety.

Since humans have been using water in its various forms, at various temperatures, and in conjunction with many different substances for health and healing for thousands of years, much of the information on the effects of hydrotherapy treatments has been anecdotal. It was handed down initially through oral history and then later written down. No doubt there has been much trial and error in the application and results of hydrotherapy treatments through the centuries. Earlier practitioners of hydrotherapy may not have known the science behind a particular treatment and why it worked for a particular condition; they just knew that it worked.

With the development of modern scientific research methods, anecdotal evidence was no longer considered valid. Although written records have historically shown hydrotherapy treatments to be effective, Western thought did not consider them to be medicine because they had not been proven scientifically. Instead, hydrotherapy was relegated to the realm of folk medicine. Recently, however, there has been an increase in the interest in and use of alternative medicine, including massage therapy, traditional Chinese medicine, acupuncture, shiatsu, and, of course, hydrotherapy. Because of this interest, Western science has undertaken research into the effectiveness of these treatments.

Water of the Earth, Water of the Body

Water is the most abundant substance in the world. It is also the most abundant substance in the human body. Depending on age and gender, 45 to 75 percent of adult bodies consist of fluids. Lean muscle mass contains more water than adipose (fat) tissue. Adipose actually repels water, so people who have more adipose tissue have less water content in their bodies than those with more lean muscle mass. Infants have the highest percentage of water, up to about 75 percent of body mass. The amount decreases until about age 2. Until puberty, water makes up about 60 percent of body mass in both boys and girls. Since adult women generally have more adipose tissue than men, about 55 percent of women's body mass is water and about 60 percent of adult men's body mass is water. See ▶Figure 2.1 for the breakdown of water content in the bodies of adults, children, and infants.

Water needs to be taken in to ensure the proper health and functioning of the organs and systems of the body. However, people are instinctively drawn to water for more than just replenishing their fluids. There is a connection between living creatures and the water of the Earth. The fluids of the body have a remarkable resemblance to seawater. In fact, the fluids of the body can be thought of as an "inner ocean." Body fluids and the ocean both consist primarily of water, and many of the same chemical components are found in each.

CHEMISTRY OF THE BODY

An **element** is a substance that cannot be split into a simpler substance by ordinary chemical means. Elements are the building blocks of all matter, living and nonliving. Each element is designated by a chemical symbol, which is one or two letters of the name of the element in English, Latin, or another language.

A **mineral** is an inorganic element that occurs naturally in the Earth's crust. Minerals can dissolve in water as water comes into contact with the Earth's crust, or they can be absorbed by growing plants. When animals and humans eat plants, they ingest the minerals, which become part of their bodies. Minerals can also come into the body by drinking mineral water, and extremely small amounts can enter by soaking in mineral baths or by the

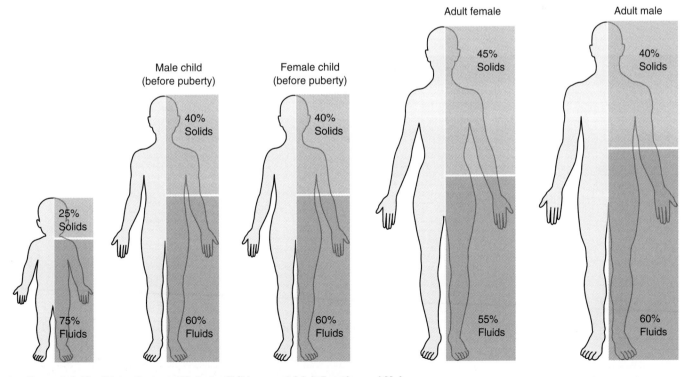

▶ **Figure 2.1 The Water Content of Infants, Children, and Adult Females and Males**

application of muds to the surface of the body. When humans eat animals, or products the animals make, such as milk, they absorb the minerals from the animals' tissues and products.

There are about seventy minerals dissolved in seawater (the seven most common are shown in ▶Table 2.1) and about twenty-six minerals in the human body (see ▶Table 2.2). The concentration of each mineral, however, can vary greatly between seawater and the human body and between different parts of the body. For example, the concentration of sodium and chlorine in seawater is much higher than in body fluids. The concentration of calcium is much higher in the bones of the body than in any body fluid.

Ions, electrolytes, pH, hydration—all of these are terms used in the spa and bodywork professions. But what exactly do they mean? And why are they important? Believe it or not, they all have to do with chemistry. Many of the effects of hydrotherapy and spa treatments are due to chemical reactions. All the processes happening in the body are also due to chemical reactions (the term for all these chemical reactions is **metabolism**). So to understand the effects of spa and hydrotherapy on the client and the client's metabolism, it is necessary to understand the chemistry of the body.

Atoms

As previously stated, all matter is made up of elements. Each element is made up of **atoms**, the basic unit of matter that retains the characteristics of the element (see ▶Figure 2.2). The dense center of an atom is its **nucleus**, and it is made up of positively charged **protons** and uncharged **neutrons**. Negatively charged **electrons** travel around the nucleus in a sort of "cloud."

Each element has a characteristic number of protons, neutrons, and electrons in its atoms. That is what differentiates each element from the others. For example, each hydrogen atom has one proton and no neutrons in its nucleus and one electron orbiting around its nucleus. All atoms of carbon have six protons, six neutrons, and six electrons. The number of electrons in the atoms of an element will always be the same as the number of protons; the negatively charged electrons and the positively charged protons balance each other and the total charge of the atom is zero (see ▶Figure 2.3).

In order to interact with one another, atoms of each element have a certain way of gaining, losing, or sharing electrons. The end result of this interaction is the formation of either **molecules** or **ions** (**electrolytes**). When two or more atoms share electrons, they form a molecule. A molecule can consist of two atoms of the same element, such as oxygen, or atoms of different elements, such as hydrogen and oxygen, as in water. When the formula of a molecule is written, it shows the number of atoms of each element that are in the molecule. A molecule of oxygen is O_2 (see ▶Figure 2.4a), and a molecule of water is H_2O (see ▶Figure 2.4b).

TABLE 2.1		
The Seven Most Common Minerals in Seawater		

Element	Symbol	Percentage of Total Elements
Chlorine	Cl	55.04
Sodium	Na	30.61
Sulfur	S	7.69
Magnesium	Mg	3.69
Calcium	Ca	1.16
Potassium	K	1.10
Bromine	Br	.19
Other compounds and trace minerals*		.52

*Examples of trace minerals are aluminum (Al), chromium (Cr), cobalt (Co), iron (Fe), flourine (Fl), iodine (I), manganese (Mn), and selenium (Se).

(Charton, 2001; Pernetta, 1994)

TABLE 2.2

The Twenty-six Minerals Found in the Human Body

Element	Symbol	Percentage of Total Body Mass
Oxygen	O	65
Carbon	C	18.5
Hydrogen	H	9.5
Nitrogen	N	3.2
Calcium	Ca	1.5
Phosphorus	P	1
Potassium	K	.35
Sulfur	S	.25
Sodium	Na	.2
Chlorine	Cl	.2
Magnesium	Mg	.1
Iron	Fe	.005
Trace minerals*		.2

*Examples of trace minerals are aluminum (Al), boron (B), chromium (Cr), cobalt (Co), copper (Cu), flourine (Fl), iodine (I), manganese (Mn), and zinc (Zn).

(Tortora and Derrickson, 2006)

Ions

If an atom either gains or loses electrons, it becomes an ion, which is also known as an electrolyte (*electrolytes* and *ions* are terms that can be used interchangeably). An ion is an atom that has either a negative or positive charge because it does not have the same number of protons and neutrons. An ion is symbolized by writing its chemical symbol with the number of its positive or negative charges. For example, Na^+ is a sodium ion that has lost one electron; Ca^{2+} is a calcium ion that has lost two electrons; Cl^- is a chloride ion that has gained an electron. A positively charged ion is called a **cation**; a negatively charged ion is called an **anion**. ▶ Table 2.3 shows common ions in the body.

A **chemical bond** holds atoms together. When atoms share electrons, as in a molecule, the bond is called a **covalent bond.** Covalent bonds are extremely strong, so it takes a great deal of energy to break them. The solid components of the human body, such as skin, bones, and muscle, all have covalent bonds between the atoms. **Ionic bonds** form from the attraction of a cation and an anion. An example is NaCl (table salt). The cation Na^+ is attracted to the anion Cl^-.

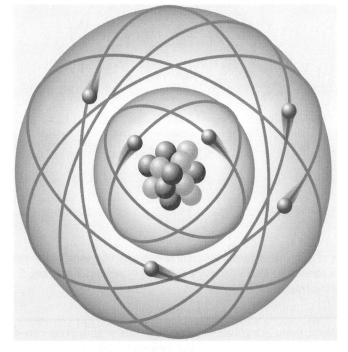

▶ **Figure 2.2** An atom; in the nucleus, the red circles are protons and the blue circles are neutrons. Circling the nucleus are electrons. *(Robin Hunter © Dorling Kindersley)*

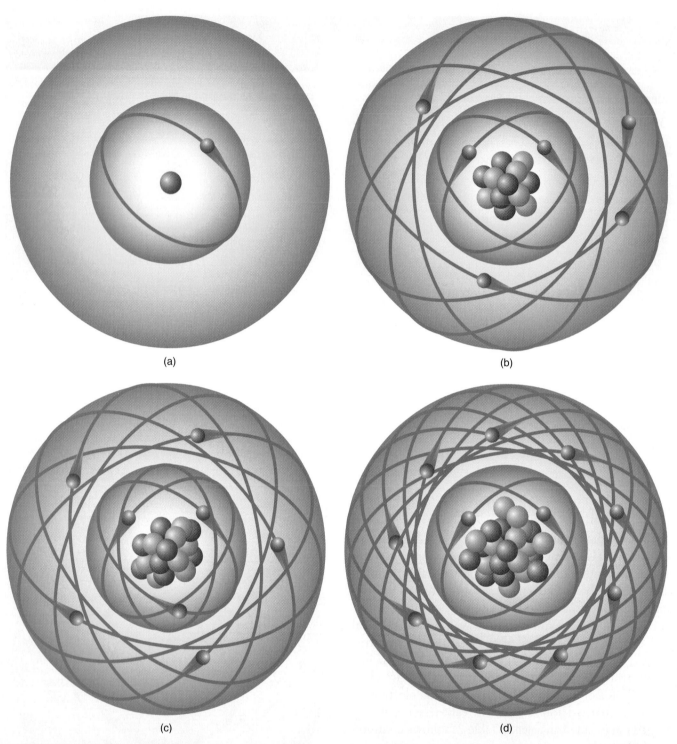

(a)

(b)

(c)

(d)

▶ **Figure 2.3 a) Atomic Structure of Hydrogen (1 proton, 0 neutrons, 1 electron) b) Atomic Structure of Carbon (6 protons, 6 neutrons, 6 electrons) c) Atomic Structure of Oxygen (8 protons, 8 neutrons, 8 electrons) d) Atomic Structure of Sodium (11 protons, 12 neutrons, 11 electrons)** *(Robin Hunter © Dorling Kindersley)*

Most ionic compounds exist as solids with a structured arrangement of ions (e.g., salt crystals). In the human body, most ionic bonds are found with the elements calcium and phosphorus in the teeth and bones, where they give the tissue a great deal of strength.

Most of the rest of the ions in the body are dissolved in body fluids. Ionic compounds that dissociate, or come apart, into cations and anions in a solution are called electrolytes. Electrolytes are so called because their solutions can conduct electricity. As the ions move around in the

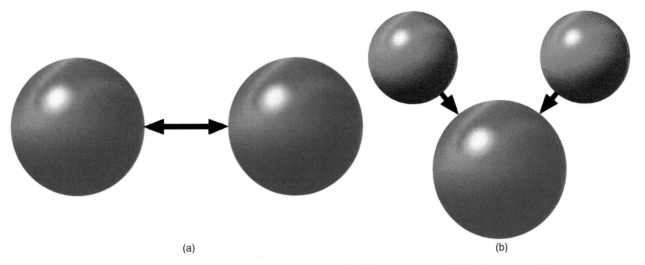

(a)   (b)

▶ **Figure 2.4 a) Oxygen Molecule (2 oxygen atoms) b) Water Molecule (1 oxygen atom and 2 hydrogen atoms)** *(Bernstein & Andriulli, Inc.)*

solution, they are creating an electrical current. Some molecules can also be positively or negatively charged. These electrolytes are extremely important to metabolism and the health of the body. The four main functions of electrolytes are to:

▶ control the movement of water between different areas of the body
▶ assist in maintaining the acid-base balance necessary for normal metabolism
▶ carry electrical current for nerve impulses and muscle contraction
▶ perform as part of the enzymes needed for metabolism

All the minerals of the body that are in body fluids are in ionic form. Therefore, most of the electrolytes of the body are, indeed, minerals. Replenishing electrolytes really means replenishing minerals. The most common ways that minerals, as electrolytes, are lost from the body are through perspiration and the elimination of wastes from the body through urination and defecation. If the body is in homeostasis, it is able to maintain electrolyte balance by replacing lost minerals from foods and liquids and by drawing minerals out of storage in bone tissue.

pH

pH is a major factor in spa products and services. The pH of the skin is of utmost importance, as well as that of products that are applied to the skin and hair. Maintaining pH balance is significant in many aspects of spa and hydrotherapy treatments. But what, exactly, is pH?

Acids and **alkalis** (also known as **bases**) are normal byproducts from the body's chemical reactions. However, body processes are quite sensitive and need to operate within very narrow limits of acidity and alkalinity because they are easily disrupted outside these limits. The **pH scale** (see ▶Figure 2.5) shows a solution's acidity or alkalinity. The scale has demarcations from 0 to 14 and is based on concentrations. The lower end of the scale (0 to 6) represents acidity. The upper end of the scale (8 to 14) represents alkalinity. A pH of 7 is neutral. Each number on the scale is a factor of 10. In other words, a pH of 5 is 10 times more acidic than a pH of 6; a pH of 13 is 100 times more alkaline than a pH of 11.

TABLE 2.3			
Common Ions in the Body			
Cations		**Anions**	
Name	**Symbol**	**Name**	**Symbol**
Calcium ion	Ca^+	Chloride ion	Cl^-
Hydrogen ion	H^+	Fluoride ion	F^-
Potassium ion	K^+	Hydroxide ion	OH^-
Sodium ion	Na^+	Phosphate ion	PO_4^{3-}
Magnesium ion	Mg^+	Sulfide ion	S^{2-}

(Tortora and Derrickson, 2006.)

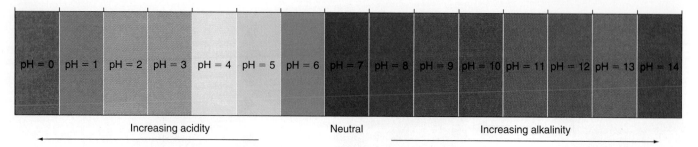

Increasing acidity   Neutral   Increasing alkalinity

▶ **Figure 2.5 pH Scale**

Each body fluid has its own particular pH, and it is important for that pH to be maintained. For example, normal pH of blood is 7.35 to 7.45. **Acidosis** is a blood pH below 7.35, and the main effect is depression of the central nervous system, possibly leading to coma and death. **Alkalosis** is a blood pH above 7.45, and the main effect is overexcitability of the central nervous system, possibly leading to muscle contractures and tetany (muscles that cannot stop contracting). The body has many mechanisms to keep pH within normal homeostatic levels, and when the body is healthy, pH levels stay relatively constant (see ▶Table 2.4 for a listing of the pH levels of common substances and parts of the body).

TABLE 2.4	
pH of Common Substances and of Different Parts of the Body	
Substance/Body Part	**pH**
Gastric juice (HCl found in the stomach)	1.2–3.0
Vinegar	3.0
Orange juice	3.5
Tomato juice	4.2
Skin	3–5
Coffee	5.0
Saliva	6.35–6.85
Milk	6.8
Distilled water	7.0
Blood	7.35–7.45
Cerebrospinal fluid	7.4
Bile	7.6–8.6
Lye	14.0
(Tortora and Derrickson, 2006)	

EBB AND FLOW OF BODY FLUIDS

Spa and hydrotherapy treatments can be applied to the entire body, or to just specific regions of the body, depending on the treatment being used. For instance, heat can be applied to the back to loosen tight muscles or to the front to alleviate abdominal cramps. A mud wrap, on the other hand, involves applying mud to the client's entire body, then wrapping the client completely. A hot foot bath can be sedating to the entire body, even though only the feet are submerged in the water. Whether the treatments are applied locally or generally, many of them work by impacting the fluid systems of the body. Understanding how body fluids work is essential to understanding how spa and hydrotherapy treatments work.

Blood, Interstitial Fluid, and Lymph

Most of the body's cells are embedded in tissues and thus are stationary. They can neither move around to get oxygen and nutrients nor move away from wastes they produce (carbon dioxide, heat, and other metabolic wastes) or from changes in pH. Instead, three fluids interact to ensure the health of these stationary cells: blood, interstitial fluid, and lymph (see ▶Figure 2.6).

Blood carries oxygen from the lungs and nutrients from the digestive tract to the tissue cells. Interstitial fluid (fluid surrounding the cells) acts as a medium for exchange between the blood and the cells: oxygen and nutrients travel from the blood through interstitial fluid into the cells; carbon dioxide, heat, other metabolic wastes, and products made by the cells such as enzymes and hormones move from the cells into the interstitial fluid. Some of the interstitial fluid, and the substances it contains, enter the blood that is carried away from the cells while some interstitial fluid continually drains into lymphatic vessels and becomes lymph. After being filtered through lymph nodes (to remove cellular debris and **pathogens** (disease-causing organisms such as bacteria, viruses, and fungi), lymph returns to the blood and becomes part of the cycle again.

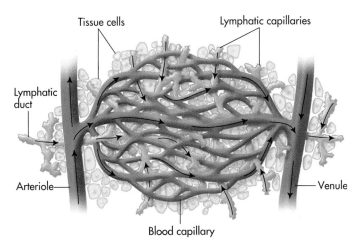

Figure 2.6 Relationship of Blood, Interstitial Fluid, and Lymph
Cells are embedded in tissues and thus are stationary. Blood, interstitial fluid, and lymph interact to ensure the health of stationary cells within the body's tissues.

Homeostasis of the body depends, in great part, on the continual movement of the blood, interstitial fluid, and lymph, and on having the correct amount of each of these fluids. That is why water intake is so important. For example, if not enough interstitial fluid drains into lymphatic vessels, an excessive amount of interstitial fluid can accumulate, resulting in edema (swelling of tissues). If there is not enough fluid in the blood, **hypotension** (low blood pressure) can result. **Fluid balance** means that various parts of the body have the amount of water and solutes (dissolved particles) they need to function properly. Fluid

balance depends mainly on electrolyte balance so the two are interconnected.

Water is attracted to charged particles such as electrolytes. As electrolytes move through the different parts of the body, water will follow. This can be thought of as electrolytes "drawing" water with them. If more water is needed in a particular area, the body has mechanisms to move it there directly, or the body can move water indirectly by moving electrolytes. An example is what occurs when blood volume decreases, such as blood loss from an injury. When blood volume decreases, there is a chance that blood pressure will dip dangerously low. To increase blood volume, the body secretes several hormones. One, antidiuretic hormone (ADH), causes the movement of water molecules from the urine back into the bloodstream. The other, aldosterone, causes the movement of Na^+ from the urine back into the bloodstream. As the Na^+ moves, water is drawn with it. Both mechanisms result in an increase in blood volume and, if not too much blood has been lost, blood pressure will return to normal.

Independent of charges that particles may or may not have, water will also travel from an area of higher concentration of solutes to an area of lower concentration of solutes. This is called **osmosis.** In ▶Figure 2.7, a dilute solution is separated from a concentrated solution by a membrane selectively permeable to water. "Selectively permeable" means that only certain particles or molecules are allowed through. In this case, the membrane will allow only water molecules, not the solutes, through. As seen by the arrow, water will travel through the membrane until

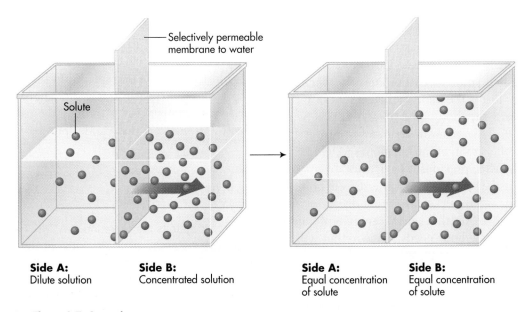

Side A:
Dilute solution

Side B:
Concentrated solution

Side A:
Equal concentration
of solute

Side B:
Equal concentration
of solute

Figure 2.7 Osmosis
Osmosis is the term that describes water moving from an area of low solute concentration to an area of higher solute concentration.

there is an equal concentration of solutes on both sides. The higher the concentration of solutes, the faster and more strongly osmosis will occur.

Body Water Gain and Loss

Throughout a given day, the human body generally gains and loses water. **Hydration** describes the state in which the body has enough fluids. If the body does not have enough fluids, it is in a state of **dehydration.** Replacing fluids to counteract dehydration is called **rehydration.**

There are three main ways the body gains water each day:

▶ ingested liquids absorbed through the digestive tract; this equals about 1600 mL
▶ ingested foods that contain water (such as fruits, vegetables, and meat) absorbed through the digestive tract; this equals about 700 mL
▶ water created through the body's metabolic reactions; this equals about 200 mL.

All of this adds up to about 2500 mL of water that the body gains each day.

There are four main ways the body loses water each day:

▶ urination; this equals about 1500 mL
▶ evaporation from the skin; this equals about 600 mL
▶ exhalation from the lungs (exhaled air contains water vapor); this equals about 300 mL
▶ elimination of feces from the digestive tract; this equals about 100 mL

All of this adds up to about 2500 mL of water that the body loses each day (see ▶Figure 2.8 for more detail on daily body water gain and loss).

As can be seen, body fluid gain and loss should be equal each day; body fluid volume remains constant when the amount of water lost is the same as the amount of water gained. This means that body fluid homeostasis is being maintained. The body has many mechanisms to ensure this. One example is the action of the hormones ADH and aldosterone, as discussed previously. They work together to retain water to make sure blood volume stays in homeostatic ranges, and, as a result, urine output decreases. On the other hand, if a greater than normal amount of fluid is taken in, more than the body needs, urine output will be more than usual to eliminate the excess fluid.

Sometimes body water gain and loss are not equal and the body's fluid homeostasis is challenged. For example, excessive fluid loss, perhaps through sweating, diarrhea, or high urine output, can result in dehydration and loss of minerals. If fluids are replaced by drinking only plain water, then body fluids will become more dilute. This dilution attracts

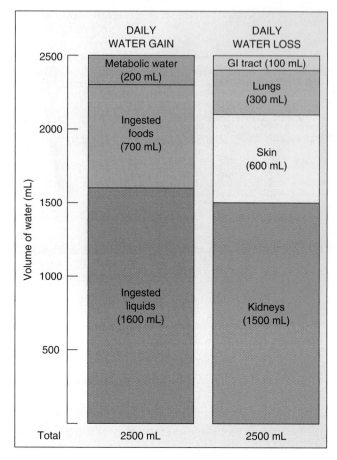

▶ **Figure 2.8 Daily Body Water Gain and Loss**

Na^+ in the blood, and Na^+ moves from the blood into interstitial fluid, then into the cells. Through osmosis, water follows the Na^+ and enters the cells as well, causing them to swell dangerously. This can lead to a condition called *water intoxication,* which is characterized by convulsions, coma, and, possibly, death. To prevent this, electrolytes should always be replaced when drinking fluids to rehydrate.

Electrolytes can be replaced in several ways. One of the simplest is to take in a small amount of salt when drinking fluids. Another way is through the use of commercial electrolyte packets that can be purchased and added to

DID YOU KNOW?

Alcohol inhibits the secretion of ADH. That is why urine output increases when drinking alcoholic beverages, which may lead to dehydration. In fact, the effects of a hangover are really the effects of dehydration. This is one of the reasons why spa and hydrotherapy treatments, especially those involving heat that can cause the loss of body fluid through perspiration, should not be performed on clients who have been drinking.

drinking water. A third way is drinking commercial beverages that already have electrolytes in them; there are many of these currently on the market. Yet another way is through eating fruits and vegetables that have varying amounts of minerals in them. For example, bananas are high in K^+, which is why they are often offered to those participating in sports events such as charity walks and triathlons.

Since spa and hydrotherapies involving the use of heat may cause clients to perspire and subsequently lose fluids and electrolytes, it is important to have water readily available for them during and after the treatment. It would also be helpful to offer something to help replace electrolytes, such as fruit juices or pieces of fruit and vegetables—bananas, oranges, melon, cucumber, or watercress, for example.

BODY SYSTEMS

The human body is a marvel of design and function. Humans can live in the Arctic, the desert, the mountains, and the tropics. Because of all the mechanisms the body uses to maintain homeostasis, with certain adaptations, people not only survive but thrive in these widely varying environments. Additionally, the body is able to heal itself from many types of injuries, traumas, and illnesses (although if severe enough, medical intervention may be needed). To understand how this is possible, it is necessary to take a closer look at the body.

Western scientists have separated the body into eleven systems. Each system is composed of organs that have related or common functions (see ▶Figures 2.9–2.19).

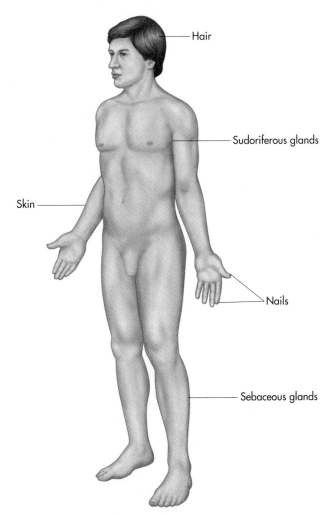

Integumentary System

Organs: Skin, hair, nails, sudoriferous (sweat) glands, sebaceous (oil) glands

Functions: Protects the body; helps regulate body temperature; eliminates some wastes; plays a role in vitamin D synthesis; detects sensations such as touch, warmth, cold, pain

▶ **Figure 2.9 The Integumentary System**

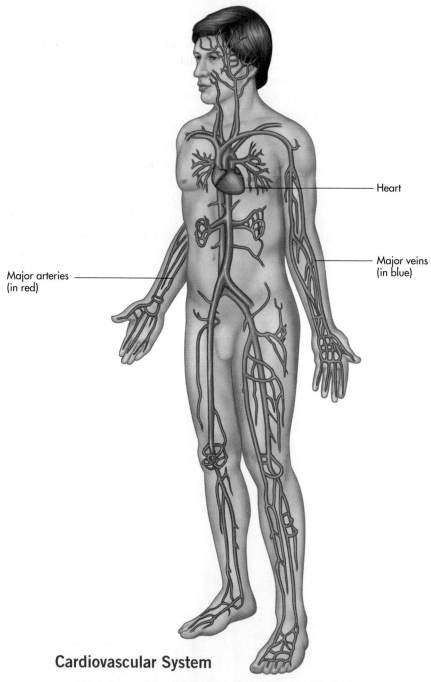

Heart

Major veins
(in blue)

Major arteries
(in red)

Cardiovascular System

Organs: Blood (the liquid portion is called *plasma;* there are three types of blood cells: red blood cells called *erythrocytes,* white blood cells called *leukocytes,* and platelets called *thrombocytes*), heart, blood vessels

Functions: Blood carries oxygen (via red blood cells) and nutrients to cells and transports carbon dioxide, wastes, and heat away from cells; helps regulate acid-base balance, temperature, and water content of body fluids; defends against disease (via white blood cells) and blood loss (via platelets); heart pumps blood through blood vessels

▶ **Figure 2.10 The Cardiovascular System**

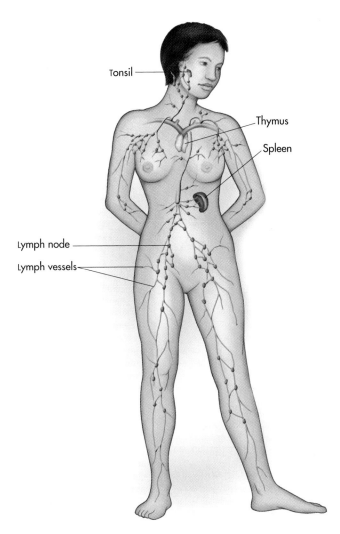

Tonsil

Thymus

Spleen

Lymph node

Lymph vessels

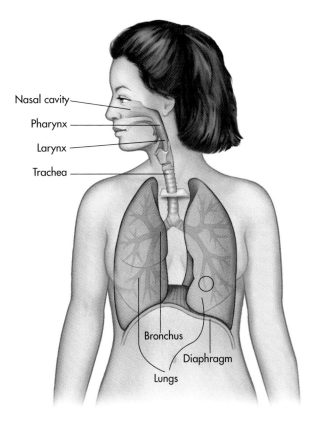

Nasal cavity

Pharynx

Larynx

Trachea

Bronchus

Diaphragm

Lungs

Respiratory System

Organs: Lungs and air passageways (pharynx or throat, larynx or voice box, trachea or windpipe, and bronchial tubes)

Functions: Transfers oxygen from inhaled air to the blood, and carbon dioxide from the blood to exhaled air; helps regulate acid-base balance of body fluids; sound production

▶ **Figure 2.12 The Respiratory System**

Lymphatic and Immune System

Organs: Lymphatic fluid, lymphatic vessels, lymphatic tissue (spleen, thymus, lymph nodes, tonsils)

Functions: Returns proteins and fluids to the blood; filters cellular debris out of lymph before it is returned to the blood; protects against disease-causing organisms

▶ **Figure 2.11 The Lymphatic System**

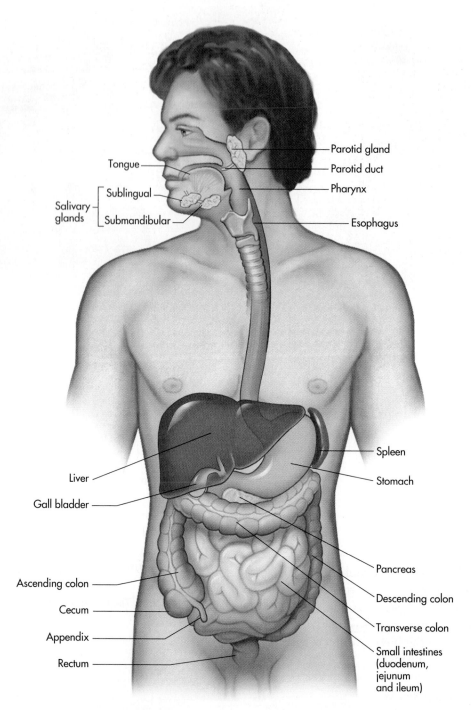

Digestive System

Organs: Mouth, esophagus, stomach, small intestine, and large intestine; accessory structures and organs include salivary glands, liver, gallbladder, and pancreas

Functions: Breakdown of food; absorption of nutrients; elimination of solid wastes

▶ **Figure 2.13 The Digestive System**

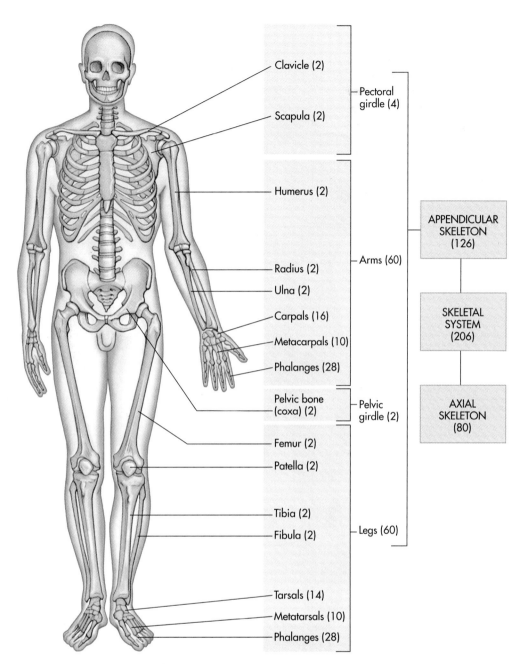

Clavicle (2)
Scapula (2)
Pectoral girdle (4)

Humerus (2)

Radius (2)
Ulna (2)
Carpals (16)
Metacarpals (10)
Phalanges (28)
Arms (60)

Pelvic bone (coxa) (2)
Pelvic girdle (2)

Femur (2)
Patella (2)

Tibia (2)
Fibula (2)
Legs (60)

Tarsals (14)
Metatarsals (10)
Phalanges (28)

APPENDICULAR SKELETON (126)

SKELETAL SYSTEM (206)

AXIAL SKELETON (80)

Skeletal System

Organs: Bones, joints, associated cartilage
Functions: Supports and protects the body; aids body movements; blood cell formation; mineral and lipid storage

▶ **Figure 2.14 The Skeletal System**

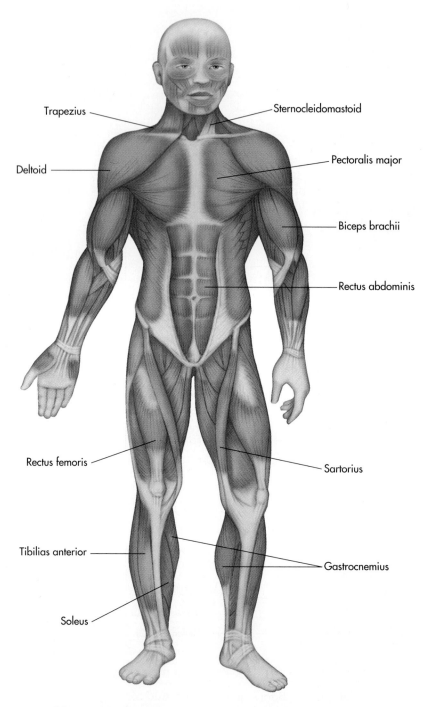

Trapezius
Sternocleidomastoid
Deltoid
Pectoralis major
Biceps brachii
Rectus abdominis
Rectus femoris
Sartorius
Tibilias anterior
Gastrocnemius
Soleus

Muscular System

Organs: Skeletal muscles (each muscle is a separate organ); called skeletal muscles because they are attached to bones of the skeleton

Functions: Produces body movements; stabilizes body positions; generates body heat

▶ **Figure 2.15 The Muscular System**

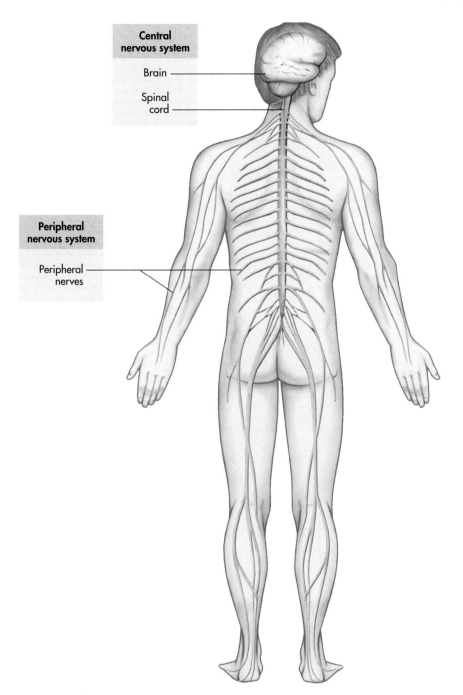

Central
nervous system

Brain

Spinal
cord

Peripheral
nervous system

Peripheral
nerves

Nervous System

Organs: Brain, spinal cord, nerves, and specialized
sense organs such as the eyes and ears

Functions: Detects changes in the body's internal
and external environment; interprets the changes;
responds by generating nerve impulses that cause
muscular contractions or glandular secretions

▶ **Figure 2.16 The Nervous System**

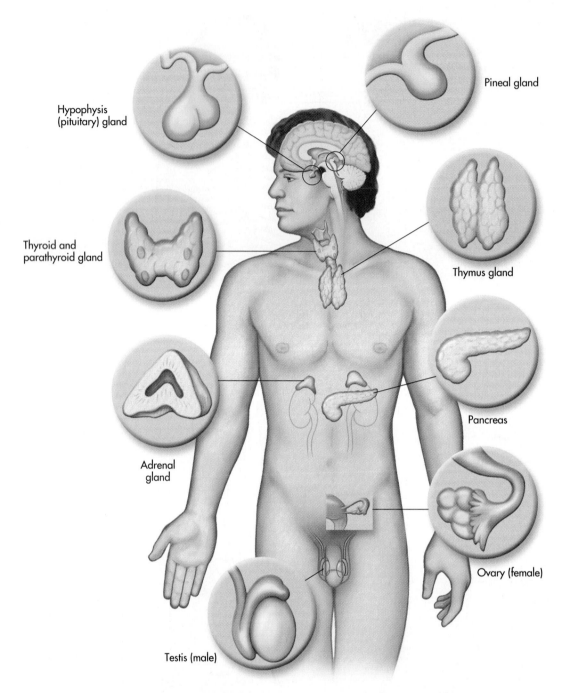

Hypophysis (pituitary) gland

Pineal gland

Thyroid and parathyroid gland

Thymus gland

Adrenal gland

Pancreas

Ovary (female)

Testis (male)

Endocrine System

Organs: Hormone-producing glands: hypothalamus, pituitary gland, pineal gland, thymus, thyroid gland, parathyroid glands, adrenal glands, pancreas, ovaries, testes

Functions: Regulates body functions by releasing hormones, which are chemicals transported in the blood to a particular organ or tissue

▶ **Figure 2.17 The Endocrine System**

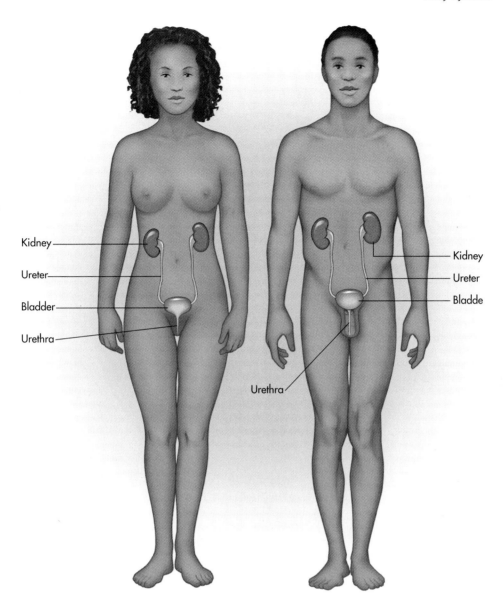

Kidney

Ureter

Bladder

Urethra

Kidney

Ureter

Bladde

Urethra

Urinary System

Organs: Kidneys, ureters, urinary bladder, urethra

Functions: Produces, stores, and eliminates wastes in urine; regulates volume and chemical composition of the blood; helps maintain acid-base balance of body fluids; maintains body's mineral balance; helps regulate red blood cell production

▶ **Figure 2.18 Male and Female Urinary Systems**

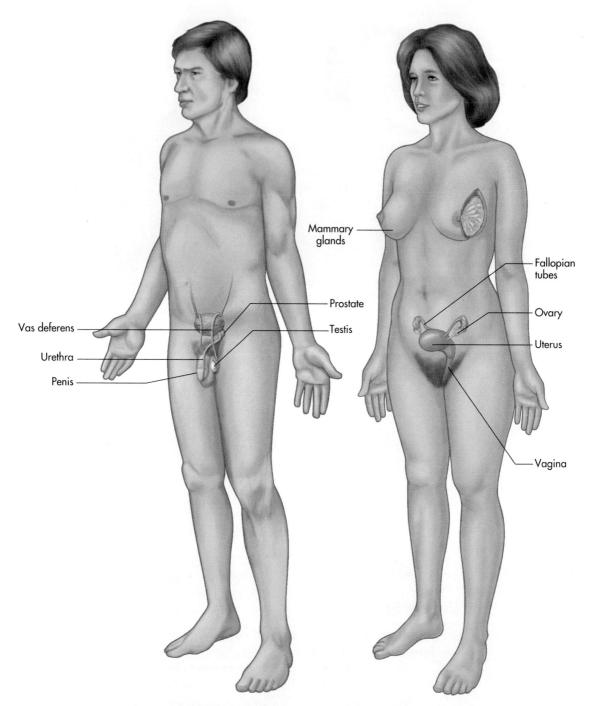

Mammary glands

Fallopian tubes

Ovary

Prostate

Uterus

Vas deferens

Testis

Urethra

Penis

Vagina

Reproductive Systems

Organs: In males: testes, epididymis, ductus deferens, penis; in females: ovaries, uterine tubes,
uterus, vagina

Functions: Sperm and egg production; hormone release for regulation of reproduction and other body
processes

▶ **Figure 2.19 Male and Female Reproductive Systems**

A CLOSER LOOK AT FOUR SYSTEMS

All 11 body systems work together, of course, to ensure the smooth functioning of the body. No system functions alone; each system is interconnected with the others. For example, blood, part of the cardiovascular system, flows to every organ in the body. Nerves within the nervous system go to the muscles and organs of all the other systems. Immune cells, part of the lymphatic system, are on patrol in the tissues of all the organs of the body.

Spa and hydrotherapy treatments can have an effect on all the systems of the body, even when applied to only part of the body. This further shows how all the systems of the body work together. But even though the entire body is reaping the benefits of these treatments, and giving the client an overall sense of well-being, four systems are affected most directly. These four systems are discussed in detail.

Integumentary System

The skin is the part of the body on which spa and hydrotherapy treatments have their first and most immediate impact. The function of the skin is to separate the body's internal environment from the external environment. It is the largest organ of the body, covering about 22 square feet, and the heaviest, weighing about 10 to 11 pounds. Associated with the skin are glands, muscles, and nerves.

The functions of the skin include:

▶ protecting the body from the external environment
▶ receiving sensations
▶ acting as a blood reservoir
▶ regulating body temperature
▶ playing a role in vitamin D synthesis
▶ participating in excretion and absorption

It is the skin's structure that allows it to perform these varied functions. See ▶Figure 2.20 for a visual representation of the layers of the skin.

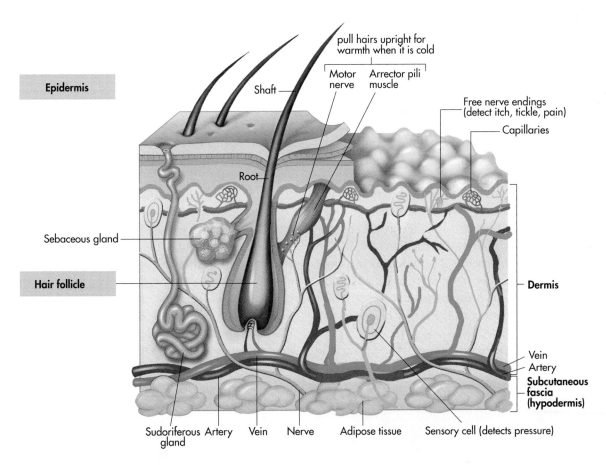

▶ **Figure 2.20 The Three Layers of The Skin**
It is vital to understand the parts and functions of the skin as this is where spa and hydrotherapy treatments have their initial and most immediate impact.

There are two parts to the skin: the epidermis and the dermis. The **epidermis** is the superficial aspect of the skin, forming the surface of the body. It has many layers of densely packed cells and is avascular, which means it does not contain any blood vessels. The deeper layers of cells are continually dividing and migrating toward the surface of the skin. As they travel upward, they fill with keratin, a waterproof, protective substance that kills the cells. Thus the top-most surface of the skin is composed of waterproof dead cells that are continually being sloughed off, taking bacteria and other pathogens with them. In the deep layers of the epidermis, another type of cell participates in immune responses, providing further protection from pathogens that are able to enter the skin from the outside.

Sebaceous (oil) glands secrete oil that coats most of the body and its hairs, keeping them from drying out and making them supple and soft. Oil also plays an important role in the body's defense. The pH of the skin ranges from three to five and is due to acids in the oil. This acidity kills most of the bacteria and other disease-producing organisms that land on the skin.

The skin, then, provides protection from the external environment by being an effective barrier; not only are the top skin cells hard to penetrate, there are also many ways the skin protects underlying tissues from disease-causing organisms.

The skin is able to receive many different sensations because of the various types of cells in the deep layers of the epidermis that are part of the nervous system. These cells detect sensations such as pain, warmth, cold, touch, and vibration.

Underneath the epidermis is the **dermis.** This layer is made of connective tissue that is composed of protein and adipose tissue. Blood vessels, nerves, **sudoriferous (sweat) glands,** sebaceous glands, and hair follicles are all embedded in the dermis. Underneath the dermis is the **subcutaneous layer** or the **hypodermis.** The subcutaneous layer is not part of the skin; rather it serves to anchor the skin to underlying structures such as muscles and bones. Blood vessels in the dermis connect to the larger blood vessels in the subcutaneous layer.

The skin has the function of being a blood reservoir because of the blood vessels in the dermis. When more blood is needed elsewhere in the body, such as in mus-cles that are contracting during exercise, certain skin blood vessels will **vasoconstrict,** or decrease in diameter, so less blood will flow through them, and more blood will flow to blood vessels in the muscles. When the exercise ceases, these skin blood vessels will **vasodilate,** or become larger in diameter, so that more blood will flow in them once again.

The skin helps with body temperature regulation, or **thermoregulation,** with both sudoriferous glands and the blood vessels in the dermis. When the body is warm and needs to cool, the sudoriferous glands are stimulated; the evaporation of perspiration takes a great deal of heat away from the body. Blood has a high water content, and water absorbs and transports heat readily. To cool the body, certain blood vessels in the dermis vasodilate. This increases blood flow to the skin, where the heat in the blood can radiate to the environment. This increased blood flow to the skin is what gives the skin its characteristic red color when warm. When the core of the body is cooling, skin blood vessels vasoconstrict so that the warm blood will be shunted to the core to keep it warm.

One aspect of some spa and hydrotherapy treatments is to actually induce a "flushing" action of the blood in the affected area, which involves the phenomena of vasoconstriction and vasodilation. Vasodilation floods the region with blood, bringing in necessary oxygen and nutrients; vasoconstriction pushes the blood out of the region, taking with it waste products.

In order for the body to produce Vitamin D, UV rays in sunlight need to activate a precursor molecule found in the skin. Once this molecule is activated, enzymes from the liver and kidneys modify it into an active form of Vitamin D that can help increase the absorption of calcium from the digestive tract into the blood.

The skin plays a minor role in absorption and a somewhat larger role in excretion. Because of the overall structure and properties of the skin, not many substances are able to exit or enter the body. Only a few substances are able to be absorbed through the skin, including oxygen and carbon dioxide; certain drugs; fat-soluble substances, such as vitamins A, D, E, and K; and some small ions. Water, wastes, and small molecules are excreted through the skin in perspiration. In fact, up to 10 percent of the body's metabolic wastes are eliminated through perspiration.

Since spa and hydrotherapy treatments are placed directly on clients' skin, they can interact with the skin's acid mantel and affect its pH. They can also draw impurities out of the skin, hydrate it, and remove the top layer of dead skin cells. Exfoliation treatments are designed to assist in the removal of dead skin cells. Blood flow just under the surface of the skin and deeper can be affected by applying hot and cold treatments, and muscles, connec-

DID YOU KNOW?

The acidic film of oil is also known as the skin's "acid mantel."

tive tissue, and joints can benefit from treatments applied at the body's surface. Of course not all spa and hydrotherapy treatments do all of these things. It is important that treatments are chosen based on clients' specific needs and wants, as well as with consideration as to what would not be healthy for them. Throughout the succeeding chapters, treatment choices will be explained in detail that includes benefits, indications, and contraindications along with the treatment procedure itself, allowing practitioners to have the information they need to offer their clients the best possible therapy.

Cardiovascular System

Since the cardiovascular system responds quickly to changes in both external and internal temperature, it is important to have an understanding of its complexity when performing spa and hydrotherapy treatments. There are three major parts to the cardiovascular system: the blood, the heart, and the blood vessels. *Cardio* is from the

Greek *kardio,* meaning "heart"; *vascular* is from the Latin *vasculum* meaning "small vessel," so it is easy to see how this system got its name.

Blood consists of plasma (the fluid portion), red blood cells, white blood cells, and platelets. Red blood cells, or erythrocytes, carry O_2 and some CO_2; the rest of the CO_2 dissolves in the plasma. Many types of white blood cells, or leukocytes, protect against disease by killing pathogens. White blood cells also produce antibodies, which are specialized proteins that also help protect against disease. Platelets, or thrombocytes, are part of the clotting process, which protects against blood loss. Proteins, electrolytes, nutrients, hormones, O_2 and CO_2, and waste products are also in the blood (see ▶Figure 2.21 for a visual representation of the components of the blood).

As discussed previously in "Ebb and Flow of Body Fluids," one of the functions of blood is to transport red blood cells, white blood cells, and platelets throughout the body.

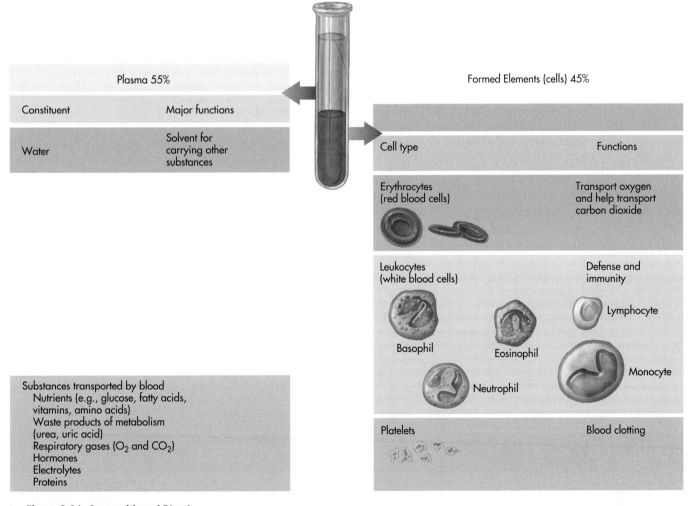

▶ **Figure 2.21 Composition of Blood**
Blood consists of plasma (the fluid portion), red blood cells that carry O_2 and some CO_2, white blood cells that protect against disease by killing pathogens, and platelets that are part of the clotting process to protect against blood loss.

The blood also helps regulate the body's pH, temperature, and water content of cells. It has chemicals that buffer acids and bases so that the pH of the blood stays within the homeostatic range of 7.35 to 7.45. Blood transports heat away from cells to the surface of the body (discussed in the section on the integumentary system). This heat is produced by cells as they carry out the chemical reactions involved in metabolism. By being part of the fluid movement between cells, interstitial spaces, and the lymphatic system, blood helps control the amount of water inside cells.

Certain spa and hydrotherapy treatments can promote health and well-being through their effects on the blood. For example, cold treatments that are tonifying can stimulate the body to increase its metabolism, which, in turn, can stimulate the increased production of leukocytes and cause them to work more efficiently. Mild heat can, to a limited extent, accelerate the clotting process.

The heart consists of cardiac muscle that contracts to pump blood to the lungs and out to the rest of the body.

The heart is unique in that it does not need nerves from the nervous system in order for its muscle to contract. It has its own conduction system that generates nerve impulses that travel through the heart and makes its chambers contract in a synchronized manner. Even though the heart does not need nerves to stimulate it to contract, nerves do go to the heart from both the parasympathetic and sympathetic nervous systems. Parasympathetic impulses keep the heart at its resting heart rate, which is normally somewhere in the range of sixty to seventy-five beats per minute (it is different for everyone). Sympathetic nerve impulses stimulate the heart to beat harder and faster, as occurs during exercise or certain stressful situations. The parasympathetic and sympathetic divisions of the nervous system are discussed in more detail in the following section.

People who have or have had certain heart conditions may not be good candidates for some hydrotherapy treatments. Extreme temperatures are stressful on the body and can stimulate the heart to beat harder and faster. A client with a healthy heart would be able to tolerate this, but a client who has heart issues may not be able to withstand the stress. For this type of client, the temperatures would need to be modified; the heat and cold would need to be milder. Or, in some cases, treatments with heat and cold would need to be avoided and other spa therapies could be offered instead (Werner, 2008).

The third component of the cardiovascular system is the blood vessels. Arteries are the blood vessels that carry oxygenated blood away from the heart. The only exception to this classification is the pulmonary arteries, which travel from the heart to the lungs. They are the only arteries in the body to carry deoxygenated blood. Veins are the blood vessels that return deoxygenated blood to the heart.

Arteries branch extensively, becoming smaller and smaller until they become arterioles. Arterioles are very small and have very thin walls. They extend into tissues and divide into capillaries, which are microscopic in size. Capillaries are where substance- and gas-exchange (the process by which cells take up oxygen and give up carbon dioxide) occurs between the cells and the blood. Capillaries join into slightly larger vessels called venules, which exit tissues. Venules continue joining together into smaller, then larger veins. All the veins end up draining into the superior and inferior vena cava, which empty into the right atrium of the heart (see ▶ Figure 2.22 for a visual of blood vessels and the capillary connection).

Arteries are buried deep within the tissues of the body. Many veins are also deep within the tissues. However, there are also superficial veins, some of which can be seen through the skin. Treatments involving heat and cold affect the superficial veins first. As discussed previously, heat causes blood vessels to dilate, and cold causes them to vasoconstrict. If the treatment is of a lengthy duration, the deeper arteries and veins can also be affected as the heat and cold penetrate deeper into the tissues.

Nervous System

The spinal cord and brain make up the central nervous system (CNS). All the nerves that communicate with the brain and spinal cord make up the peripheral nervous system (PNS). Cranial nerves communicate directly with the brain; spinal nerves communicate directly with the spinal

---

DID YOU KNOW?

Blue whales, the largest animals on earth, have a resting heart rate of six beats per minute. The average hummingbird's heart rate is 1,200 beats per minute.

DID YOU KNOW?

There are about 60,000 miles of blood vessels in the human body. That's long enough to go around the Earth 2½ times!

cord. The spinal cord and brain also communicate with each other. This communication encompasses detecting sensations from the body and the external environment, sending the information via nerve impulses into the CNS (which assesses and integrates the information), then transmitting nerve impulses from the CNS out to effectors—muscle tissue and glands—that respond to the nerve impulses. The peripheral nerves that send nerve impulses into the CNS are called *sensory* nerves because they detect sensations. Another term for them is *afferent* nerves; *afferent* is from Latin and means "to bring to." The peripheral nerves that carry nerve impulses away from the CNS to effectors are called *motor* nerves because they send impulses out to muscle tissue to make it contract or relax, and/or to glands to make them increase or decrease their secretions. Another term for motor nerves is *efferent* nerves; *efferent* is from Latin and means "to carry outward." Most peripheral nerves contain both sensory and motor nerves.

The PNS is further divided into the somatic nervous system (SNS), which controls skeletal muscles and voluntary movements, and the autonomic nervous system (ANS), which controls the cardiac muscle of the heart, the smooth muscle in organs, and glandular secretions. The ANS itself has two divisions: the parasympathetic branch, which is responsible for maintenance of the body's

daily functions; and the sympathetic branch, which overrides the parasympathetic branch during emergencies and exercise (see ▶Figure 2.23 for a visual representation of the full nervous system).

Emergencies and exercise place stress on the body, and the body responds by readying itself for action. Some of these responses are noticeable, such as an increased heart rate and tensed muscles. Other body responses that are equally important but not noticed are pupil dilation (to see better), increased transport of blood sugar to cells (for energy), and increased blood pressure (to better facilitate substance exchange between the blood and the cells).

Thirty-one pairs of spinal nerves emerge from between the vertebrae on both sides of the spinal column and from the sacrum and coccyx. Each section of the spinal cord from which a pair of spinal nerves arises is

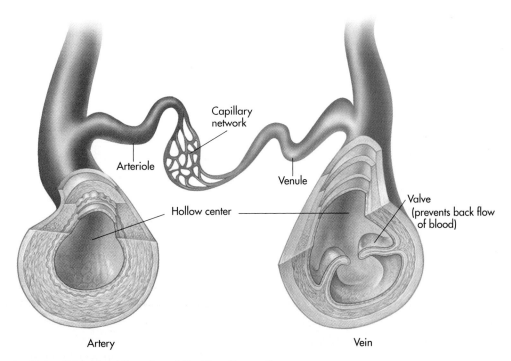

▶ **Figure 2.22 Blood Vessels and Capillary Connection**
Blood Vessels carry oxygenated blood to and from the heart. Blood vessels branch and reduce in size until they divide into capillaries, where oxygen and carbon dioxide are exchanged between the cells and the blood.

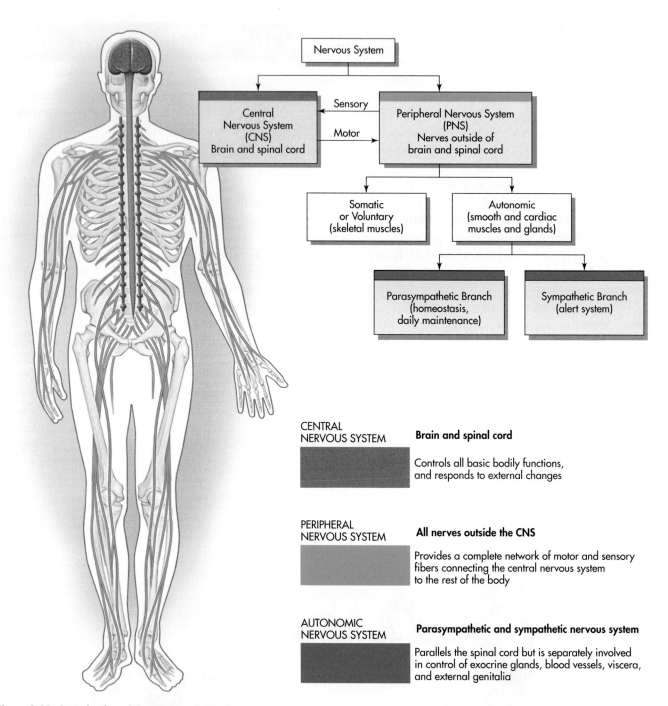

▶ **Figure 2.23 Organization of the Nervous System**
The nervous system includes the central, peripheral, and autonomic subsystems.

called a *segment* (see ▶Figure 2.24). There are eight pairs of cervical nerves (C1–C8), twelve pairs of thoracic nerves (T1–T12), five pairs of lumbar nerves (L1–L5), five pairs of sacral nerves (S1–S5), and one pair of coccygeal nerves (Co1). Twelve pairs of cranial nerves emerge from the brain, and they are labeled CN I through CN XII.

The spinal cord not only sends information from sensory nerves up to the brain, it also communicates within itself. For instance, a sensation can come into a spinal segment from one side of the body, travel up and down the spinal cord to other segments, and cause nerve impulses to travel along motor nerves from different segments and out to effectors far from where the sensation originated. Because of this, some spa and hydrotherapy treatments, especially those involving heat and cold, applied in one region of the body can produce a reaction in a different part of the body.

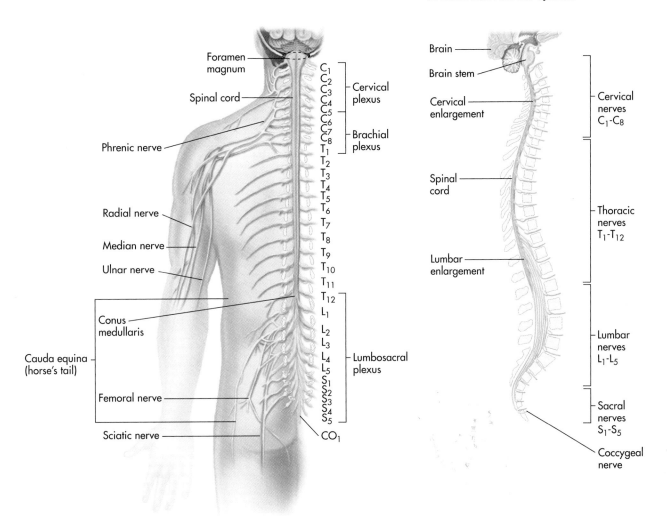

▶ **Figure 2.24 The Spinal Cord**
Each of 31 pairs of spinal nerves emerges from a segment of the spinal cord.

Spa and hydrotherapy treatments can have other effects on the nervous system. For example, many treatments are soothing and cause clients to be in deeper parasympathetic mode. This adds to their sense of well-being. Cold slows nerve impulse conduction and so can be used as an analgesic. As will be seen in Chapter 8, in aromatherapy, scent molecules travel up into nasal passages and stimulate impulses along a nerve that goes directly into the brain.

Lymphatic and Immune System

The lymphatic and immune system is composed of lymph; lymphatic vessels; specialized leukocytes called lymphocytes; and structures and organs that contain lymphatic tissue, including lymph nodes, lymphatic nodules (lymphatic tissue that is not as structured as lymph nodes, such as the tonsils), the thymus gland, and the spleen (see ▶ Figure 2.25).

As discussed previously in "Ebb and Flow of Body Fluids," one of the major functions of the lymphatic system is to drain excess interstitial fluid. Once interstitial fluid enters lymphatic capillaries, it is called *lymph*. The lymphatic capillaries drain into lymphatic vessels, which have nodes situated on them that filter out pathogens and cellular debris. The lymphatic vessels drain lymph into larger and larger vessels. There are, in fact, many more lymphatic vessels than there are veins, and superficial lymphatic vessels are closer to the surface of the body than superficial veins are. Eventually, lymph drains into two large veins near the neck. Instead of the complete circuit formed by the cardiovascular system, the lymphatic system drains only one way—from the cells to the blood.

Another major function of the lymphatic and immune system is, of course, to carry out immune functions. If pathogens make it through the body's skin and mucous membranes and penetrate more deeply into tissues, the lymphocytes go into action. Mature lymphocytes are inside the lymph nodes, the spleen, and lymphatic nodules. Lymphatic nodules are masses of lymphatic tissue located

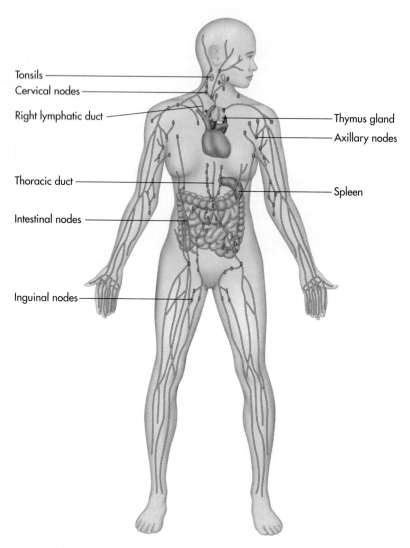

▶ **Figure 2.25 The Lymphatic System**
The lymphatic system runs from head to toe throughout the body to drain
lymph to the blood and carry out other immunity functions.

throughout the mucous membranes of the respiratory, digestive, urinary, and reproductive tracts. Since all these tracts lead outside the body, lymphatic nodules protect against pathogens trying to enter from these routes. When lymphocytes come into contact with pathogens, they respond by cloning themselves until there are large numbers of them. Some cloned lymphocytes then leave the lymphatic tissue and travel throughout the body's tissues killing pathogens as they find them. Other cloned lymphocytes stay in the lymphatic tissue and produce antibodies. These antibodies then leave the lymphatic tissue and circulate in body fluids. When they find pathogens, they inactivate them so that other leukocytes can kill them.

Spa and hydrotherapy treatments can affect the lymphatic and immune system in several ways. In addition to cold treatments that can stimulate the body to increase its metabolism, which in turn can stimulate the increased production of leukocytes and cause them to work more efficiently, it has

been found that massage therapy itself causes the body to create more leukocytes (Benjamin and Tappan, 2005). The rest and relaxation that can occur while receiving spa and hydrotherapy treatments allow the body to repair cells and put resources toward building the immune system, instead of toward dealing with stress. Exfoliation through dry brushing and other manual exfoliation methods encourages the flow of lymph in the superficial lymphatic vessels (this is discussed in detail in Chapter 5, "Exfoliation").

BODY TEMPERATURE HOMEOSTASIS

Metabolism of the Body

Metabolic rate is the overall rate at which metabolic reactions use energy for processes such as cell division, nerve impulse conduction, muscle contraction, and protein synthesis—in short, everything and anything the body needs to keep functioning. Energy that is "left over" from these processes and is not needed by the body is released as heat. So the heat that the body produces comes from all of its metabolic reactions.

Many factors affect metabolic rate, and a person's metabolic rate can change throughout a 24-hour period. For instance, exercise, stressful conditions, the release of certain hormones, ingestion of food, and fever all increase metabolic rate. Sleep and warm environments decrease metabolic rate. A child's metabolic rate is about twice that of an elderly person's rate. Women, unless they are pregnant or nursing, usually have a lower metabolic rate than men.

Thermoregulation

Shell temperature is the temperature at the body's surface, or in the skin. **Core temperature** is the temperature deep in the body underneath the skin. Usually shell temperature is 1° to 6°F lower than core temperature. When the body is in homeostasis, the rate of body heat production equals the rate of body heat loss, and core temperature remains constant at about 98.6°F (37°C). The body has homeostatic mechanisms to maintain core temperature within acceptable ranges.

As discussed in the section on the integumentary system, thermoregulation (▶Figure 2.26) is temperature regulation in the body. The body has an internal thermostat located in the brain. Receptors in the skin and brain continually monitor body temperature. When core body temperature drops to below normal, these receptors send this information to the internal thermostat, which responds in three ways to bring body temperature back up:

▶ Nerve impulses are sent to blood vessels in the skin to cause them to vasoconstrict. This decreases warm blood flow to skin (where the heat in the blood would normally radiate away from the body). Instead, the blood is moved to the core of the body to keep it warm.

▶ Nerve impulses are sent to skeletal muscles to cause them to contract and relax rapidly in a repetitive cycle called *shivering*. Most of the heat of the body is generated by muscular contraction, and maximum shivering can increase the rate of heat production up to four times that of normal heat production.

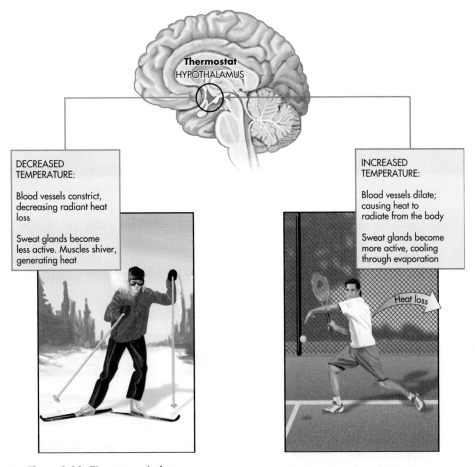

DECREASED TEMPERATURE:

Blood vessels constrict, decreasing radiant heat loss

Sweat glands become less active. Muscles shiver, generating heat

Thermostat
HYPOTHALAMUS

INCREASED TEMPERATURE:

Blood vessels dilate; causing heat to radiate from the body

Sweat glands become more active, cooling through evaporation

Heat loss

▶ **Figure 2.26 Thermoregulation**
The body's internal thermostat within the brain, the hypothalamus, is responsible for thermoregulation by responding to receptor messages about the body's core temperature.

▶ Nerve impulses are sent to the glands, causing them to secrete hormones that cause cells to increase their metabolism, which increases heat production.

The end result is an increase in core body temperature.

When core body temperature rises above normal, receptors in the skin and brain send this information to the internal thermostat, which evaluates the information and responds to bring body temperature back down. It sends nerve impulses to the sweat glands, which stimulates them to secrete perspiration. The evaporation of perspiration cools the body. Skin blood vessels vasodilate; more blood will be brought to the skin where the heat in the blood will radiate away from the body. The end result is a decrease in core body temperature.

Mechanisms of Heat Transfer

As discussed previously, maintaining normal body temperature depends on the ability to lose heat to the external environment at the same pace it is produced by metabolic reactions. There are four ways heat is transferred away from the body:

▶ **Conduction:** transfer of heat to objects in direct contact with the body—clothing, jewelry, chairs, and so on. At rest (not exercising), about 3 percent of body heat is lost this way. The body can also gain heat through conduction, such as soaking in a hot tub.

▶ **Convection:** transfer of heat resulting from the movements (currents) of air or water. Convection works in tandem with conduction. When cool air and cool water swirl around the body, they draw heat away from it. The faster the air or water moves, the faster the rate of convection. At rest, about 15 percent of body heat is lost this way.

▶ **Radiation:** transfer of heat in the form of infrared rays from warmer to cooler objects without contact. When the environment is cooler than the body, waves of heat radiate away from the body. At about 70°F, 60 percent of heat is lost in a resting person. However, if the environment is warmer than body temperature, the body will absorb heat through radiation.

▶ **Evaporation:** transfer of heat away from the body to the environment as perspiration changes from liquid to vapor. Evaporating water takes with it a great deal of heat. Evaporation is the main way the body keeps from overheating during exercise. Under extreme conditions, up to three liters of perspiration can be produced per hour, removing quite a bit of heat from the body. The higher the humidity in the environment, however, the lower the rate of evaporation. That is why it is easy for the body to overheat in humid climates. At rest, about 22 percent of heat is lost this way.

Spa and hydrotherapy treatments that involve heat and cold make use of these methods of heat transfer; more information is presented in Chapter 4.

Summary

Spa and hydrotherapy treatments are effective because they work with the body's metabolism and its systems, such as the integumentary, cardiovascular, nervous and lymphatic, and immune systems. To be able to offer clients the best possible options for their needs, an understanding of basic chem-

istry and how the body functions is essential. Since there are many treatments that use heat and cold, knowing how the body regulates its temperature and how it loses excess heat is also useful. In the world of spa and hydrotherapy treatments, a little science knowledge truly goes a long way.

Activities

1. Briefly explain the relationship between ions and minerals.

_____

_____

_____

2. Draw a picture that shows the interaction among blood, interstitial fluid, cells, and lymph. Use arrows to show how the fluids move.

3. Explain the physiological reason why spa and hydrotherapy treatments, especially those involving heat, should not be performed on clients who have been drinking alcohol.

_____

_____

_____

4. Think back to a time when you perspired a great deal. Besides water, was there something else you craved? What types of foods did you want? Why do you think you wanted those foods?

_____

_____

_____

5. Give two examples of how spa and hydrotherapy treatments can affect each of the following systems:

Integumentary

_____

_____

Cardiovascular

_____

_____

Nervous

_____

_____

Lymphatic and Immune

_____

_____

Study Questions

1. What percentage of the adult body is made up of fluids?
   a. 25–55%
   b. 30–60%
   c. 45–75%
   d. 60–90%

2. What is the term for an inorganic substance that is found in the Earth's crust?
   a. element
   b. vitamin
   c. mineral
   d. molecule

3. Which of the following is an acidic pH?
   a. 5.0
   b. 7.0
   c. 9.0
   d. 11.0

4. The term for the methods the body uses to maintain temperature is
   a. thermoregulation
   b. homeostasis
   c. vasoconstriction
   d. conduction

5. The fact that certain hydrotherapy treatments applied in one area of the body can cause a reaction somewhere else in the body is due to which body system?
   a. digestive
   b. skeletal
   c. urinary
   d. nervous

6. What is the term for the transfer of heat in the form of infrared rays from warmer to cooler objects without contact?
   a. evaporation
   b. conduction
   c. radiation
   d. convection

7. What is the homeostatic pH range for blood?
   a. 5.35–5.45
   b. 6.35–6.45
   c. 7.35–7.45
   d. 8.35–8.45

8. Which of the following is a function of electrolytes in the body?
   a. control the movement of water
   b. help maintain acid-base balance
   c. transmit nerve impulses
   d. all of the above

9. What is the definition of edema?
   a. swelling of tissues
   b. low blood pressure
   c. contracted muscles
   d. elevated heart rate

10. Osmosis involves the movement of water from a
   a. low concentration of solutes to high concentration of solutes
   b. liquid to a gaseous state
   c. high concentration of solutes to a low concentration of solutes
   d. solid to a liquid state

11. The term for the process of replenishing fluids is
   a. dehydration
   b. rehydration
   c. hydration
   d. overhydration

12. Which of the following will replenish electrolytes?
   a. excessive urination
   b. sweating profusely
   c. eating fruits and vegetables
   d. receiving cold hydrotherapy treatments

13. Which of the following is a function of the integumentary system?
   a. transmitting sensations into the CNS
   b. pumping blood throughout the body
   c. providing movement of body structures
   d. eliminating wastes from the body

14. Which of the following accurately describes an effect of spa and hydrotherapy treatments on the body?
   a. Cold treatments can stimulate the immune system to work better.
   b. Heat treatments cause vasoconstriction of blood vessels.
   c. Mild heat inhibits the clotting process.
   d. Cold treatments in one area of the body never have an effect on another area.

15. Which of the following will decrease metabolic rate?
   a. stress
   b. warm environment
   c. fever
   d. eating food

16. During profuse sweating, water intoxication can result if the person
   a. eats too many fruits and vegetables
   b. drinks fluids and electrolytes
   c. drinks only plain water
   d. eats and drinks nothing

17. If a client has heart issues, what is appropriate in terms of spa and hydrotherapy treatments?
   a. Increase the temperature of heat treatments.
   b. Alternate between decreasing and increasing the temperature for cold treatments.
   c. Use milder temperatures for both heat and cold treatments.
   d. Keep the temperatures of heat and cold treatments the same as for any other client.

18. How many pairs of spinal nerves are there?
   a. 21
   b. 25
   c. 31
   d. 36

19. An effect of cold treatments is that they
   a. stimulate the clotting process
   b. have an analgesic effect
   c. cause vasodilation
   d. decrease metabolism

20. To increase the body's temperature, nerve impulses will cause
   a. blood vessels in the skin to vasoconstrict
   b. muscles to contract and relax rapidly
   c. glands to secrete hormones that will increase metabolism
   d. all of the above

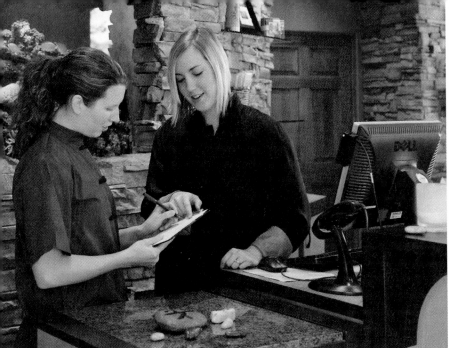

We are what we repeatedly do.

— Aristotle

LEARNING OBJECTIVES

After studying this chapter, the reader will have the information to

1. Discuss aspects of the spa experience.
2. Discuss why clear communication with clients is necessary for spa and hydrotherapy treatments.
3. Explain the various features of what it means to work in a spa.
4. Explain the universal precautions, hygiene, and sanitation necessary for spa and hydrotherapy practice.
5. Differentiate between the terms *indication* and *contraindication*.
6. Outline ways to help clients choose the best treatments for themselves.
7. Describe the considerations for incorporating spa and hydrotherapy treatments into a bodywork practice.

KEY TERMS

Antiseptics	Cross-contamination	Indication	Sanitation
Capital expenditures (expenses)	Disinfectants	Local (zonal, regional)	Systemic (general)
Code of Conduct	Esthetician	Microorganisms	Universal (standard) precautions
Contraindication	Independent contractor	Overhead	

SUCCESSFUL SPA AND HYDROTHERAPY PRACTICES

Although there is great diversity in spa settings, successful spa and hydrotherapy practices have the following in common: practitioners and spa staff need to have an awareness of what the experience means, know how to communicate effectively with clients, and be experts in helping choose the best treatments for clients. Successful spa and hydrotherapy practitioners also understand and use universal precautions and hygiene as well as rigorous sanitation methods.

There are two major options for practitioners who are interested in performing spa and hydrotherapy treatments:

▶ choosing to work in a spa setting, either as an employee or independent contractor
▶ choosing to work in private practice, either in one's own business or as part of a treatment office

There are considerations unique to each option; they can serve as guidelines for practitioners who are undecided about which path they want to follow.

ELEMENTS COMMON TO ALL SPAS

The Spa Experience

People visit spas, and want spa treatments, for a variety of reasons. Some may view spas as a place to pamper themselves and try something new. Others may see spas as places of relaxation and rejuvenation. Others may see them as wellness and life-transforming centers. Whatever the reason, spa goers, and those who want spa and hydrotherapy treatments, are usually heavily invested in having a "spa experience." This experience extends beyond the treatment itself to include the setting and all of the people encountered from the moment of arrival to time of departure.

Even though a spa experience probably means something different for everyone, some common expectations exist. One is excellent customer care. This includes being treated courteously and with respect, whether on the telephone or in person. Therefore, any questions should be answered thoroughly and pleasantly. If staff members do not know the answers, they should say so and make every effort to find out. In general, communication should be designed to put the client at ease. This is especially important for people experiencing spa and hydrotherapy treatments for the first time.

Another common expectation is that the spa or private practice office atmosphere will be warm, welcoming, and safe. Spa and hydrotherapy treatments provide a respite from the demands of everyday life, so the spa or office should be clean and tastefully decorated and convey health and healing. Many spas now choose natural materials and earth tones to emphasize the connection between wellness and natural elements. A welcoming atmosphere is also created by spa staff and private practitioners who smile and greet clients promptly, escort them where they need to go, help them with anything they need, and say good-bye as they leave.

Practitioners performing the treatments should be knowledgeable, skillful, confident, and well-groomed—that is, professional. They need to be well informed about all the services, packages, promotions, and retail products offered by the spa. Clients expect their practitioners to be properly trained for all the treatments they perform. Clients are trusting their bodies to these practitioners, so the treatments should be done smoothly and competently. The client should be the practitioner's first priority, and the client should feel this. (Most clients instinctively know when the practitioner is not focused on them.)

Another common expectation is that the experience will be special and out of the ordinary (▶Figure 3.1). Clients want something different from their everyday lives. This "specialness" can come in many different forms: offering hibiscus tea before or after a treatment or performing an exfoliation that combines ground espresso beans with dark chocolate shavings. It might be in the names of the signature treatments each spa or practitioner offers or in the color of the uniforms the spa staff wears. It could be the location of the spa itself. Often it is the combination of many different factors that adds up to a unique and extraordinary experience for the client.

Communication

The ability to communicate well is an important part of being a bodywork and spa professional. Practitioners need to be able to put clients at ease and inspire confidence. This begins the very moment the practitioner greets the client. Good eye contact, a firm handshake, and a smile are typical American ways to make a good first impression. However, in some cultures, it is considered respectful for practitioners to avert their eyes and refrain from touching the client right away. It is important for practitioners to learn how best to greet clients in the particular settings in which they are working, and then greet their clients accordingly.

The client interview should always be done privately, preferably in the treatment room with the door closed. Since intake forms are not always used in spa environments, the practitioner needs to ask appropriate questions quickly and efficiently so as to not take away time

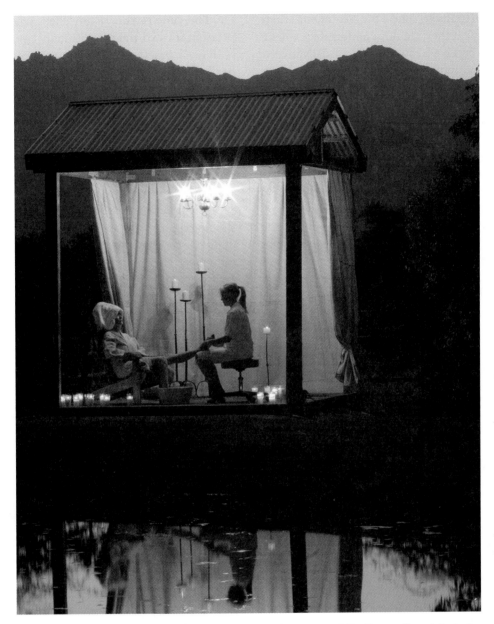

▶ **Figure 3.1** The practitioner, the ambiance, and the treatment itself can all contribute to helping the client experience something different from his or her everyday life.

from the treatment itself. It is important for the practitioner to listen carefully and make eye contact (if appropriate) while the client talks, and ask for clarification as needed. Practitioners need to remember that the client expects to feel special (Rhines, 2007).

Practitioners need to answer the client's questions as completely as possible. Going to a spa and receiving spa and hydrotherapy treatments may be a totally new experience for the client, who may be feeling excited and apprehensive at the same time. The treatment needs to be explained in depth and include:

▶ benefits, indications, contraindications
▶ how the treatment is performed

▶ what results the client can expect
▶ how the client can expect to feel after the treatment

Some spa and hydrotherapy treatments involve a certain amount of nudity for the client. For example, a client may have mud from a mud wrap rinsed off with a special shower installed above the treatment table and is either totally nude or covered only minimally for this process. Other treatments may involve only minimal coverage of the breasts, genitals, and buttocks throughout the treatment. Even though practitioners are used to this, they should still have some awareness of how unexpected it may be for a new client. Clients need to be tactfully informed about their possible levels of nudity during the treatment and given the opportunity to refuse the treatment if there is anything with which they are not comfortable. Clients may also choose to receive treatments that usually involve minimal coverage but request more conservative draping; it is up to the practitioner to modify draping as necessary to make the client feel at ease.

Sometimes clients want treatments that would not be the best ones for them. For example, a client may have spent the morning sunning out by the pool and then arrives for an afternoon spa treatment, an exfoliation, with a bad sunburn. Unfortunately, the scheduled treatment is now not possible because it would be painful and damaging to the client's skin. It is up to the practitioner to explain this clearly and tactfully to the client. Most clients will accept the expertise of the practitioner and allow themselves to be directed to another treatment more appropriate under the circumstances, or to reschedule the appointment. If clients insist on receiving treatments that are not in their best interests or could even be harmful to them, the practitioner who is employed in a spa should consult the spa supervisor for support to help manage the situation. If this occurs in the practitioner's private practice, the client can simply be asked to leave.

Occasionally clients arrive inebriated or under the influence of drugs for a spa or hydrotherapy treatment. It is very risky for clients who are under the influence to receive spa and hydrotherapy treatments for the following reasons:

▶ Some substances used in the treatments may react differently with alcohol and other drugs.
▶ Clients are not able to perceive temperature changes and the amount of pressure being applied to their body accurately and so cannot give true feedback to the practitioner.
▶ Alcohol causes the body to increase urination, which may cause dehydration. Some spa and hydrotherapy treatments are also dehydrating, particularly those involving the use of heat; using these treatments on someone who has been drinking can increase dehydration even further, possibly dangerously so.
▶ Client behavior can be unpredictable, placing both the client and the practitioner in danger.

For all these reasons, it is the responsibility of the practitioner and the spa or private office to refuse treatment to those clients under the influence. If working in a spa, practitioners may need their supervisor's support to help manage the situation. If practitioners are in private practice, they have the right to ask the client to leave and call law enforcement if necessary.

The same is true for any client who behaves inappropriately toward the practitioner. Even though spas and bodywork practices cultivate an atmosphere of health and healing, some clients assume that, at the least, it is okay to make suggestive remarks to their practitioner or that, at the most, sexual services are available. Almost every practitioner in every spa and bodywork setting has had to deal with inappropriate behavior at one time or another. In a spa, practitioners may call on their supervisor for help. In private practice, they can ask the client to leave and call law enforcement if necessary.

Any practitioner who is considering working in a spa should research the spa's policies and procedures for handling clients who are abusive, inappropriate, or under the influence. The practitioner should determine what support is available, and how it is implemented. This information is best acquired before a troublesome situation arises.

The International SPA Association has developed a **Code of Conduct** that delineates spa guest responsibilities and rights (▶Box 3.1): "To enjoy your spa experience to the fullest, observe the Code of Conduct, act responsibly and be aware that common sense and personal awareness can help ensure your satisfaction, comfort and safety, as well as that of others." This Code of Conduct is specifically for spas and hotels, but the responsibilities and rights can certainly be extended to all massage therapy and bodywork practices.

BOX 3.1

International SPA Association Code of Conduct

AS A SPA GUEST, IT IS YOUR RESPONSIBILITY TO:
1. Communicate your preferences, expectations and concerns;
2. Communicate complete and accurate health information and reasons for your visit;
3. Treat staff and other guests with courtesy and respect;
4. Use products, equipment and therapies as directed;
5. Engage in efforts to preserve the environment; and
6. Adhere to the spa's published policies and procedures.

AS A SPA GUEST, YOU HAVE THE RIGHT TO:
1. A clean, safe and comfortable environment;
2. Stop a treatment at any time, for any reason;
3. Be treated with consideration, dignity and respect;
4. Confidential treatment of your disclosed health information;
5. Trained staff who respectfully conduct treatments according to treatment protocols and the spa's policies and procedures;
6. Ask questions about your spa experience; and
7. Information regarding staff training, licensing and certification.

The Code of Conduct is officially endorsed and prepared in partnership by International SPA Association and Resort Hotel Association.

WHAT IT MEANS TO WORK IN A SPA

Spas can be exciting and energizing places to work. To remain competitive, most are continually looking for new treatments to offer and so look for the latest innovations. Spas always need enthusiastic professionals with positive attitudes, who like people, and are willing to work hard and learn new things. Practitioners in spas are regarded as experts by the clients so the practitioners need to be able to assist clients in choosing the best treatments for their needs. Clients expect practitioners to have knowledge of all spa services, packages, promotions, and retail products.

Sales and Profits

Although spas can generate a great deal of money, quite a bit of it is necessary for startup and continuing expenses. The typical spa has a large overhead. **Overhead** is the term for all the ongoing expenses of operating a business. Examples of overhead expenses include:

- marketing costs
- rent or mortgage payments
- utilities
- equipment maintenance
- business licenses and permits
- business name registration
- commercial liability insurance
- employee payroll

In addition to overhead, spas have **capital expenditures,** or **expenses.** This is money spent to upgrade, such as decorating costs and buying new equipment and supplies.

Thus, practitioners not only need to be able to perform treatments well, they are also expected to participate in selling the treatments and associated products. This is done through educating the client not only about the benefits of single treatments, but also the benefits of receiving multiple treatments. For example, if a client may have initially wanted only a body wrap, the practitioner could explain how accompanying exfoliation and massage treatments will enhance the effects of the body wrap. Additionally, there could also be products the client can purchase and use to continue experiencing the effects of the spa treatments. By being skilled at performing treatments, marketing, and working well with clients and colleagues, practitioners can enjoy a long and healthy career in the spa industry and be offered opportunities for advancement, such as into spa management and practitioner training.

Expectations of Spa Staff

Not everyone, however, has the temperament to work in a spa. It is important to consider what the work environment is like and whether it is a good fit. Many factors make up the spa work setting, and spas work best when these factors interact and function smoothly. Practitioners who work in spas should understand:

- that they are part of a team, and that their actions impact everyone else on the team
- what their roles on the team are
- who the other team members are as well as what their roles are
- how all team members work together

Spa staff needs to be able to personify and promote the spa's vision, be flexible, and be willing to learn new skills.

A chain of command ensures that the team in the spa environment works smoothly and efficiently. It is different in every spa, of course, but spa staff usually has an immediate supervisor (see ▶Figure 3.2). The supervisor's role is to make sure practitioners are on time and perform the treatments for which they are scheduled and to problem solve issues that may arise. These issues can be anything from a towel shortage to unruly clients. The supervisor also addresses disciplinary issues with practitioners and gives them feedback about their performance.

The supervisor may either be the spa manager or report to the spa manager. Spa managers not only oversee spa

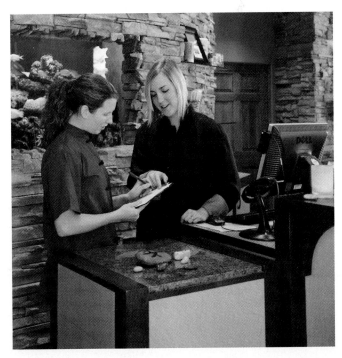

▶ **Figure 3.2** Spa supervisor interacting with a staff member.

staff, they see to it that all the supplies and equipment are maintained, as well as track the number of spa visits, the revenue generated by the spa, and the expenses the spa incurs. All of this information is sent to higher management.

The most employable spa professionals are those who have training in more than one modality, and practitioners are expected to represent all their training and experience accurately. It is unethical, and in many states illegal, to perform treatments in which the practitioner has no training.

One of the benefits of working in a spa is that practitioners usually receive training in all the treatments offered. It is expected that practitioners participate in this training even if they have completed a program of study at a school. Every spa has its own signature treatments as well as protocols for how all treatments should be given. Spas have invested a lot of time and money in these and want to ensure that all treatments are given to all clients the same way. This way, the clients always know exactly what they will be receiving regardless of the practitioner, and the spa knows exactly what is being performed.

Practitioners are expected to be punctual and have a professional appearance. This most likely involves:

▶ wearing a uniform, which needs to be clean and presentable
▶ no visible tattoos or facial piercings
▶ neatly groomed hair and nails

There is usually a seniority system for both available shifts and client booking. Those who have the least amount of seniority get the last choice of shifts. This could involve working late into the evening and/or on weekends. Practitioners may also be expected to work before and after hours of operation to help maintain the treatment rooms. The length of shifts varies with each spa. They could be in two-, three-, or four-hour blocks of time, with breaks, up to eight or more hours per day. Some spas require practitioners to be on-site for their entire shift; some require practitioners to come in only for their booked treatments but be available to come in with short notice.

Customer service is the number one priority. To meet the needs of clients, spa employees may be expected to work more often than just their regular shifts. For example, they may have regular shifts during the week plus be on-call other days.

Spa practitioners are also expected to work with their scheduled appointments; refusing to work with a particular client is generally not acceptable. Practitioners need to set aside personal feelings and be professional. If, however, there is a safety issue, such an abusive or inebriated client, practitioners do have the right to decline the treatment. Their supervisors should provide support and step in to manage uncomfortable and dangerous situations.

In some areas of the country, spa work is seasonal. During the high season, when the spa is doing most of its business, there is more demand for practitioners. During the low season, when business is much slower, some practitioners may be laid off. For example, spas in the northern part of the United States will have summer as a high season, and winter as a low season. Spas in the Southwest have a winter high season and a summer low season. It is usually the practitioners with lowest seniority who are laid off first. When interviewing for a spa position, it is important to ask about the spa's high and low seasons and what the spa's policy is regarding practitioners during their low season (Sohnen-Moe, 2008; Trieste, 2003; Wiedner, 2007).

Workforce Structure

There are two major workforce structures spas use. One of the most common is that practitioners are employees; another possibility is that practitioners are **independent contractors.** ▶ Table 3.1 shows how employees and independent contractors differ.

Pay rates can vary greatly from spa to spa. Some spas pay by the hour, some by a percentage of the cost of the treatment performed. Some spas pay lower amounts for some treatments and higher amounts for other treatments that are considered specialties. For example, there may be one pay rate for a mud wrap but a higher pay rate for an Ayurvedic wrap treatment. In some spas, practitioners may earn a commission on services and retail sales or have a combination of an hourly wage plus commission. Many times there are incentives and rewards for selling products and services. Practitioners should make sure to find out the pay structure, rates, raise policy, and sales expectations, if any, and opportunities for career advancement in any spa for which they are interested in working.

In many spas, but not all, gratuities are expected from guests. Independent contractors will receive the money directly from the client, whereas employees may either receive the money directly from the client or it is added onto their paychecks.

Whether a practitioner becomes an employee or an independent contractor for a spa, it is important that a contract be signed between the practitioner and the spa. For employees, this contract should clearly and specifically outline:

▶ the work schedule
▶ pay rates

TABLE 3.1

Employees versus Independent Contractors

Work Features	Employees	Independent Contractors
Amount of Work/Benefits	Can be full time (qualify for benefits) or part time (do not qualify for benefits)	Can be full time or part time; do not receive benefits in either case
Pay	Can be hourly or by treatment	Pay to spa either monthly room rental fee or percentage of cost of treatment performed
Costs of Treatments	Set by spa	Set by mutual agreement between spa and contractor
Client Payment for Treatments	Clients pay spa for treatments	Clients directly pay contractor
Wages	Set by spa: income taxes, Social Security, Medicare deducted from paycheck	Responsible for paying own taxes, Social Security, Medicare
Schedule	Set by spa	Set by contractor
Booking of Treatments	All booked by spa	May be booked by contractors, spa, or both
Equipment and Supplies	All provided by the spa	Contractor uses own; with mutual agreement, could use spa's equipment and supplies
On-Site Requirement	May or may not be required on-site for full shift: • If required on-site for full shift may be paid wage lower for time not booked than for time performing treatments; may also be required to perform other duties (facility maintenance) when not booked • If required on-site during shift for booked treatments only paid for treatments performed	Only required on-site for booked treatments; receive no pay for being on-site with no treatments booked

A practitioner must consider many differences before deciding whether to become a traditional spa employee or an independent contractor.

(Sohnen-Moe, 2008)

▷ amount of sick time and vacation time
▷ whether the spa pays for the employee's professional liability insurance
▷ any health care plan options

For independent contractors, the contract should include the monthly rental rate or percentage of each treatment paid to the spa and the days and times the independent contractor is choosing to work. Basically, contracts should include the employee's or independent contractor's responsibilities and the spa's responsibilities. All expectations and duties should be written in very clear language.

Spas may also have other policies and procedures of which the employee or independent contractors need to be clearly aware and should get in writing. For example, practitioners may be required to sign a confidentiality agreement and agree to not take clients with them should they leave the spa. The employee or independent contractor should know what the spa's leave-of-absence policy is as well as its policy for dealing with difficult or inebriated clients.

There are many benefits to working in a spa. Aside from the teamwork and camaraderie of coworkers and the opportunities to trade information, support, and treatments with other professionals, worker's compensation is available for employees injured on the job. Investment retirement plans may be a possibility. Other aspects of the spa's facility may be available to practitioners, such as a weight room, and there may be discounts on the spa's services. Opportunities for further training and continuing education, either on-site or by receiving reimbursement for courses completed, are also possibilities (Trieste 2003; Wiedner 2007).

Supplies and Equipment

Spas can choose from a variety of equipment and supplies and they can differ greatly in what they use for treatments. Spa staff members are expected to become familiar with and proficient at using what the spa has; each spa will provide its staff with proper training. However, certain pieces of equipment and certain categories of supplies are likely to be encountered at any establishment.

Supplies

Supplies can be everything from substances used during treatments to footwear given to clients to wear in showers. Even though there are broad categories of supplies, it is important for practitioners to remember that each

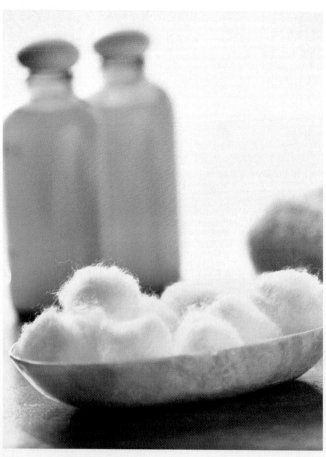

(John Davis © Dorling Kindersley)

spa has its own line of signature treatments and products, and it is important for spa practitioners to become knowledgeable about these.

▶ **Linens.**   These can include sheets used during treatments, face rest covers, blankets, towels, washcloths, plastic sheeting using during certain treatments (e.g., wraps), robes, or staff uniforms (these may be laundered on-site or practitioners may be expected to launder their own). Practitioners will be instructed in the spa's protocols for handling the linen, such as where clean ones are kept and how to dispose of used linens.

▶ **Substances.**   These are applied to the client's body or used as aromatherapy during the various treatments and can include muds, clays, seaweed, peat, creams, gels, exfoliation substances (salt, sugar, ground coffee, etc.), essential oils, herbs and other plants (for herbal infusions), and paraffin. Practitioners will be instructed in the safe use, handling, storage, and disposal methods of each substance used within the spa.

▶ **Supplies needed during the performance of treatments.**   These can include plastic wrap to cover paraffin after it has been applied to the client's body, disposable undergarments for clients, disposable spatulas to mix substances, and so forth.

▶ **Toiletries.**   These are offered for client cleanliness and convenience. They can include body washes, bath scrubbies and shower footwear, deodorant, shampoo, hair conditioner, hair spray, hair gel, combs, cotton swabs, and cotton balls. It may be the responsibility of practitioners to make sure these items are readily available for client use, or it may be a duty of other spa staff.

▶ **Cleaning supplies.**   These are necessary for hygiene and sanitation and can include rubbing alcohol, bleach and other sanitizers, and disinfectants.

Another item spas should have readily available for staff to use is disposable gloves when there is danger of contamination from coming in contact with any body fluids. This is discussed in more detail later in this chapter under "Universal Precautions, Hygiene, and Sanitation."

Equipment

Equipment encompasses everything from small brushes used in facial exfoliations to hydrotherapy tubs and Vichy showers. What follows are some examples of the equipment practitioners may use while working in a spa.

▶ Small equipment. This includes bowls used for treatment substances, spatulas, eye pillows, stones for hot and cold stone treatments, music CDs, and table warmer pads.

▶ Hot towel cabi (▶Figure 3.3). These store rolled moist towels at a temperature of about 175°F. Many have a built-in UV sanitizer that keeps the towels hygienic until they can be used.

▶ Paraffin unit (▶Figure 3.4). This safely melts paraffin and keeps it at the temperature required for application to the body (125 to 130°F). Paraffin treatments are discussed in more detail in Chapter 6.

▶ Hydrocollator (▶Figure 3.5). These are stainless steel tanks filled with water that is 160 to 165°F. The pads

are made of canvas and filled with heat-absorbing clay. Once heated, the pads are applied to the body and the heat penetrates to loosen tight muscles.

▶ Wet table (▶Figure 3.6A). This type of table has a drain in it. Clients lie on the table for treatments

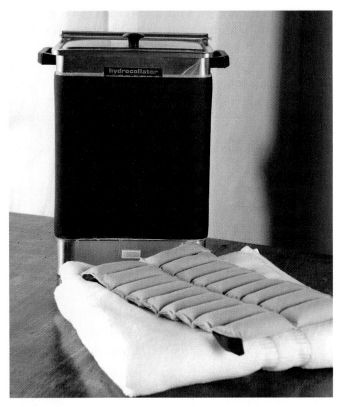

▶ **Figure 3.5** Hydrocollator and hydrocollator pads provide a local application of heat to loosen tight muscles.

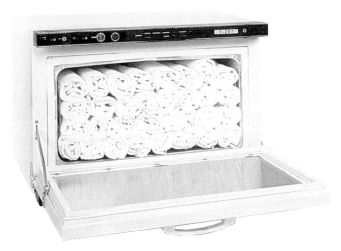

▶ **Figure 3.3** Hot towel cabi. *(Photo courtesy of YCC Products, Inc.)*

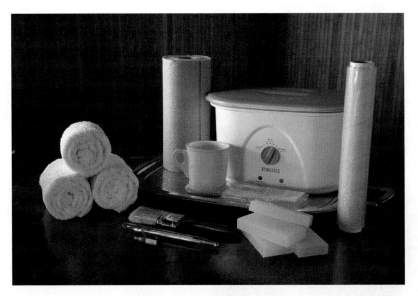

▶ **Figure 3.4** A heavy-duty professional paraffin heater is recommended over those sold for home use. Professional units are generally better made and will last longer.

involving substances that need to be rinsed off, such as muds and seaweed. Rather than have the client go to a separate shower facility, the practitioner rinses the client off, using a Vichy shower (see next entry) or other water source, while the client is on the table.

▶ Vichy shower (▶Figure 3.6B). This shower has multiple nozzles that hang above the client. The practitioner controls the temperature, pressure, and amount of water used to rinse off the client.

▶ Hydrotherapy tub (▶Figure 3.7). This tub is used for hydro massage. It is specially designed with jets and an underwater pressure hose that can be directed to areas of tension on the client's body.

UNIVERSAL PRECAUTIONS, HYGIENE, AND SANITATION

As with all services that involve human-to-human contact, practitioners need to be aware of the dangers of pathogen transmission. Pathogens are disease-causing organisms such as fungi, yeast, molds, viruses, and bacteria. Sometimes the term **microorganism** is used instead of pathogen. Microorganisms are any life forms that are microscopic. Because practitioners are working with clients who are in varying degrees of undress, the risk of passing pathogens from practitioners to clients, and from clients to practitioners, is great. There is also a risk of practitioners transferring pathogens from one client to another. Pathogens

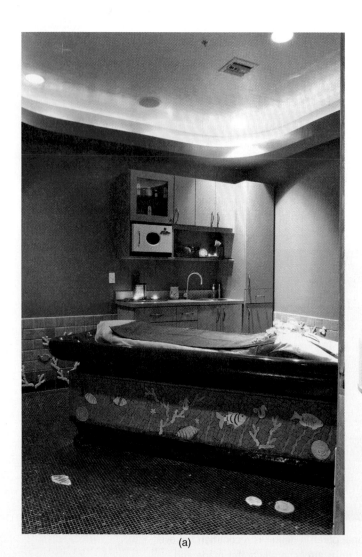
(a)

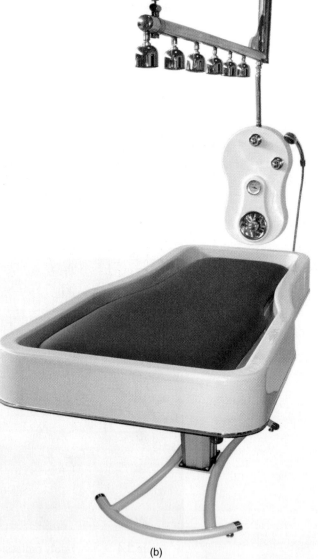
(b)

▶ **Figure 3.6** **a)** Wet tables are ideal for treatments involving substances that need to be rinsed off the client's body. **b)** Athlegen Neptune Wet Table and Vichy Shower. *(Athlegen Neptune Wet Table and Vichy Shower)*

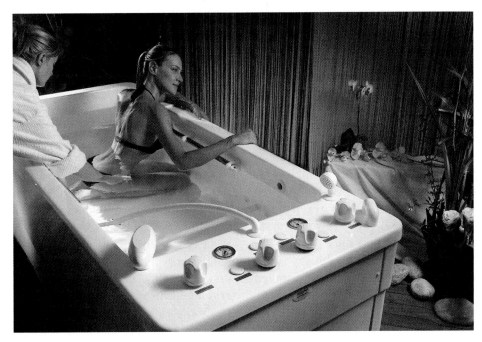

▶ **Figure 3.7** Hydro tubs have jets and an underwater hose to provide hydro massage to specific areas on the client's body. *(Image courtesy Stas Doyer Hydrotherapy)*

can also be found on supplies and equipment, as well as in any of the substances used in spa and hydrotherapy treatments. This is important to note since many pathogens grow in dark, warm, damp places, which makes spa and hydrotherapy treatment settings especially vulnerable to mold growth and disease transmission.

The danger of client exposure to pathogens, whether through equipment, supplies, water, and/or other human beings, needs to be guarded against with utmost diligence. Hygiene and **sanitation** encompass practices that ensure good health and cleanliness and need to be an integral part of spa and bodywork practice routines. They involve the use of **disinfectants**, which are applied to nonliving objects to destroy microorganisms. **Antiseptics**, on the other hand, kill microorganisms on living tissue.

Universal (standard) precautions are protocols established by the Centers for Disease Control and Prevention (CDC) to reduce the chance of spreading contagious diseases within health care settings. These protocols are designed to protect both the patient and the health care provider. They are required to be followed when health care providers are performing medical procedures that involve puncturing or penetrating the body, and/or when dealing with body fluids. The reason these are called universal precautions is that they are applied universally to all patients, not just to some. Since *universal* is sometimes misunderstood to mean that these precautions protect patients and health care providers from all pathogens universally and perfectly, which they do not, the term *standard precautions* is sometimes used instead.

For health care providers, these precautions include:

▶ wearing protective equipment such as masks, gowns, gloves, goggles, and face shields
▶ specific methods of disposal for needles and other sharps and for linens
▶ specific decontamination techniques for instruments and supplies as well as for blood spills
▶ frequent and thorough hand washing

Not all universal precautions that apply to the health care profession apply to the spa and bodywork profession. Several, however, are particularly relevant. Although practitioners may not regularly come into contact with body fluids, there is always the possibility that blood, mucus, saliva, urine, and semen from clients can contaminate linens and equipment and can come in contact with practitioners' skin and clothing.

Each area of the country has different regulations pertaining to hygiene and sanitation procedures in the spa and bodywork environment. The following sanitation and hygiene guidelines are useful for spa and bodywork practitioners. However, practitioners should check with their state and local municipalities to see exactly what is required of them by law.

1. Take care of personal hygiene by bathing daily.
2. Keep nails short and clean, and do not wear nail polish. Long nails and cracked nail polish provide places for pathogens to grow. Long nails can also injure the client.

3. Do not wear rings, bracelets, or wristwatches during treatments. These have a lot of small crevices that will provide places for pathogens to grow.

4. Wear a clean uniform or clean clothing each day. If the uniform or clothing comes in contact with body fluids, it needs to be changed immediately.

5. Thoroughly wash hands, forearms, and elbows, and dry them before and after each treatment. Hands should also be washed during the treatment if warranted, such as after application of a body wrap substance or after touching a contaminated surface such as a dirty towel. The process involves using soap, hot water, and paper towels. Liquid soap in a pump dispenser is best since bar soap can become contaminated by direct contact. Paper towels are more sanitary because they are disposed of after one use. Cloth towels that are used repeatedly become a haven for germs.

   Massage soapy hands (making sure to include the areas between the fingers), forearms, and elbows for thirty seconds; then rinse them until all lather is gone. Wipe dry with paper towels, and use the paper towels to turn off the taps to prevent recontamination.

6. Disposable gloves should be worn any time the practitioner has a cut or broken skin, such as from a wound, on the hands, when handling contaminated linens, or when cleaning any equipment that has come in contact with body fluids.

7. Do not perform treatments when ill because of the danger of passing on pathogens to clients and coworkers.

8. Do not perform treatments under the influence of alcohol or recreational drugs. These impair judgment and increase the chance of making poor decisions about infection control. (Fritz, 2008; Salvo and Anderson, 2004)

Practitioners should also note that in some areas of the country, state laws or employers may require or highly recommend that practitioners be vaccinated against certain diseases such as rubella, tuberculosis, poliomyelitis, and hepatitis. Research should be done by practitioners to determine the immunization requirements for their particular municipalities or find out from the spas in which they are interested in working.

Just as important as personal hygiene is proper sanitation for equipment and supplies. As with personal hygiene and sanitation requirements, each area of the country has different regulations pertaining to sanitation procedures. Practitioners should check with their state and local municipalities to see exactly what is required of

them by law. Additionally, each spa has its own protocols for cleaning and maintaining its equipment, supplies, and treatment areas and trains practitioners accordingly.

It is important that everything—linens, equipment, floors, tables, countertops, and so on—is cleaned between clients. Many good antibacterial sprays and disinfectants are on the market; practitioners should research them to find the ones that work the best for them.

Rubbing alcohol is a good, all-purpose disinfectant and antiseptic because it can be wiped over the skin and other surfaces, evaporates quickly, and destroys a wide variety of pathogens. Rubbing alcohol is most useful when combined with water; seventy percent isopropyl alcohol is, in fact, more effective than ninety-five percent alcohol. Seventy percent isopropyl alcohol is inexpensive and easy to obtain. There are, of course, many other sanitizers and disinfectants available as well.

Some clients may have chemical sensitivities; therefore, using "green" or environmentally safe products is highly recommended. Citrus products made from citrus essential oils such as orange, lemon, or grapefruit are highly recommended. These disinfectants are safe, nontoxic, and environmentally friendly. Other natural products and commercial cleaning agents are also available. Manufacturers' instructions on all products should be followed to ensure they disinfect properly.

Whatever other disinfectants are used, household bleach should also be kept on hand. It is mandated by the CDC as part of universal precautions for cleaning up blood and other body fluid spills in health care settings, and it is the most effective disinfectant available. Since it is inexpensive and easy to obtain, it should be used for body fluid decontamination in the spa and bodywork setting. Practitioners should also have disposable gloves readily available to wear to clean up surfaces and linens contaminated by body fluids (see Clinical Alert box).

Guidelines

The following guidelines are especially useful for those practitioners in private practice:

1. Follow all manufacturers' instructions to clean and maintain equipment properly. Improperly maintained equipment can endanger client and practitioner safety, as well as be potential havens for pathogens.

2. Use only clean linens, face rest covers, bolster and pillow covers, and towels. They should be used on only one client and laundered between uses. Wash them in hot water with detergent, and then dry them in a dryer with hot air. Wool blankets, as long as they do not come in contact with the client's

skin, can be dry cleaned every two weeks. Washable wool blankets are better; they can be laundered with hot water and detergent, and hot-air dried between uses.

3. Uniforms or other clothing used while performing treatments should be laundered separately from linens, equipment covers, and towels. They should be washed in hot water with detergent, and hot-air dried between wearing.

4. The insulating sheet used for wraps (rubber, plastic, Mylar, etc.) should be sprayed with alcohol or another disinfectant and allowed to dry after each use before folding and storing. It can also be washed with soap and water, but it should still be sprayed with the disinfectant after washing.

5. All bowls, basins, and foot tubs should be washed in warm, soapy water and rinsed after each use, then sprayed with alcohol or other disinfectant and allowed to dry before storing.

6. Equipment such as massage tables and wet tables need to be cleaned and disinfected after each use (see ▶Figure 3.8).

7. Any wet areas such as floors, especially in shower areas, and countertops, as well as any wet equipment such as showerheads and hoses need to be cleaned and disinfected daily.

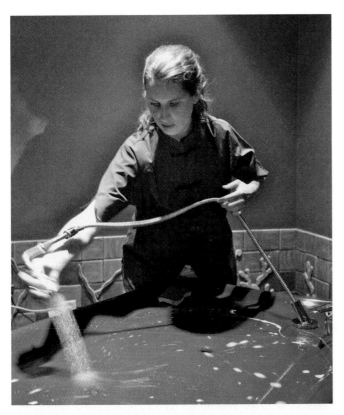

▶ **Figure 3.8** Massage tables, wet tables, and other equipment need to be cleaned and disinfected after each use.

8. **Cross-contamination** is the spread of pathogens from one person to another via substances. This can occur if massage lubricant or spa materials become contaminated and are reused. To prevent this, use closed dispensers for massage lubricant. Open jar containers can be used, but practitioners should never remove lubricant from the jar, place it on the client's skin, and then reach back into the jar for more lubricant. Instead, practitioners should use a small, clean spatula to remove enough lubricant for one treatment and place it on a disposable container such as a paper disc. After the treatment, the spatula should be washed in warm, soapy water, rinsed and dried, and then sprayed with alcohol or another disinfectant.

All spa and hydrotherapy treatment substances should be removed from containers with a clean spatula or spoon for each treatment. *No hands dipping in!* Only enough for one client should be removed; unused portions should be discarded after the treatment. The spatula or spoon should be washed as just described.

CLINICAL ALERT

If any of the linens, coverings, or towels should become contaminated with body fluids, practitioners should wear disposable gloves to remove them from the treatment area and place them in a secure container separate from containers that hold other used linens. The contaminated items should be laundered separately from any other items. Hot water, detergent, and one-fourth cup of chlorine bleach should be used, and then the linens should be hot-air dried. This procedure should also be used for contaminated uniforms or other clothing worn to perform treatments.

Practitioners should wear disposable gloves to wipe up any body fluids that come in contact with equipment, the floor, or other surfaces. Paper towels should be used and then discarded in a secure container separate from other waste. The area should then be cleaned with soap and water, using disposable paper towels that are discarded in the separate, secure container. Next, the area needs to be disinfected with a solution of water and chlorine bleach in a 10:1 solution (i.e., 10 parts water to 1 part bleach). After cleaning and disinfecting the area, the disposable gloves should be removed and discarded in the separate, secure container, and practitioners should thoroughly wash their hands using soap and water.

9. Replace bowls, other utensils, and equipment as soon as they show signs of wear. Cracks and crevices in the surfaces of these items are ideal for pathogen growth. (Fritz, 2008; Salvo and Anderson, 2004; Williams, 2007)

In the following chapters, a section called "Hygiene" is included after every treatment. It provides specific methods for cleaning and disinfecting the equipment and supplies used for each treatment.

HELPING CLIENTS CHOOSE THE BEST TREATMENTS

So many spa and hydrotherapy treatments are available to clients that it is sometimes difficult for clients to choose which one they want. Sometimes the treatment a client really wants to experience is not one the client should receive, or perhaps a treatment that the client does not know about would suit the client's needs perfectly.

It is the responsibility of practitioners to be knowledgeable about all therapies they perform. They need to know the benefits, indications, and contraindications, as well as how to perform the treatment. An **indication** is a reason to perform a treatment. In other words, there is some factor or body condition that would be relieved by the application of a particular treatment. An example is dry skin as an indication for an exfoliation treatment. A **contraindication** is a factor or body condition that prohibits the administration of a treatment; administration of the treatment would, in fact, make the factor or body condition worse. For example, if a client is dehydrated from lying in the sun all morning, a heat treatment would be contraindicated because of the possibility of increasing the client's dehydration. Contraindications can be **systemic** or **general**, meaning that the client should not receive the treatment at all. An example is a client with a flare-up stage of rheumatoid arthritis, involving the majority of the joints. A heat treatment would be a systemic contraindication because heat would make the inflammation in the client's joints worse. Other contraindications can be **local, zonal,** or **regional,** which means that the treatment should not be applied in certain areas of the body but may be applied to the rest of the body. For example, if a client has a skin rash on one arm, mud should not be applied in the area of the skin rash, but it can be applied to the rest of the client's body.

Questions to Ask Clients

Another crucial aspect of helping clients decide which treatment is best for them is information from the clients themselves. With this information, practitioners can com-

municate with clients about different options in an informed manner.

There are a few ways practitioners can get vital information from clients. They can have clients fill out a pretreatment form (also called an intake form), conduct a pretreatment interview, or do a combination of both. Whatever method is used, it is important that certain pieces of information about the client's health, vitality, and medical history be established before any treatment is performed. For example, if the client has a condition that is contraindicated for a particular treatment, practitioners need to know so the client's condition is not made worse by receiving the treatment. On the other hand, the client may have a condition that would be alleviated by a specific treatment, and without the pretreatment form and interview, practitioners may never think to suggest it (see ▶Figure 3.9).

The following questions should be asked to get as complete a picture of a client's health and medical history as possible and to have a good framework for designing the treatment session. Many of these questions can be asked on an intake form. Follow up by asking the client for clarification as needed.

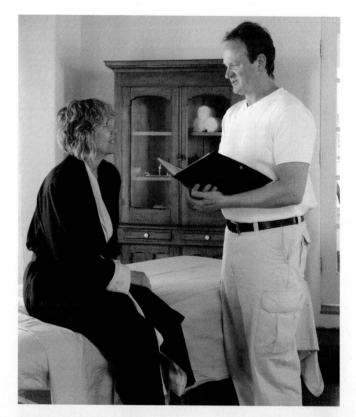

▶ **Figure 3.9** A pretreatment interview is an effective way for a practitioner to get information directly from a client to help determine which treatments would be best (or not advisable) for each individual client.

▶ **Do you have any medical conditions?** This can include chronic and acute conditions. Heart conditions, uncontrolled high blood pressure, varicose veins, and diabetes mellitus, for example, are contraindications for local and systemic heat therapies and contrast therapies (therapies that alternate between heat and cold applications). Pregnancy is a contraindication for certain therapies and the use of certain essential oils. (All therapies in each chapter of this book include indications and contraindications that can be used to design a pretreatment form.)

Be sure to ask about any medications the client may be taking. For example, if a client is taking an analgesic (pain reliever), this could interfere with the ability to give accurate feedback about temperature and pressure; heat and contrast therapies would, therefore, be contraindicated. Also, certain essential oils inhibit the actions of certain medications.

▶ **Do you have any allergies?** Clients can be allergic to any and all spa and hydrotherapy treatment substances including muds, peat, clays, ginger, essential oils, and sea products, including seawater. It is best if the client notes any allergies on an intake form so there is written documentation. People can develop allergies throughout their lives; therefore, every time a client arrives for a treatment, the practitioner should check for any updates.

A common allergy is one to shellfish. Clients who are allergic to shellfish and/or iodine should *never* receive thalassotherapy treatments. Clients may not realize that an allergy to shellfish and/or iodine also means allergies to sea products, so it is important for the practitioner to discuss this with clients. Another well-known allergy is one to nuts. Clients with nut allergies should not receive treatments with nut-based oils or exfoliants.

Clients may not be aware of allergies they have. Before any treatment is performed, the substance should be applied to a small area on the client's skin, usually the forearm, to see if there is an allergic reaction.

▶ **Do you have any areas of inflammation, rashes, or other skin conditions?** Inflamed areas are contraindicated for heat treatments. Inflammation, rashes, or other skin disorders may cause certain other treatments to be contraindicated, such as exfoliations (especially salt glows), ginger fomentation, and seaweed. On the other hand, there are treatments that can be soothing for some skin conditions, such as a mud poultice or wrap.

CLINICAL ALERT !

Allergic reactions run a wide gamut. They can be as simple as a few localized hives and itching all the way up to a full-blown anaphylactic reaction, which interferes with the client's ability to breathe.

If a client has an allergic reaction, the most important thing the practitioner should do is to stay calm and stop the treatment immediately. The substance should be removed and the client thoroughly rinsed off. If the client's condition worsens, for example, if numerous hives, impaired breathing, and/or widespread inflammation develop, emergency care, such as calling 911, should be initiated immediately.

▶ **Have you had a spa or hydrotherapy treatment before?** If there is no prior experience, then the client may need explanations of all treatments. It is important that practitioners answer all client questions as completely as possible. For example, the client may really want a wrap until the practitioner explains that minimal draping is involved, and so the client may opt for a facial mask instead.

If the client has had spa and hydrotherapy treatments before, practitioners should ask the client what the results were and whether the client liked it.

Perhaps the client is looking to repeat a great experience or perhaps try something new. If the client did not have good results or did not like the treatments, a different treatment should be suggested.

Practitioners should also let clients know that some spa and hydrotherapy treatment products have odors to them, just so the client is prepared. Muds, peat, and clay have an earthy aroma; seaweed smells like the ocean. Practitioners can let the client smell the substances, and, if the odor is displeasing, the client may choose another treatment.

▶ **How often do you get sick? How fast do you recover?** If the client is robust and not prone to illness, and provided there are no other contraindicated conditions, the client can receive just about any treatment. If, however, the client is in fragile health, then heat and cold treatments would need to use less extreme temperatures or are contraindicated. Sedating treatments may be more beneficial; invigorating treatments could possibly deplete the client further.

▶ **What are your desired goals for the treatment?** Does the client want softer, smoother skin? An exfoliation treatment followed by a seaweed wrap could be suggested. Does the client have a specific area of discomfort, such as some muscle tension in the back? A paraffin treatment followed by massage on the area might be the best treatment. If the client has some sinus congestion, an inhalation treatment with eucalyptus essential oil could be performed.

► **What are you doing after the treatment session?** Is it okay for the client to feel sedated afterwards, or does the client need to be energized? This can determine which treatments to suggest. For example, if the client is making a high-powered presentation later in the day, a mud wrap that makes the client feel sleepy is not the best choice; a salt glow with peppermint essential oil may be better.

► **What is your temperature tolerance?** Clients who have a low tolerance to hot temperatures may not be the best candidates for heat treatments or would need the temperatures lowered. Likewise, clients who have low tolerance to cold temperatures may not be the best candidates for cold treatments or would need the temperatures raised. Contrast applications may not be chosen either, unless the temperatures were modified. (Fritz, 2008; Rhines, 2007; Venclik, 2007; Williams, 2007).

Considerations for Package Treatments

Practitioners should also give some thought to combining treatments into packages that they can offer their clients. The effectiveness of individual treatments can be enhanced by pairing them with other treatments. Spas already do this; owners and managers discovered a long time ago that this appeals to clients and is a great way to generate more revenue. As individual practitioners learn the various therapies presented in this book, they can be thinking about which treatments go best with one another.

It is essential that treatments are combined in packages that are safe and useful to the client. There are several ways to do this, such as by themes or by needs. An example of a theme package could be a desert botanical series—salt glow with desert mineral salts, prickly pear wrap, and a chaparral inhalation treatment. Another example could be a fruit and flower theme—a sugar glow exfoliation enhanced with orange and grapefruit essential oils and a rose petal immersion bath. An example of a package that is need based could be one for softening and smoothing the skin—a back exfoliation, a foot scrub, and then a mud wrap. Another example could be for someone needing the rejuvenation that thalassotherapy gives, such as a sea salt scrub coupled with a seaweed wrap. ►Figure 3.10 shows a spa menu with examples of spa packages.

The package possibilities are almost endless. However, there are a few cautions to keep in mind. Generally, heat treatments should not be added to heat treatments because there is danger of burning the client. For example, a paraffin treatment should never be performed over the same area where a ginger fomentation was just done. A ginger fomentation on the back should not be followed with a full body mud wrap since the mud is a heating treatment. However, depending on the client's tolerance to heat, paraffin could be applied to the feet, and a ginger fomentation performed on the client's shoulders coupled with a back exfoliation. These individual local heat treatments on different areas of the body are safer than heat treatments applied to the same area, or multiple systemic heat treatments.

Extra consideration should be given when choosing multiple treatments for clients with sensitive skin. For example, a vigorous exfoliation followed by a ginger fomentation or mud wrap may be too stimulating to the client, and instead of being relaxed and soothed, the client may end up feeling irritated and in pain. A gentler exfoliation may be in order.

When presenting package options to clients, it is important to find out if the client has sensitivities or allergies to any or all of the substances in all aspects of the treatments. No matter how wonderful the package may sound, it is of no use or, worse, dangerous to a client who has an adverse reaction to the treatments.

INCORPORATING SPA AND HYDROTHERAPY TREATMENTS INTO A BODYWORK PRACTICE

For practitioners who are in private practice or work in a massage therapy and bodywork office, some factors to consider before deciding to offer spa and hydrotherapy treatments are:

► legal constraints
► scope of practice
► which treatments to perform
► costs of implementing new treatments
► where to purchase supplies and equipment
► marketing the new treatments

There are many options for offering spa and hydrotherapy treatments. Private practitioners and bodywork offices may want to start small by adding just a few treatments that can be performed in a dry room, such as dry brushing or wraps. Depending on the success of these, they may choose to expand further and add Vichy showers and hydro tubs, or they may choose to offer many specialty treatments.

Spa Packages

Refresh
Enliven your senses with an invigorating salt glow and relaxing massage. You'll be left velvety smooth and delightfully tranquil.

Alpine Herbal Steam Therapy
Conditioning Body Scrub
Swedish Massage
Brine Light Therapy

2 1/2 hours   *$167*

Escape
Steam under the stars...play with colorful muds...receive a head to toe massage...then a nap by the sea...you're not in Tucson anymore.

Rasul Ceremony – Terra Sigillata or Bali Paradise
Swedish Massage
Brine Light Therapy

3 hours   *$203*

Sports Events
Enjoy this reprieve after any sport. A great way to relieve fatigue and muscle stress.

Alpine Herbal Steam Therapy
Soft Pack Treatment – Warm Moor Sport Treatment
Therapeutic Massage
Brine Light Therapy

3 hours   *$207*

Executive Break
Stress is one of the key underlying causes of modern illness, so when the stress and strains of everyday life start to take a hold, it's time to take action. In just a few hours you'll be back on top...feeling, looking and performing better than ever.

Alpine Herbal Steam Therapy
Conditioning Body Scrub
Custom Massage
Spa Lunch
Eminence Custom Facial
Spa Pedicure
Brine Light Therapy

5 1/2 hours   *$322*

Deluxe Pampering Package
Take time to be pampered, leave everything behind, step into our luxurious environment and experience this very special package.

Alpine Herbal Steam Therapy
Pantai Luar Treatment
Swedish Massage
Spa Lunch
Pantai Herbal Facial Treatment
Spa Manicure and Pedicure
Brine Light Therapy

6 hours   *$466*

Retreat
Experience paradise with the love of your life - a lavish treat for two. Share a day of spa therapies with that very special person.

Rasul Ceremony for Two – Terra Sigillata or Bali Paradise
Swedish Massage for Two
Spa Lunch for Two
Alpine Herbal Steam Therapy for Two
Signature Facials for Two
Brine Light Therapy for Two

5 hours   *$600 for Two*

6884 East Sunrise Drive, Suite 150, Tuscon, Arizona 85750
Hours of Operation
Monday - Saturday 9am - 7pm   Sunday 10am - 5pm
Make an appointment 520-615-9608
Gift Certificates and Memberships available at the Spa and Online
www.touchoftranquility.com

▶ **Figure 3.10** The effectiveness of individual treatments can be enhanced by packaging them with other treatments. This allows clients to enjoy a more thorough and beneficial spa treatment. *(Image courtesy of Touch of Tranquility Spa)*

No matter which path practitioners and private office owners choose, it is important that they make well-informed decisions. The failure rate of new businesses and those that expand too quickly is astronomical. Realistic views of costs and income possibilities are essential, and so are organized business and development plans. A business coach may be able to help with making the best decisions.

When deciding whether to spend the time and effort to branch into spa and hydrotherapy treatments, it might be useful to consider some of the pros and cons (See Box 3.2).

Legal Considerations

If a practitioner in private practice or a massage and bodywork treatment center wants to expand into offering spa and hydrotherapy treatments, careful research and preparation need to be done first. It is much better to spend the time and effort necessary to determine what local and state regulations exist regarding spa and hydrotherapy treatments than to invest the time and money for equipment, and so on only to discover that the owners have not met certain legal requirements or, worse yet, that the treatments are not allowed by law in the owners' locality.

Depending on the region in which the private practice or center is located, there can be state and municipal zoning, licensing, and sanitation laws to follow. These laws and regulations will be different for every locality. For example,

▶ An area may allow massage therapy to be performed in the practitioner's home, but not spa and hydrotherapy treatments because of sanitation concerns.

▶ A massage and bodywork office needs to be reclassified as a spa and install a shower in order to perform even the simplest spa and hydrotherapy treatments in a dry room.

Practitioners and treatment center owners who want to install showers, baths, or wet rooms need to check to see if local, regional, and state regulations allow them. If so, owners should also keep in mind that there will also be specific requirements to meet the Americans with Disabilities Act, as well as codes for health, hygiene, and sanitation. If practitioners have home practices and want to have clients use their home showers and baths, they, too, would need to check local regulations to see if this is allowed, and which municipal codes need to be met.

Regulations are not necessarily always clear, and sometimes it is difficult to wade through the legalese of statutes and zoning codes. The first place practitioners and owners can start their research is with their municipal licensing office. Internet research is also a possibility since most local, regional, and state licensing and regulating bodies post their laws and regulations online. Working with legal counsel would also be a proactive step in ensuring that the private practice or treatment center meets all requirements.

Practitioners also need to be aware that following all the legal steps necessary to incorporate spa and hydrotherapy treatments into their practice or a massage and bodywork office can be time consuming. Even if legally allowed, a facility may still be required by the municipality to acquire building permits to remodel or expand to offer spa and hydrotherapy treatments. There will also be inspections of the addition, as well as to ensure that all treatments; treatment rooms; and facilities for showers, baths, hydrotherapy tubs, and wet rooms meet zoning codes and health and sanitation standards. There can be inspections for the structure, electrical wiring, plumbing, and the equipment itself. Sometimes all the inspections can be made by one city or county representative; most often, each inspection needs to be done by a different person.

Depending on the municipality's workload, these inspections may take a long time to schedule and carry out. Practitioners need to not only plan for costs and time required to build and install equipment, but also time for inspections. Many business owners have been surprised, to say the least, that their time frames for expansion had to be greatly altered (Sohnen-Moe, 2008).

Scope of Practice

Practitioners should never go beyond their scope of practice. They need to understand their municipality and state

BOX 3.2

Pros	Cons
Many easily incorporated treatments	Extra set up and clean up
Treatments blend well with bodywork	Extra preparation time
More options for clients	Extra equipment to purchase, clean, and store
Variety in work routines	Initial costly investment
Opportunities for creativity	
Cost efficient (profit is higher than the investment of time and money)	

regulations regarding the treatments they want to perform. For example, in some areas of the United States, massage therapists cannot perform exfoliations or wraps or apply facial masks. They need to be trained and licensed as an **esthetician** or cosmetologist to do them. Or perhaps they can perform manual exfoliations and apply masks but cannot do deep pore cleaning and extractions. Likewise, they may need to be trained and licensed as an aromatherapist to use essential oils with their clients.

Practitioners and treatment center owners should find out the exact legalities under which they can perform treatments. Some indications for spa and hydrotherapy treatments may be considered medical conditions, and local or state regulations may decree that they can be performed only under the direct supervision of a physician. They may want to carefully consider the wording of indications and benefits of treatments described in all marketing materials, and make them sound more as if the treatments are for relaxation and rejuvenation. If owners or practitioners prefer not to do this, they may consider having a physician on staff, forming a professional relationship with health care centers in their area, or requiring their clients to have a prescription for the treatments they receive.

Starting Off Small: Dry Rooms

Many of the spa treatments mentioned in this book can easily be added to a bodywork menu in settings where there is no access to a shower. The treatments are easily incorporated into and blend well with bodywork. These services can be offered along with a basic massage, shiatsu, or reflexology treatment or offered as stand-alone treatments. An added benefit is that many of the techniques and natural substances used in spa and hydrotherapy treatments have physiological effects that address a client's therapeutic needs. Alone or in conjunction with bodywork, spa and hydrotherapy treatments can be a way for clients to relax and restore.

The following treatments are suitable for a dry room, and the list can be used as a template for adding to a treatment menu:

Exfoliations

▶ Exfoliations are treatments that brighten the skin by removing dead skin cells. Exfoliations can be done using dry brushes; mitts; loofahs; abrasive cloths (for applying friction); and natural substances, such as salt, sugar, cornmeal, and coffee, that are abrasive. Natural substances such as yogurt, milk, and papaya contain acids and enzymes and also act as natural exfoliants because they contain enzymes that dissolve dead skin cells (Chapter 5 is devoted to exfoliation).

▶ One way to start is by offering 30- and 60-minute dry-brushing routines.

▶ Initial costs include the dry brushes or other exfoliation tools. Manual exfoliations using natural substances such as salt and sugar glows could then be added.

▶ Additional costs include the purchase of the exfoliants (this cost would be ongoing), nonmetal bowls, and possibly essential oils to enhance the treatments (Chapter 8 discusses essential oils).

Compresses and Ginger Fomentation

▶ A compress is a towel or soft cotton cloth folded two or three times until it reaches the desired thickness, then it is soaked in hot or cold water and applied to a specific area of the body to relieve conditions such as muscle tension or mild edema. Hot compresses are also called fomentations; ginger fomentations are applied specifically to relieve deep muscle tension, among other things. Compresses are relatively easy to apply and can be very effective. (More information on these treatments can be found in Chapter 4.)

▶ Initial costs include towels—approximately six will be needed, basins to hold the water, a heating source for hot compresses and ginger fomentation such as an electrical hot plate, and a muslin bag or cheesecloth for the ginger.

▶ Ongoing costs would be for ice for the cold treatments, if there is not a ready supply, and fresh ginger.

Hot Foot Bath

▶ This is an excellent treatment to help clear chest and sinus congestion and to warm clients for other treatments such as a heating (cold sheet) wrap. Clients place their feet in a foot tub or large basin filled with hot water while wrapped in a sheet and blanket. To enhance the heating effect, dry mustard powder can be added to the foot bath. A cool washcloth can be applied to the client's forehead. The overall result is that blood is drawn downward, thereby relieving chest and sinus congestion (hot foot bath is outlined in detail in Chapter 4).

▶ Initial costs are for a foot tub or large basin, a wool blanket, sheet, washcloth, and a pool thermometer.

▶ An ongoing cost would be for optional dry mustard powder.

Wraps

▶ Many different types of wraps can be performed. Cold sheet wraps (Chapter 4); mud and peat wraps (Chapter 6); seaweed wraps (Chapter 7); and herbal wraps (Chapter 8) are all options for practitioners to explore.

▶ Initial costs include exfoliation tools or ingredients for a scrub (wraps work better if the client's skin is exfoliated first); muslin or other all-cotton sheets; insulating sheets (rubber, plastic, or Mylar, etc.); wool blankets; large- and medium-sized towels; textured washcloths or bath scrubbies for each individual client (to remove wrap residue); a small nonmetal bowl; and for body wrap substance removal in a dry room, a basin for warm water, a crock pot, or a towel cabi (see Figure 3.3).

▶ Ongoing costs would be for the body wrap substances. Many muds and seaweeds come in gel and crème form for practitioners and private offices that do not have a shower available for clients to wash off body wrap substances and do not want to use the Dry Room Substance Removal Technique (outlined in Chapter 5). The crèmes and gels usually do not require removal from the client's skin at the end of the body wrap treatment.

Poultices

▶ Poultices are soft, moist masses of a substance that are applied either directly to the body or encased in a clean cloth. They are excellent local treatments that can help alleviate a variety of symptoms. Generally, cold poultices are used to withdraw heat from an inflamed or congested area, and hot poultices are used to relax spasms, reduce pain, and draw out infection or insect venom (more information can be found in Appendix 1).

▶ Initial costs include poultice cloths, poultice substance (such as mud, peat, or seaweed), and washcloths to remove poultice residue from the skin.

▶ Ongoing costs would be for poultice substances.

Paraffin

▶ Paraffin is hot wax applied locally to the body for deep, penetrating heat into tight and aching muscles and joints. It can be painted on, or clients can dip their hands or feet into it (paraffin treatments are discussed in Chapter 6).

▶ Initial cost is for the paraffin heating unit (see Figure 3.4). A heavy-duty professional unit is recommended over those sold for home use. Professional units are generally better made and will last longer. Another cost is for the blocks of paraffin. A paintbrush and ceramic cup will need to be purchased if painting on the paraffin. For both the painting and dipping methods, plastic wrap and towels are also necessary.

▶ Ongoing costs would be for blocks of paraffin and plastic wrap.

Baths and Showers

▶ Since dry room treatments are designed for practices in which clients do not have access to showers or baths, practitioners may choose to recommend certain baths and showers for clients to perform at home. They can give clients samples of salts, muds, and seaweeds. (Showers are discussed in Chapter 4; baths are discussed in Chapters 4, 6, 7, and 8.)

▶ Ongoing costs would be the substances and whatever practitioners need to package them.

There are other items practitioners would need to consider purchasing as well as the items listed for each treatment. These include:

▶ rubbing alcohol, bleach, and other disinfectants to ensure safe, hygienic, and sanitary practices
▶ spatulas
▶ extra nonmetal bowls
▶ extra sheets
▶ bathrobes
▶ disposable undergarments for clients to wear during treatments

Practitioners may choose to purchase only one or two muds, peats, clays, salts, or seaweeds at first, and then decide to have a number of different types on hand. They may also decide to invest in essential oils to have these available for treatments.

Most supplies can be purchased at local stores, beauty supply stores, natural foods stores (for herbs, ginger, some muds, clays, and seaweed), and through the internet. When practitioners consider what to buy, it is important that they remember that the supplies and equipment need to be able to withstand multiple treatments. Something may seem like a bargain initially but turns out not to be if it has to be replaced often. For example, towels that are inexpensive initially may end up being quite expensive in the long run if they are so thin that they wear out after just five or six treatments. Thicker, plusher towels that cost more at first are more cost effective because they can last for twenty-five to thirty treatments.

The following websites can be explored for supplies:

▶ Massage Warehouse and Spa Essentials—www.massagewarehouse.com
▶ Universal Companies (all types of spa supplies)—www.universalcompanies.com

► Ahava (Dead Sea mud)—www.ahava.com
► Torf Spa (organic moor mud from Europe)—www.torfspa.com

Practitioners should note that some spa and hydrotherapy supply businesses do not sell to individuals. They sell only to large spas or companies and require a contract and a commitment to buying large amounts of products.

No matter where practitioners buy their equipment and supplies, they should keep receipts for all items purchased. These are business expenses that can be deducted from income taxes.

Practitioners and private office owners will need to market their new spa and hydrotherapy treatments, which will be an additional expense. There are many advertising options:

► posting a flyer in the office announcing the new treatments
► sending mailers to all clients
► displaying the new treatments on a website

The treatments need to be added to the practice's menu as soon as possible to make clients aware of them, and the practitioner will need to create new brochures.

Sometimes clients are unfamiliar and possibly uncomfortable with receiving the new treatments, and they may even be uncomfortable with the concept of hydrotherapy and spa. They may think of spa treatments as only being cosmetic and superficial, as "beauty treatments" rather than restorative and therapeutic modalities. Educating clients is an important way to introduce them to spa and hydrotherapy treatments. This can be done by giving them a menu of the expanded services and explaining the health benefits of each. Practitioners should be sure to answer any questions clients have about the treatments.

One way to encourage clients to take advantage of expanded services is to give them complimentary mini-treatments. A foot scrub, aromatherapy facial massage, or hot ginger fomentation, for example, can be easily integrated into a bodywork treatment. If a client has a buildup of dry skin, practitioners can offer an exfoliation treatment. Having gift certificates available for all the services is a definite plus. Mother's Day, Father's Day, Valentine's Day, anniversaries, birthdays, and bridal showers are all special occasions for which a spa or hydrotherapy treatment may be the perfect gift.

Expanding Further

Massage and bodywork practitioners who start off small may decide to expand further into the spa arena. One way to do this is to incorporate other types of treatments, such as manicures, pedicures, hair styling, and esthetician services. Treatment menus can be expanded even further by offering hydrotherapy. Shower, bath, and hydrotherapy tub facilities may be installed, if they are legally allowed. This could be as simple as a shower clients can use to rinse off substances applied during dry room treatments, all the way up to specialized rooms that have wet tables and Vichy showers.

Costs for installing baths, showers, and wet tables can vary. Baths and hydrotherapy tubs can cost anywhere from under $1,000 up to $5,000 or more, depending on the equipment options chosen. Wet tables can be as simple as having a drain and a nearby water source with a hose and can cost just under $1,000. A more elaborate setup could involve using wall-mounted handheld showers, which also cost just under $1,000. Upgraded wet tables and Vichy showers can cost into the $10,000 range. Additionally, there would be special plumbing needs and sanitation requirements.

The following websites can be explored for wet-room equipment:

Water Werks—vichyshower.com
Innovative Spa—innovativespa.com
SpaEquip—spaequip.com
Spa Elegance—spaelegance.com

There would be ongoing costs for maintenance and hygiene, plus sizeable water bills. Costs for supplies would increase, and there would be a need for more staff, causing greater payroll expenses.

As can be seen, the expenses for wet rooms can be considerable. Although they allow for many more treatment possibilities, it is important to make the investment "worth it." Careful consideration needs to be given to how many treatments would need to be performed, and the price of the treatments, to offset the initial outlay. Practitioners debating whether to expand into the day spa business need to have sound, written business and development plans and follow them carefully.

Summary

Practitioners can explore many different options when choosing to perform spa and hydrotherapy treatments. They may choose to work in an established spa, or they may decide to incorporate treatments into their private practice or into a massage and bodywork treatment center. Whatever method they choose, they need to be mindful of the factors that ensure safe and successful practices. These factors include an understanding of what creates a meaningful spa experience, communicating well with clients, being able to help clients choose the best treatments for them, and following universal precautions and hygiene and sanitation practices.

Practitioners who are debating whether to work in a spa need to be aware of the roles in sales and marketing that spa staff play as well as other expectations of them. They need to have an understanding of the spa's workforce structure and to determine for themselves whether working in a spa is the right choice for them.

Practitioners who are in private practice or working in a massage and bodywork practice and want to incorporate spa and hydrotherapy treatments should recognize and understand all the parameters involved. These include legal requirements, scope of practice issues, and necessary expenditures, to name a few. There are many different ways treatments can be included, but it is important to have organized and well thought-out business and development plans to ensure as smooth a transition as possible.

Activities

1. List five expectations of spa staff.

   _____
   _____
   _____
   _____
   _____

2. Name three components of professional appearance.

   _____
   _____
   _____

3. List five relevant questions a practitioner should ask the interviewer when applying for a position with a spa.

   _____
   _____
   _____
   _____
   _____

4. Make your own list of pros and cons of working for a spa.

   Pros   **Cons**

   _____   _____
   _____   _____
   _____   _____
   _____   _____
   _____   _____

5. Briefly explain at least ten sanitation and hygiene guidelines for massage and bodywork practitioners.

   _____
   _____
   _____
   _____
   _____
   _____
   _____
   _____
   _____
   _____
   _____
   _____

6. List six questions you can ask clients to help determine their best treatment option.

_____

_____

_____

_____

_____

_____

7. Using the information presented in the section "Helping Clients Choose the Best Treatments," design a client intake form for spa and hydrotherapy treatments.

8. List five factors a practitioner needs to consider before offering spa and hydrotherapy treatments in a private practice.

_____

_____

_____

_____

_____

9. Describe three methods practitioners in private practice can use to market spa and hydrotherapy treatments.

_____

_____

_____

10. Envision your perfect spa setting, and describe it in detail. What would you name your spa? Where would it be located? How would the treatment rooms look? How would you decorate the waiting area? What types of treatments would you offer? Include a menu of services with descriptions of treatments, length of treatments, and prices. Which special features would your spa have? To whom would you market your spa? How would you market it?

_____

_____

_____

_____

_____

_____

_____

_____

Study Questions

1. Which of the following demonstrates the best way practitioners help clients choose spa and hydrotherapy treatments?
   a. respecting client privacy by avoiding questions about medical history
   b. giving the treatment the client requests, even if there are contraindications
   c. offering the client discounts on treatments that would be ineffective for the client
   d. determining whether the client has any skin rashes or allergies

2. Which of the following is an example of practitioners using universal precautions?
   a. asking clients about their HIV status
   b. changing linens between each client
   c. washing up blood spills with soap and water
   d. performing treatments when ill

3. An expectation of spa staff is to
   a. handle all client issues on their own
   b. perform treatments in any manner they choose
   c. be flexible regarding work schedules
   d. participate only minimally in product sales

4. Part of the definition of independent contractors is that they
    a. set their own schedules
    b. receive payment from the business owner
    c. have taxes taken out of their pay by the spa owner
    d. use only the treatment center's equipment

5. Which of the following is a legal consideration for offering spa and hydrotherapy treatments?
    a. checking municipal zoning laws to see if the therapies are allowed
    b. complying with the Americans with Disabilities Act facility requirements
    c. dealing with inspections for electricity, plumbing, and structural features
    d. all of the above

6. What is the term for a condition that would be made worse by the application of a treatment?
    a. indication
    b. contamination
    c. contraindication
    d. benefit

7. If a client is uncomfortable with minimal draping during a treatment, the practitioner should
    a. reassure the client that everyone feels that way
    b. explain that that is what the treatment requires
    c. refuse to do the treatment
    d. adjust coverings until the client is comfortable

8. Which of the following may a practitioner in a spa be expected to learn how to use?
    a. Vichy shower
    b. paraffin unit
    c. hydrotherapy tub
    d. all of the above

9. Which of the following is a practitioner most likely to do when working in a spa?
    a. use cleaning supplies
    b. complete payroll
    c. order supplies
    d. supervise other practitioners

10. Which of the following would be the best way for the practitioner to design a client's treatment session?
    a. rely on intuition
    b. ask questions about medical history
    c. perform the same ones on everyone
    d. remember that everyone needs to be relaxed afterward

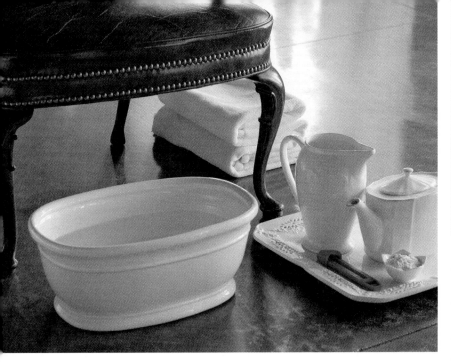

Hydrotherapy

LEARNING OBJECTIVES

After studying this chapter, the reader will have the information to

1. Explain the properties of water and how and why they make hydrotherapy so effective.

2. Describe the mechanical, chemical, and thermal effects of hydrotherapy treatments.

3. Outline the four main variables in hydrotherapy.

4. Discuss indications, contraindications, and considerations for local (zonal, regional) and systemic heat applications; local (zonal, regional) and systemic cold applications; and contrast applications.

5. Explain how cold affects the body; distinguish between the effects of a local and a systemic cold application.

6. Explain how heat affects the body; distinguish between the effects of a local and a systemic heat application.

7. Delineate the supplies needed, rationale, indications, contraindications, treatment procedure, hygiene, and after-treatment care for single cold compress.

8. Explain how and why cryotherapy is used.

9. Delineate the supplies needed, rationale, indications, contraindications, treatment procedure, hygiene, and after-treatment care for hot compress.

10. Delineate the supplies needed, rationale, indications, contraindications, treatment procedure, hygiene, and after-treatment care for ginger fomentation.

11. Delineate the supplies needed, rationale, indications, contraindications, treatment procedure, hygiene, and after-treatment care for hot foot bath.

To understand water is to understand the cosmos, the marvels of nature, and life itself.
— Masaru Emoto in *The Hidden Messages in Water*

12. Delineate the supplies needed, rationale, indications, contraindications, treatment procedure, hygiene, and after-treatment care for heating (cold sheet) wrap.

13. Delineate the supplies needed, rationale, indications, contraindications, treatment procedure, hygiene, and after-treatment care for alternating or contrast compress.

14. Describe the therapeutic effects of and contraindications for hot, warm, tepid, and cold showers.

15. Define balneology, and describe the therapeutic effects of and contraindications for hot, warm, tepid, and cold baths.

16. Explain why and how inhalation treatments, steam baths, and saunas are used.

17. Explain why and how hydrotherapy tubs, flotation tanks/sensory deprivation tanks or rooms, Hubbard tanks, and whirlpools/Jacuzzis® are used.

18. Describe Watsu® and Water Dance.

KEY TERMS

Affusion	Diaphoresis	Hyperemia	Reflex (consensual response)
Balneology	Fluxion	Hypertension	Retrostasis
Buoyancy	Fomentation	Hypothermia	Revulsive
Cold plunge	Heat capacity	Immersion bath	Systemic (general) application
Compress	Heat cramps	Local (zonal or regional) applica-	Systemic (general) response
Counterirritant	Heat exhaustion	tion	Tonic
Cryotherapy	Heat stroke	Local (zonal or regional) response	Tonifying
Derivation	Hydrostatic pressure	Neuropathy	Vascular disorders

Authors' Note: Most content in Chapter 4 has been adapted from Barron, 2003; Benjamin and Tappan, 2005; Crebbin-Bailey, Harcup, and Harrington, 2005; Fritz, 2008; Nikola, 1997; O'Rourke, 1995; Sinclair, 2008; and Williams, 2007.

WHAT IS HYDROTHERAPY?

Hydrotherapy is one of the oldest natural medicines. Early civilizations made use of its healing properties by bathing in seawater, local streams, and mineral springs. The ancient Greeks and Romans knew the hygienic and restorative value of bathing on a regular basis—one of the simplest ways to maintain health and well-being. These early bathing practices, as well as Roman methods of waste removal, are the forerunners of modern sanitary practices.

European spas have long made ample use of hydrotherapy, and spa menus in the United States currently offer many different options. These can include mineral baths, water massage such as Watsu®, whirlpool baths and Jacuzzis®, hot tubs, jet or percussion showers, Vichy showers, steam rooms, and saunas. Additional hydrotherapy

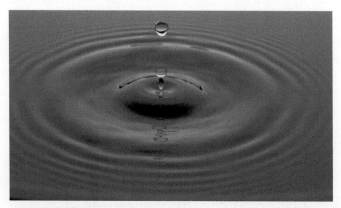

(Don Farrall/Getty Images, Inc.—Photodisc.)

treatments are found not only at spas but can also be easily integrated into the private practices of massage therapists and other bodyworkers. These include hot and cold **compresses** (hot compresses are also called **fomentations**), ginger fomentations, cold sheet wraps, and hot foot baths. There are also simple hydrotherapy treatments that practitioners can recommend that clients do at home for themselves, such as showers and baths at various temperatures, medicated baths, and simple inhalations.

In order to understand how to choose the most effective treatment to give to a client or recommend that the client perform at home, it is essential to understand how hydrotherapy works. Understanding the properties of water, the effects of hydrotherapy on the body, and how heat and cold affect the body gives the practitioner a foundation on which to build.

PROPERTIES OF WATER

Water has properties that make hydrotherapy effective. First, it is the most effective solvent known. More substances dissolve in water than in any other liquid. Substances that do not dissolve in water will be suspended in it. Because water can dissolve or suspend so many different substances, it is an ideal medium for hydrotherapy treatments. Salts, ginger, and certain herbs are examples of substances that dissolve in water. Clays, on the other hand, do not dissolve in water but are, instead, suspended in it.

Water can also participate in chemical reactions. In order to release the therapeutic properties of certain substances, such as ginger and herbs, the addition of water, and perhaps heat, may be necessary. The water and heat can help break apart the chemical bonds in the substances and be the method of transfer of the substances to the body.

Since water is a lubricant, it provides glide when exfoliation substances are applied to the body. Exfoliation treatments remove the top layers of dead skin, and a certain amount of friction is necessary to do this. The glide that water provides decreases the friction to a therapeutic level, protecting the skin (Tortora and Derrickson, 2006).

Water is readily available and easily applied. Towels and sheets can be soaked in it for certain compresses and body wrap applications. Ice therapies can be administered directly to specific parts of the body, steam baths use water in vapor form, and, of course, baths and showers are the earliest form of hydrotherapy.

Buoyancy is the power of a fluid to exert an upward force on a body placed in it. The human body has almost the same density as water so it floats easily in water. The buoyancy of water depends on its density, and density depends on the amount of minerals in it. The more minerals, the denser the water; the denser the water, the easier it is to float in it. The oceans are 3 percent saline, which make them especially easy to float in. The Dead Sea in Israel, though, has about ten times more salt than seawater and is about 33 percent saline. This makes possible an experience of almost complete weightlessness.

Even in waters that do not have a high mineral content, buoyancy is possible to a certain extent. Non–weight-bearing exercise, such as water aerobics, makes use of this feature, and some rehabilitation techniques after surgeries or injuries are also done in water to keep weight off healing tissues.

When water is contained, it exerts equal pressure or force against all sides of the container, which is called **hydrostatic pressure.** When people are immersed in the water, the water will exert hydrostatic pressure equally on their bodies as well. The denser the water and the deeper into the water, the higher the pressure exerted. The force exerted against the muscles increases blood circulation and lymphatic flow, as well as awareness of body movements. It also causes the heart to beat harder and faster, creating a bit of a cardiac workout. This is how water aerobics strengthens the heart. The principle of hydrostatic pressure applies to all baths, but especially to whirlpools, hydrotherapy tubs, and Hubbard tanks (all discussed later in the chapter).

One of the most important properties of water with regard to hydrotherapy is that it has a high **heat capacity.** This means that in comparison to most other substances, water can absorb or release a large amount of heat without much change in its own temperature. Water can exist in three states: liquid, solid, and vapor (gas). At 32°F (0°C), water freezes and becomes solid, or ice; at 212°F (100°C), water boils and becomes vapor; between 32°F and 212°F water exists as a liquid (Diracdelta Science and Engineering Encyclopedia, 2006.) ▶ Table 4.1 gives descriptions of water at different temperatures.

TABLE 4.1

Water Temperatures

Temperature Ranges in Degrees

Description	Fahrenheit	Celsius
Boiling (becoming a vapor)	212	100
Dangerously hot	125+	52+
Painfully hot	110–124	43–51
Very hot	105–109	41–42
Hot	100–104	38–40
Warm	92–99	34–37
Tepid (lukewarm)	86–91	30–33
Neutral	80–85	27–29
Cool	65–79	18–26
Cold	55–64	13–17
Very cold	33–54	0–12
Freezing (becoming a solid)	32	0

Water temperature can have all different effects on the body; it is important to have a basic understanding of the temperatures at which water freezes and boils, and the temperatures in between.

When any substance changes states, it either takes in or gives up heat (McConnell, 2001). This is why cold therapies and ice therapies can be so potent in their effects: they are excellent at drawing heat from the body. This is also why they need to be monitored carefully. If too much heat is drawn from the body too quickly, it can cause damage to tissues and be painful for the client. Heat therapies are powerful because they are excellent at transferring heat, and substances within the heat such as ginger or herbs, to the body. This is also why serious burns can occur with heat and steam treatments; they need to be monitored carefully as well.

Heat Transfer

Because of water's high heat capacity, it has the ability to transfer large amounts of heat to and from the body twenty-five times faster than air (Curtis, 2002). There are three main ways water transfers heat, and these methods are foundational for certain spa and hydrotherapy treatments. (These are also three of the same four processes the body uses to transfer heat to the external environment, as discussed in Chapter 2.)

▶ Conduction: transfer of heat through direct contact. As water contacts the body, heat will move

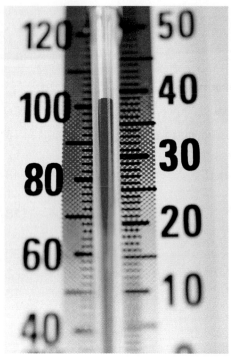

(Corbis RF)

from whichever is warmer to whichever is cooler. For example, when a hot compress is applied to the body, the heat will transfer from the compress to the body. When a cold compress is applied to the body, the heat will transfer from the body to the compress. The heat transfer will happen for as long as there is a difference in temperatures. Once the temperatures are equal, no further transfer will occur.

▶ Convection: transfer of heat due to the movements (currents) of air or water. Convection works with conduction. When warm air and warm water swirl around the body, they bring heat to it. Examples are hot baths, steam saunas, and steam baths. When cool air and cool water swirl around the body, they draw heat away from it. Examples are being in a room that is cooler than the body, cool baths, and ice bath plunges. Again the heat transfer will happen for as long as there is a difference in temperature, and it stops when the temperatures become equal.

▶ Radiation: transfer of heat in the form of infrared rays without contact. Dry saunas and infrared heat lamps use radiation to bring heat to the body. The heat from sunlight is due to infrared radiation. The body will also lose heat due to radiation any time it is in an environment that is cooler than body temperature. An example is, again, just being in a room that is cooler than the body (Miller, 2008).

THE EFFECTS OF HYDROTHERAPY TREATMENTS

There are many different types of hydrotherapy treatments, and each has its own particular way of affecting the body. These effects, though, can be grouped into three broad categories: mechanical, chemical, and thermal. Sometimes a treatment can affect the body in just one way, but, more often, a hydrotherapy method has more than one effect.

Mechanical

Water impacts the body physically, which can be thought of as a mechanical effect on the body. Buoyancy from floating in baths, flotation tanks, Hubbard tanks, Jacuzzis®, and whirlpools is a mechanical effect. An **affusion** (water applied to the body through a hose) applied at a low pressure could be a soothing treatment, whereas a vigorous whirlpool bath can be very stimulating; both of these are mechanical effects of water on the body.

Hydrostatic pressure provides a great deal of mechanical resistance against muscles and associated joints and bones. This is important for rebuilding muscle and increasing joint range of motion following injuries or surgeries. Also, hydrostatic pressure can perform a "pumping action" on blood and lymphatic vessels, thereby encouraging flow of both blood and lymph. Fluid flows from an area of higher pressure to an area of lower pressure. As discussed previously, the deeper into the water a part of the body is, the higher the hydrostatic pressure placed on it. Therefore, blood and lymph will flow to the lower pressure body areas that are in shallower water, or out of the water completely. This usually means blood and lymph flow upward toward the heart. The heart responds by beating more strongly to pump out the blood it receives, but it does not beat faster; this results in overall strengthening of the heart, which is another mechanical effect of hydrotherapy.

DID YOU KNOW?

Jacuzzi® is the last name of the man who developed Jacuzzis®. Candido Jacuzzi and his brothers owned Jacuzzi Brothers, a company that manufactured hydraulic aircraft pumps. In 1943, Candido's son developed rheumatoid arthritis, and in 1948, Candido developed a submersible bathtub pump so his son could have soothing whirlpool treatments at home in between therapeutic hydrotherapy treatments at the local hospital. Jacuzzi Brothers marketed the pump starting in 1955.

Chemical

Although it may not be thought of this way, water is a chemical, and it plays a role in chemical reactions in certain spa and hydrotherapy treatments. In treatments that use substances with water, it is through chemical reactions that the healing properties of the substances are released. Examples are ginger used in fomentations, muds and seaweed used in body wraps, and herbs used in poultices. These substances then react chemically with the body to affect blood flow, decrease muscle spasms, or soothe the skin.

Thermal

Hydrotherapy is at its most powerful when the water is above or below body temperature. The greater the difference in the temperature between the body and the treatment being used, the greater the effect of the treatment. Therefore, it is important to understand how heat and cold affect the body, which is why temperature is one of the variables in hydrotherapy.

FOUR MAIN VARIABLES IN HYDROTHERAPY

There are four main variables in hydrotherapy. These variables should be factored into every hydrotherapy treatment to ensure the therapeutic effect of the treatment, and the health and safety of the client.

Temperature

The first variable is temperature (see ▶Table 4.2). The greater the difference between the body's temperature and the temperature used in the treatment, the greater

TABLE 4.2
Hydrotherapy Application Temperatures

Application	Temperature (°F)
Hot water	100–104
Warm water	92–100
Tepid (lukewarm)	80–92
Cool	65–80
Cold	55–65
Very cold	32–55
Ice	32

Temperature is the first of four variables that affect how the body receives a hydrotherapy treatment.

the intensity of the treatment. And the greater the intensity, the greater the need to closely monitor the temperature of the treatment as both heat and cold can damage tissue and cause the client pain.

Duration

The second variable is duration (see ▶Table 4.3). At extreme temperatures (both hot and cold), the shorter the duration, the more intense, and effective, the treatment. At moderate temperatures, intensity and effectiveness increase the longer the treatment is applied. Frequency of treatment, as in successive applications, also increases the intensity.

TABLE 4.3
Duration of Hot and Cold Applications

Application	Duration
Short hot	Less than 5 minutes
Prolonged hot	More than 5 minutes
Short cold	Less than 1 minute
Prolonged cold	More than 1 minute

Duration is the second of four variables that determine how the body receives a hydrotherapy treatment.

Condition of the Client

The third variable is the condition of the client. The client's health and vitality are major considerations in determining both the type of hydrotherapy to be used and the results of the treatment. Clients who are less vital need treatments without great temperature extremes. On the other hand, clients who are healthy may have positive body responses to the stresses placed on them by treatments with wide temperature extremes. For example, an elderly client in frail health would need a shorter application of a warm compress in the tepid (80 to 92°F) range, whereas a triathlete may respond better to a longer application of a hot compress, one in the 92 to 100°F range.

Location

The fourth variable is location. Hydrotherapy treatments need to be applied where they will have the most beneficial effect for the client. Sometimes the effect is just where the treatment is placed on the body; sometimes the treatment is placed in one location so it will have an effect in another location on the client's body; sometimes an overall body treatment is indicated.

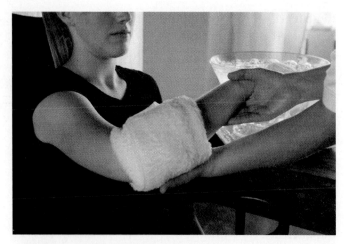

▶ **Figure 4.1** This cold compress will react locally on the client's arm.

A **local** (**zonal** or **regional**) **application** is one that is applied to just one area of the body (see ▶Figure 4.1). A **local response** to the heat or cold application is one that occurs in only the area of application. A **systemic** (or **general**) **application** is one that is applied to the entire body (see ▶Figure 4.2). A **systemic** (or **general**) **response** is one that occurs to the entire body. Local applications are capable of producing systemic responses as well as local responses, and systemic applications are capable of producing local responses as well as systemic responses.

Also, a local application is capable of producing a reaction in an area far from the site of the application. In other words, a heat application on one ankle can produce vasodilation and increased blood flow in the other ankle. This is called a **reflex** or **consensual response.** Stimulation, as in application of heat or cold, to one area of the body results in a response in another area. These reflexes are due to the structure of the nervous system. As discussed in Chapter 2, the spinal cord not only sends information

from sensory nerves up to the brain, it also communicates within itself. A sensation can come into a spinal segment from one side of the body, travel up and down the spinal cord to other segments, and cause nerve impulses to travel along motor nerves from different segments and out to effectors far from where the sensation originated (Tortora and Derrickson, 2006). This is how a hydrotherapy application in one region of the body can produce a reaction somewhere else in the body. Consensual reflexes are particularly helpful for local applications that are contraindicated for an area of the body. The treatment can be applied elsewhere and cause a response in the area of contraindication.

WAYS TO PERFORM TREATMENTS

There are many ways to perform hydrotherapy treatments. Each of the following sections includes methods practitioners can use to learn basic procedures. Once practitioners are skilled at these, they can develop more creative treatments and build their treatment menus. Practitioners who work in spas should note that each spa has its own treatment protocols and trains its practitioners accordingly. What is presented in this chapter may or may not be consistent with how individual spas perform treatments. However, practitioners will acquire foundational hydrotherapy skills, become comfortable handling supplies and equipment, and become able to knowledgeably discuss hydrotherapy treatment options with clients.

COLD THERAPIES

In a healthy person, reactions to cold applications can help strengthen the body's vitality. When cold is applied, the body reacts to it as a stress. Within limits, stresses placed on the body make it stronger by causing it to respond more quickly and efficiently with each successive stress. Over time, this can lead to a stronger heart, better respiration, more toned muscles, and increased cellular metabolism.

The factors involved in applying cold treatments include the temperature of the treatment, the temperature differential between the skin and the treatment, how long the treatment is applied, and how much blood supply the area of the body has. Generally, cold applications penetrate deeper than hot applications do. There is a risk of tissue damage with cold, so it is important that the temperature be monitored carefully when performing cold treatments on clients.

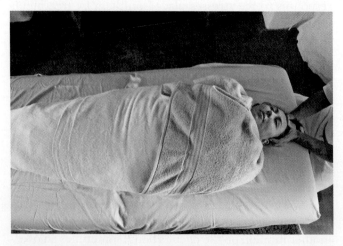

▶ **Figure 4.2** This wrap will react systemically on the client's entire body.

The body progresses through several stages when stimulated by cold:

▶ **First stage:** immediate cardiovascular response. Blood vessels in the skin vasoconstrict, the heart rate slows, and blood pressure increases slightly.

▶ **Second stage:** metabolic warming via the endocrine system. This is a thermal (warming) stage in which the tissues, responding to thyroid hormones, increase their metabolism to generate heat to combat the effects of the cold.

▶ **Third stage:** nervous and muscular system involvement. Increased nerve impulses to muscles cause them to contract slightly, increasing their tone and generating more heat for the body. Because of this increase in muscle tone, cold treatments are also referred to as **tonic** treatments. If the third stage lasts long enough, there can be a progression to a sedation stage in which a feeling of calmness develops. The length of time for the sedation stage to develop is different for everyone.

Sometimes, however, clients may not progress through all the cold response stages, and **hypothermia,** a lowered core body temperature, is a danger. The signs of this include:

▶ feeling chilled
▶ shivering
▶ gooseflesh
▶ cold hands and feet
▶ blue tinge to the lips, fingers, and ears
▶ nausea
▶ agitation and, perhaps, fear

These signs and symptoms indicate that the cold treatment is not working for the client and that the client will not be able to reach the second (warming) and third (sedation) stages. The treatment needs to be stopped immediately, and the client needs to be warmed with blankets or possibly a hot foot bath.

If the body is warmed first, there tends to be a more favorable reaction to cold treatments. The client could be warmed prior to receiving a cold treatment by exercising or by receiving a heat treatment. For clients who do not tolerate cold well, massage strokes performed on the client by the practitioner before applying the cold treatment may make the treatment more agreeable. Recall from Chapter 2 that sensations of touch are carried along nerves and up the spinal cord to the brain faster than temperature sensations are. Clients would not feel the cold as acutely as they would without the tactile stimulation first.

Local Cold Application

Examples of local cold applications include single and double cold compresses. The most immediate response is vasoconstriction of skin blood vessels and decreased lymphatic flow in the application area. Because less blood flows through the area, the area becomes blanched, or pale. The blood that was in the skin is shunted to the core of the body to keep it warm, and the hairs on the skin may also stand on end. The rate of metabolic reactions in the tissue area decreases. Nerve impulse conduction slows, resulting in an analgesic effect; this is why ice can be used as a numbing agent. Local muscle tone increases, and connective tissue becomes less pliable and more rigid. Wound healing slows because of the decreased blood flow to the area. The cold, though, increases the activities of leukocytes.

A local cold application of short duration can be very stimulating since it is an immediate shock to the body. Prolonged local applications are, instead, more numbing, although there is a risk of tissue damage when applying ice to an area of the body for an extended period of time.

Indications for local cold application include:

▶ mild edema
▶ joint inflammation (but not from an autoimmune disorder)
▶ headache
▶ low back pain
▶ sprain
▶ acute muscle strain

Systemic Cold Application

The initial effects of a short systemic cold application, such as a cold plunge or cold bath, are of a stimulating nature. However, the effects of a prolonged systemic application tend to be more sedating. ▶Table 4.4 shows the effects of short and prolonged systemic cold applications on the body.

Indications for systemic cold application include the need to:

▶ increase energy
▶ boost immune responses
▶ increase muscle tone
▶ increase stamina
▶ decrease muscle spasms

Contraindications and Considerations for Cold Application Treatments

Because of how powerfully cold can affect the body, there are certain conditions that are contraindicated for the

TABLE 4.4

Effects of Short and Prolonged Systemic Cold Applications on the Body

	Short Application	Prolonged Application
Heart	Increase in heart rate and strength of contraction	Decrease in heart rate and strength of contraction
Blood pressure	Increases	Decreases
Blood vessels	Skin blood vessels vasoconstrict; core blood vessels vasodilate	Skin blood vessels vasodilate; core blood vessels vasoconstrict
Respiration	Respiration rate increases and breathing becomes shallow	Respiration rate decreases and breathing becomes deeper
Muscle tone	Increases	Increases
Connective tissues	Little effect	Becomes less pliable and more rigid
Blood cells	Little effect	Increase in the number of erythrocytes; increase in the number and activity of leukocytes
Metabolism	Little effect	Decreases
Digestive activities	Little effect	Increase

application of cold, as well as considerations that need to be kept in mind about certain types of clients. These contraindications and considerations apply for both local and systemic cold application treatments.

Contraindications to cold application treatments are:

▶ heart conditions
▶ untreated **hypertension** or hypotension
▶ respiratory conditions
▶ numbness or loss of sensation
▶ **neuropathy** (any disorder involving nerves)
▶ **vascular disorders** (disorders affecting blood vessels)
▶ serious burns
▶ flare-up stages of autoimmune disorders such as lupus, rheumatoid arthritis, and multiple sclerosis (there is generally a great deal of pain with flare-up stages; a cold application would only be more painful and debilitating)
▶ any disorders with accompanying vascular issues or neuropathy, such as diabetes
▶ cancer
▶ high body temperature (fever)
▶ broken, bleeding, or irritated skin
▶ condition in which the person is not able to communicate or give accurate feedback about temper-

ature, such as treatments on infants, those under the influence of drugs or alcohol, or those who are unconscious

Considerations are needed for clients who are fragile physically or emotionally such as from aging or chronic disease. They may be able to receive hydrotherapy treatments, but the treatments must be modified for their particular conditions. Generally, an increase to a more moderate temperature and decrease in duration of cold treatments are warranted. The same is true for people with intolerance to cold.

▶Table 4.5 shows the indication, contraindications, and considerations for cold applications.

Treatments

Local cold treatments can take the form of showers applied to certain parts of the body; compresses; foot baths; and the use of **cryotherapy,** which is the application of ice to the body. Systemic cold treatments can take the form of a full-body shower, **immersion bath,** and **cold plunge.** Compresses and cryotherapy are explained next; showers and cold foot and immersion baths, and cold plunges are covered later in this chapter.

	Indications	Contraindications	Considerations
Local cold	Mild edema	**The following apply to local and systemic hot and cold applications:**	Clients who are fragile physically or emotionally such as from aging or chronic disease may be able to receive hydrotherapy treatments, but the treatments must be modified for their particular conditions. Generally, a decrease to a more moderate temperature and decrease in duration of heat treatments are warranted. The same is true for clients who have intolerance to cold or heat.
	Joint inflammation (not from autoimmune disorder)	Heart conditions	
	Headache	Untreated hypertension or hypotension	
	Low back pain	Respiratory conditions	
	Sprain	Numbness or loss of sensation	
	Acute muscle strain	Neuropathy	
		Vascular disorders	
		Serious burns	
		Flare-up stages of autoimmune disorders	
		Disorders that can accompany vascular issues or neuropathy such as diabetes	
		Cancer	
		High body temperature (fever)	
		Broken or irritated skin	
Systemic cold	Need for increased energy	Any condition in which the person is not able to communicate or give accurate feedback about temperature such as treatments on infants, those under the influence of drugs or alcohol, or those who are unconscious	
	Need to boost immune responses		
	Need to increase muscle tone		
	Need to increase stamina		
	Muscle spasms		
Local heat	Chronic muscle tension		
	Tight joints (from noninflammatory conditions)		
	Muscle spasms		
	Pain from old sprains and strains		
	Insomnia		
	Congestion in the sinuses or the chest		
	Congestive headache		
	Preparation of tissue for massage or other bodywork		

TABLE 4.5 (cont.)

	Indications	Contraindications	Considerations
Systemic heat	Chronic muscle tension		
	Tight joints (from noninflammatory conditions)		
	Insomnia		
	Need for relaxation and detoxification		
	Preparation of tissue for massage or other bodywork		
Alternating (local and systemic)	Chronic muscle tension	Acute inflammation is not contraindicated for local and systemic cold treatments but is contraindicated for local and systemic heat and alternating treatments	
	Tight joints (from noninflammatory conditions)		
	Muscle spasms		
	Pain from old sprains and strains		
	Abdominal cramping from premenstrual syndrome and menstruation		
	Congestion in the sinuses and chest from colds, flu, and chronic bronchitis		
	Headache		
	Preparation of tissue for massage or other bodywork		

Local Cold Treatments

Compress   Temperature (heat or cold) can be applied to any area of the body with a moist compress. A cold compress decreases pain impulses in an area; decreases local inflammation; and causes vasoconstriction of blood vessels, which decreases local blood flow. Cold compresses can be single or double depending on the purpose of the application.

The supplies for compresses can be purchased at local stores or online. These treatments can also be performed by clients at home with proper instruction from practitioners.

Double Cold Compress   Double cold compress treatment is unlikely to be performed in a spa or private practice. Instead, the following are useful treatments practitioners can recommend to their clients to perform at home.

A double cold compress consists of a cold moist cloth or towel covered completely by a dry cloth of flannel or wool. Wool works the best because of its ability to insulate. This application is sometimes called a *heating* compress because it acts by initially pushing blood and lymph away, stimulating a secondary heating response. This attracts fresh oxygenated blood back to the area, flushing out congestion and speeding up the healing process. A double cold compress is extremely effective and versatile because it can be shaped or folded for application anywhere on the body. It can even be applied before going to bed at night and left on until morning. The following are examples of two useful double cold compresses.

Throat Double Cold Compress: a simple application of a cold cloth that is thoroughly wrung out, wrapped around the neck, and then covered by a larger flannel or wool cloth. A safety pin secures the compress around the neck. It is left on the body overnight. The cold cloth alerts the body to the cold stimulus. The body responds by focusing on the area and sends warm, oxygenated blood, thus speeding up the healing process (▶Figures 4.3 a, b, and c).

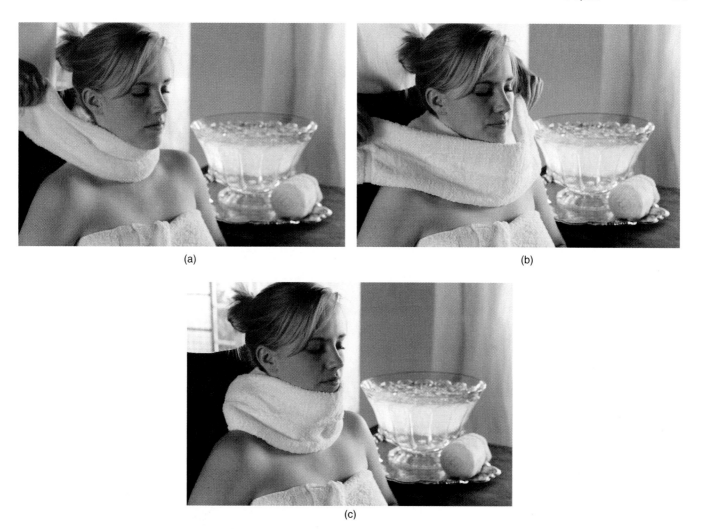

(a)

(b)

(c)

▶ **Figure 4.3** Application of a throat double cold compress.

Foot Double Cold Compress: also called the wet sock treatment. It is an old "tried-and-true" folk remedy that works wonders. Two pairs of socks are needed. The first pair should be cotton. Wet them with cold water, wring them out thoroughly and put them on the feet. The second pair can also be cotton, but wool socks are more effective at insulating. Cover the cold wet socks with a dry pair and go to bed. In the morning the wet socks will be almost completely dry. The body responds to the cold stimulus and works hard to warm the feet. A derivative action kicks in and congestion is pulled downward. This is an amazingly simple treatment that can be done at the beginning or end of a cold or flu. If done in the beginning, it may actually ward off the illness. If done during a cold or flu, it will shorten the duration of the illness; and at the end, it will combat a cold or flu that lingers.

Cryotherapy

Cryotherapy is the therapeutic use of cold (*cryo-* is from the Greek *kryos* meaning "icy cold"). In hydrotherapy, cryotherapy is also known as ice massage and is the application of ice using deep circular friction over a localized area of the body. This application of prolonged cold initially causes vasoconstriction and then vasodilation of blood vessels, causing a pumping action of blood out and into the tissues in the affected area. The application of cold also decreases pain, as do the friction and pressure of the ice moving over the skin (recall from Chapter 2 that nerve impulses from touch travel up to the brain faster than pain impulses).

There are generally four stages of sensation the client will feel when the ice is applied:

- ▶ first stage: cold stimulus
- ▶ second stage: slight burning sensation
- ▶ third stage: deep achy feeling
- ▶ fourth stage: numbness

Ice application should stop once the fourth stage is reached because it is at this stage that tissue damage can occur if the ice application continues.

TREATMENT 4.1

Single Cold Compress

Single cold compresses cause vasoconstriction, which inhibits blood flow, and they also numb pain receptors and draw heat from the body. Single cold compresses are typically performed for 20 to 30 minutes, using water that is as cold as the client can tolerate. To ensure continual cold application, single cold compresses are changed quickly because these compresses draw heat from the body and warm up quickly. Applying friction to the area first with a cool loofah mitt, ayate cloth (a cloth made from coarse natural fibers), or rough towel may make this treatment more comfortable for people with a low tolerance for or sensitivity to cold.

Rationale

A single cold compress can be applied for any or all of the following physiological effects:

- Analgesic: relieves pain
- Anesthetic: numbs nerve receptors at injury site
- Antispasmodic: relieves muscle spasms
- Antipyretic: decreases fever
- Vasoconstrictor: decreases local blood flow

Equipment and Supplies (see ▶Figure 4.4)

- Basin of cold or ice water
- Ice (as needed to keep water at the level of coolness)
- Three thick soft cloths or towels, approximately 18″ × 30″; the thicker the compress, the longer it stays cold

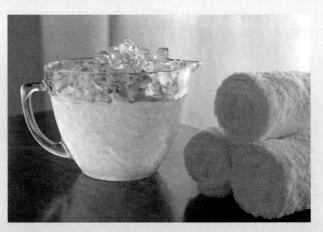

▶ Figure 4.4

Indications

- Pain relief
- Chronic muscle tension
- Muscle spasms
- Sprains and strains
- Inflammation
- Mild burns (skin is not broken or blistered)
- Congestion in the sinuses and chest from colds, flu, and chronic bronchitis
- Congestive headache
- Fever

Contraindications

- Heart conditions
- Numbness or loss of sensation in area
- Neuropathy in area
- Vascular disorder in area
- Intolerance to cold

TREATMENT 4.1 CONTINUED

Preparation

1. Cool water and place it in the basin. Position ice within easy reach for adding during the treatment.
2. Fold two towels in thirds (or to fit the size of the area being treated) widthwise and then roll them up (▶Figures 4.5 a, b, and c). Place the folded, rolled towels in the ice water (▶Figure 4.6). Leave one towel dry.

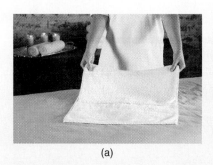 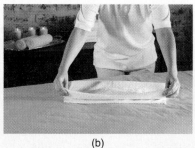 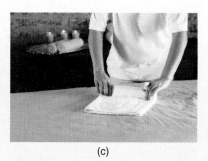

(a)	(b)	(c)

▶ **Figure 4.5**

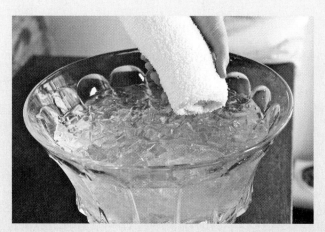

▶ **Figure 4.6**

Procedure

1. Uncover the area to be treated. Unroll (but leave folded) one towel, wring it out thoroughly, and apply it to the indicated area of the client's body (▶Figures 4.7 a, b, and c).

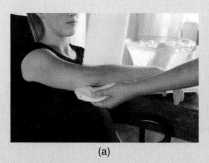 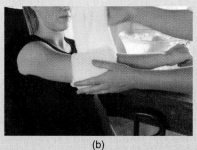 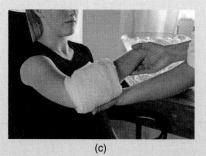

(a)	(b)	(c)

▶ **Figure 4.7**

TREATMENT 4.1 CONTINUED

CLINICAL ALERT !

Check immediately with the client about temperature. If the towel is too cold, remove it promptly and allow it to warm up a bit. Place the towel on the client again and recheck temperature. If it still too cold, remove it again and wait until the temperature is comfortable for the client. The first application should feel mildly cold to the client with the temperature gradually decreasing with each application, depending on the client's vitality and tolerance to cold.

2. The cold towel on the client should be replaced as soon as the client feels the coolness decreasing (approximately every 1 to 3 minutes). Before the towel on the client warms up completely, prepare the next cool towel for application. Wring the new cool towel out thoroughly.

3. Remove the first towel from the client's body and apply the second towel. Reroll the first towel and place it back in the basin of cold water.

4. Repeat cold compress changes as necessary for 20 to 30 minutes.

5. Using the dry towel, dry the area after the last application.

After the Treatment
Allow the client to rest for at least 20 minutes before resuming applications or performing massage. Or just let the client rest after the treatment is complete.

Hygiene
Launder the towels with hot water and detergent after each use. The basin should be washed in warm, soapy water and rinsed after each use.

Cryotherapy is especially effective at reducing swelling and congestion in tissues and in helping relieve muscle spasms. Contraindications for cryotherapy are the same as for a single cold compress:

▶ heart conditions
▶ intolerance to cold
▶ numbness or loss of sensation in the area
▶ vascular disorder in the area

The ice applied can be in the form of:

▶ self-contained ice massager: special plastic cup that can be purchased, filled with water, then frozen (see ▶Figure 4.8)
▶ an ice cup: a paper or foam cup is filled with water and frozen; the top of the cup is placed on the client while the bottom of the cup is a holder for the practitioner to use; as the ice melts, strips of cup around the top are peeled off to reveal more ice
▶ frozen can of juice
▶ cold can of soda
▶ even a popsicle

The ice should be applied in the following manner:

▶ Rub your hand over the area of the client's body where the ice will be applied; this reduces the initial shock of the cold on the client's skin
▶ Ask the client to take a deep breath, then start applying the ice using deep circular strokes and ask the client to exhale. Have the client keep taking deep breaths during the treatment. This keeps the client focused on the breath rather than the cold application and also helps the client relax.
▶ Keep the strokes continuous and smooth for approximately 5 to 15 minutes. To make sure the cold penetrates into the client's body, stay within the focus area. Use a towel to catch the drips of water on the client's skin because they can be uncomfortable.
▶ The client will progress through the four stages of sensation. Treatment is complete when the area is numb.
▶ Gently blot the area dry with the cloth or towel. Unless it is the site of a recent injury, such as a sprained ankle, massage can be applied to the area.

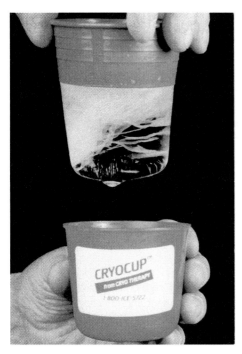

▶ **Figure 4.8** A self-contained ice massager is ideal for reducing swelling and congestion in tissues and helping relieve muscle spasms. *(Donald R. Nicolia—P.A-C/Cryo Therapy Inc.)*

Ice can be reapplied often during the first 24 to 72 hours after an acute injury, but there should be a break of at least 20 minutes between applications in order to prevent tissue damage from the ice.

Systemic Cold Treatments

Systemic cold treatments generally take the form of cold showers (discussed later in this chapter), cold baths (discussed later in this chapter), and cold plunges. The temperature for a cold plunge is usually much lower than that for a cold bath—for example, the plunges taken by members of "polar bear clubs" into icy rivers and lakes or plunges into snow or icy water after being heated in a sauna, steam room, or sweat lodge.

HEAT THERAPIES

In a healthy person, reactions to heat applications can help strengthen the body's vitality. When heat is applied, the body reacts to it as a stress, just as it does to cold therapies; the body becomes stronger by responding more quickly and efficiently with each successive stress. Over time, this can lead to a stronger heart, better respiration, more toned muscles, and increased cellular metabolism.

One of the most noticeable effects of heat applications is **diaphoresis,** or perspiration. The sweating can flush toxins from the body. However, since body fluid and salts, as well as metabolic wastes, are lost in perspiration, it is important that the client be well hydrated before, during, and after heat treatments.

Another major effect of heat application is vasodilation of blood vessels in the skin, resulting in **hyperemia** (see ▶Figure 4.9), or reddening of the skin caused by an increased blood flow to the area. This blood is warmed by the heat treatment, and the flow of blood carries heat to other parts of the body. This is how the whole body can be warmed up from a treatment such as a hot foot bath. The increased blood flow (called **fluxion**) brings more blood cells and nutrients to the area and transports cell debris and other wastes away from the area. This is an important aspect of tissue health and healing. Erythrocytes bring more oxygen to the tissues, leukocytes combat infection in the tissues by eating cell debris and pathogens, and thrombocytes can form a clot to seal off any damaged blood vessels that are leaking blood and need repair (Tortora and Derrickson, 2006).

Derivation is the process of using heat to draw blood and lymph from one part of the body to the other. Applying heat locally can have a derivative effect in another part of the body. For example, a hot foot bath can draw blood away from congested sinuses because as the blood is drawn away, the inflammation in the sinuses, and therefore the congestion, is relieved.

In addition to increasing blood flow, heat increases cellular metabolism. A law of physics, van Hoff's Law, says that for every 10°C increase in temperature, the speed of metabolic reactions increases two to three times. This higher rate of metabolism increases tissue repair. Heat

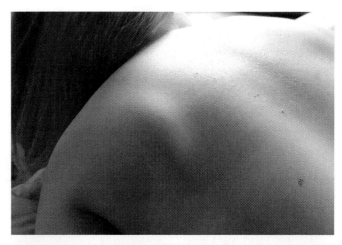

▶ **Figure 4.9** Heat applications often cause reddening of the skin, or hyperemia, because of increased blood flow to the area where heat was applied.

also stimulates the activities of leukocytes (Tortora and Derrickson, 2006).

Heat applications that do not use water, such as a heating pad, have a superficial effect, penetrating only about 1 cm into the body. Since water is a good conductor of heat, heat treatments that do use water, such as a hydrocollator pad (see ▸Figure 4.10), Thermophore pad (see ▸Figure 4.11), or certain spa and hydrotherapy treatments, penetrate about 3.5 cm into the body. Recall from Chapter 3 that hydrocollators are stainless steel tanks filled with water at 160 to 165°F. The pads are made of canvas and filled with heat-absorbing clay. The weight of the pads and their heat-retention quality (up to 30 minutes) make them ideal for local application of penetrating heat. Thermophore pads are electric heating pads covered in a fleece blend. The cover draws humidity from the air and retains it. When the pad is turned on, the heat forces moisture out of the cover and onto the body. But because Thermophore pads are lighter than hydrocollator pads, the heat from Thermophore pads does not penetrate as far into the body as the heat from hydrocollator pads does.

The more penetrating heat treatments pass through the skin and subcutaneous fat and reach down into connective tissue and muscles. As the heat warms the proteins, the connective tissue becomes more pliable. This can

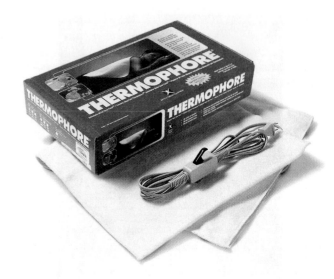

▸ **Figure 4.11** The fleece-blend cover of a Thermophore pad takes humidity from the air and forces it onto the user's body. *(Image courtesy of Battle Creek Equipment Co.)*

make joints move more freely, increasing their range of motion. As the heat warms muscle tissue, the muscle tissue also becomes more pliable and relaxed. The blood vessels in the muscle vasodilate so more nutrition is brought to the muscle, and wastes, the accumulation of which can cause muscle tension and pain, are flushed away. As the muscle tension releases, pain is alleviated. Heat, therefore, has an analgesic effect.

Local Heat Application

Local heat applications include hot compresses, ginger fomentations, and hot foot baths. Applying heat locally can have a derivative effect in another part of the body. For example, a hot foot bath can draw blood from away from congested sinuses. As the blood is drawn away, the inflammation in the sinuses, and therefore the congestion, is relieved.

Indications for local heat application include:

▸ chronic muscle tension
▸ tight joints from noninflammatory conditions
▸ insomnia
▸ congestion in the sinuses or the chest
▸ preparation of tissue for massage or other bodywork

Heat makes inflammation worse, which is why only those clients with arthritis that is not in an inflammatory stage should receive local heat treatments over the affected areas. If a client's arthritis is in an inflammatory stage, applying local heat to areas that are not inflamed may be a possibility.

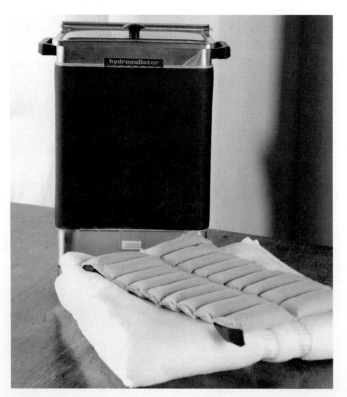

▸ **Figure 4.10** A hydrocollator and its clay-filled canvas pads are ideal for local applications of penetrating heat.

Systemic Heat Application

Systemic heat applications include full immersion baths, hot foot baths, fomentations applied to many parts of the body at once, steam baths, saunas, certain herbal wraps, mud wraps, and heating sheet wraps (sometimes called cold sheet wraps). Heating wraps have an initial cold stimulus, but the effect is to cause systemic heating within the body.

Many of the effects of a systemic heat application on the body are the same as the effects of a fever. A fever is typically triggered when a pathogen invades or there is some other tissue damage, and chemicals are released that travel to the body's internal thermostat, which is located in the brain. The thermostat then resets at a higher temperature, and core body temperature rises. Up to a point, fever is beneficial. The higher temperature increases the activities of leukocytes and interferes with some pathogens' ability to reproduce. Fever also increases heart rate, which increases the delivery of blood and, therefore, erythrocytes and leukocytes, to sites of infection faster. The heat from fever also increases metabolic reactions, which speeds the rate of tissue repair (Tortora and Derrickson, 2006).

When the body has a fever, it is under stress and not in homeostasis. Systemic heat applications use external heat as a stress to cause a reaction in the body; the goal is *not* to increase core body temperature. Rather, the goal is for the body to respond with the same effects as from a fever, without having an actual fever, to facilitate healing and health in the body. Hence, the overall effect of a general or systemic heat application is basically to induce an "artificial" fever.

In addition to increasing the activities of leukocytes and increasing cellular metabolic reactions, general heat applications cause other body reactions. One of them involves the heart. Heart rate increases initially, which also increases blood pressure. Generally, the faster the heart beats, the more blood it pumps out, and the higher the volume of blood in blood vessels, the higher the blood pressure (Tortora and Derrickson, 2006). Because of this phenomenon, *systemic heat treatments are contraindicated for clients who have cardiovascular disease or disorders* because of the risk of causing undue stress to the heart and having an adverse effect on blood pressure. In a healthy person, the heart rate and blood pressure will decrease through the course of a prolonged systemic heat application, having a sedating effect on the client. A potential risk of the sedation is the possibility that blood pressure may dip dangerously low, resulting in hypotension. If not enough blood reaches the brain, the client can feel light headed from the treatment and may need to rest for a moment after sitting up. Then the client may need assistance off the treatment table.

Respiration rate will increase. Normal respiration for an adult is about twelve to sixteen breaths per minute. A systemic heat application can cause the client's respiration rate to increase five to six breaths per minute for every degree (F) increase. Over time, however, as the treatment becomes more sedating, the client's respiration rate will fall back to normal and perhaps a little below.

Coupled with the external heat from the systemic heat treatment, heat may intensify within the client's body and cause the client much discomfort. Excessive sweating can lead to dehydration and electrolyte loss, and there is the danger of hypotension due to lowered blood volume. It is important to always make sure clients are well hydrated during treatments and to apply a cool compress during certain treatments, such as a hot foot bath, to prevent overheating. If the client is in distress, the treatment should be terminated immediately and the client cooled down.

Other risks associated with systemic heat applications are **heat cramps** and **heat exhaustion.** Heat cramps are muscle cramps that result from loss of fluid and electrolytes from the body. They can be remedied by stopping the heat treatment and replacing the fluids and electrolytes. Heat exhaustion is more serious. Symptoms include cool, moist clammy skin (due to profuse sweating), muscle cramps, dizziness, vomiting, and fainting from the loss of fluid and electrolytes. In this situation, the client's body needs to be cooled down immediately and the fluids and electrolytes replaced. Medical intervention may be necessary.

When relative humidity and heat are high, such as with moist heat applications over most of the body and in saunas, it is especially difficult for the body to lose heat. If the core body temperature starts rising, the client may go into **heat stroke.** In extreme cases, body temperature may reach 110°F, resulting in possible brain damage (death occurs at if body temperature reaches 112 to 114°F). Medical intervention is absolutely necessary. Because the person's body will not get back into homeostasis by itself, the person needs to be immersed in cool water and given fluids and electrolytes by health care professionals (Tortora and Derrickson, 2006).

Indications for systemic heat application include:

▶ chronic muscle tension
▶ tight joints (from noninflammatory conditions)
▶ insomnia
▶ need for relaxation and detoxification
▶ preparation of tissue for massage or other bodywork

Contraindications and Considerations for Heat Application Treatments

Because of how powerfully heat can affect the body, certain conditions are contraindicated for the application of heat, and considerations about certain types of clients need to be kept in mind. These contraindications and considerations apply for both local and systemic heat application treatments.

Contraindications to heat application include:

▶ heart conditions
▶ untreated hypertension or hypotension
▶ respiratory conditions
▶ numbness or loss of sensation in area
▶ neuropathy
▶ vascular diseases
▶ burns
▶ acute inflammation
▶ flare-up stages of autoimmune disorders such as lupus, rheumatoid arthritis, and multiple sclerosis; in flare-up stages of autoimmune disorder, there is generally a great deal of pain and accompanying widespread inflammation, a heat application would only be painful and debilitating
▶ any disorders that can accompanying vascular issues or neuropathy, such as diabetes
▶ cancer
▶ high body temperature (fever)
▶ broken or irritated skin
▶ any condition in which the person is not able to communicate or give accurate feedback about temperature, such as treatments on infants, those under the influence of drugs or alcohol, or those who are unconscious

Considerations are needed for clients who are fragile physically or emotionally, such as from aging or chronic disease. They may be able to receive hydrotherapy treatments, but the treatments must be modified for their particular conditions. Generally, a decrease to a more moderate temperature and decrease in duration of heat treatments are warranted. The same is true for people with intolerance to heat.

Revisit Table 4.5 to see the indications, contraindications, and considerations for heat applications.

Treatments

Local heat treatments can take the form of showers applied to certain parts of the body, compresses, ginger fomentations, and partial baths (baths in which only a part of the body is bathed such as the hands or feet). Systemic heat treatments can take the form of full-body showers, immersion baths, and the heating (cold sheet) wrap. Compresses, ginger fomentations, a particular type of partial bath called a hot foot bath, and the heating wrap are explained next; showers and other types of hot foot baths and immersion baths are covered later in this chapter.

Local Heat Treatments

Compress   Temperature (heat or cold) can be applied to any area of the body with a moist compress. Hot compresses serve to relax muscles and soften the tissues in an area, as well as cause vasodilation of blood vessels, which increases local blood flow.

The supplies for compresses can be purchased in local stores or online. These treatments can also be performed by clients at home with proper instruction from practitioners.

Ginger Fomentation   The hot, moist ginger towel treatment is a specialized hot compress—a combination heat and **counterirritant** application. A counterirritant is a locally applied agent that produces superficial inflammation in an attempt to relieve a deeper, adjacent inflammation. The hot, moist heat relaxes muscle spasms, increases circulation, and is sedating. The ginger enhances the heating effect and encourages blood flow.

Hot Foot Bath   The hot foot bath is a simple yet extremely effective hydrotherapy treatment. It can decrease internal congestion anywhere in the body. The hot water in the foot tub produces a derivative effect, drawing blood and lymph from one part of the body to another, increasing circulation and relieving the congestion caused by a headache, sinus infection, sore throat, chest cold, or flu. The addition of a cold compress applied to the head enhances the derivative effect by causing vasoconstriction of those blood vessels, thus pushing blood down toward the feet. The action of pushing blood or lymph away from an area of the body by applying cold is called **retrostasis.**

At the end of the treatment, cold water is splashed over the feet to terminate the derivative action. The hot foot bath followed by the cold splash makes it a **revulsive** treatment, which is defined as a prolonged application of heat followed by a brief application of cold.

Systemic Heat Treatments

Heating (Cold Sheet) Wrap

A heating (cold sheet) wrap is a moist body wrap that begins with a short cold stimulus that produces cooling and vasoconstrictive effects. The body reacts to the short cold stimulus with a powerful thermoregulation response that produces vasodilation and a gradual heating effect. The treatment is broken down into four stages: cooling, neutral, heating, and sweating.

Cooling Stage.   The initial cooling stage produces a **tonifying** effect by causing blood vessels to constrict and muscles to contract. Tonify means to stimulate, invigorate and strengthen. This stimulates the increased production and circulation of white blood cells that fight off disease and strengthen the body's immune response.

TREATMENT 4.2

Hot Compress

Hot compresses are excellent for relieving local muscle tightness, relaxing muscle spasms, breaking up congestion, and reducing aches and pains. A hot compress, at approximately 100°F, is left on the body for approximately 1 to 3 minutes, or until the client feels the compress cooling, then another hot compress is applied. Because the body gets used to the heat, each successive compress can be somewhat hotter than the previous one (up to 105 to 108°F). There are typically five to ten exchanges, which makes the treatment last about 30 to 60 minutes. For weak or frail clients, be sure to decrease the water temperature, decrease the length of time the compress stays on the body, and decrease the number of exchanges.

Rationale

A hot compress can be applied for any and all of the following physiological effects:

- Analgesic: relieves pain
- Fluxion: brings blood to the area
- Decongestant: breaks up mucus
- Sedative: calms muscles and nerves
- Vasodilator: increases local blood flow

Equipment and Supplies

- Stock pot, 12 quarts or larger
- Heating source, such as an electrical hot plate
- Four thick soft cloths or towels, approximately 18″ × 30″ (two to moisten, one to insulate, one to dry the client's body area after treatment)
- Insulated gloves

Indications

- chronic muscle tension
- tight joints (from noninflammatory conditions)
- muscle spasms
- pain from old sprains and strains
- insomnia
- congestion in the sinuses and chest from colds, flu, and chronic bronchitis
- congestive headache
- preparation of tissue for massage or other bodywork

Contraindications

- heart conditions
- vascular disorder in area
- numbness or loss of sensation in area
- inflammation in the area
- intolerance to heat
- broken or irritated skin
- high body temperature (fever)

TREATMENT 4.2 CONTINUED

Preparation

1. Fill the stock pot with water to about 3″ below the rim approximately 15 to 30 minutes before the scheduled treatment. Heat water to just under boiling, and then turn the heat down to medium. Be ready to turn the heat up or down according to the client's tolerance of the hot compresses.
2. Fold three towels in thirds (or to fit the size of the area being treated) widthwise, and then roll two of them up (▶Figures 4.12 a, b, and c).

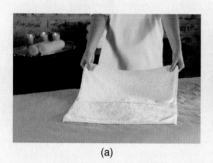
(a)

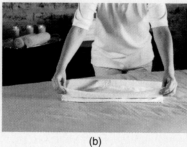
(b)

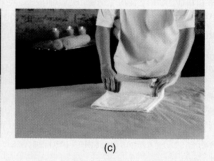
(c)

▶ **Figure 4.12**

Place the two folded, rolled towels in the hot water (▶Figure 4.13). The other folded towel will be used to insulate the compress while it is on the client's body.

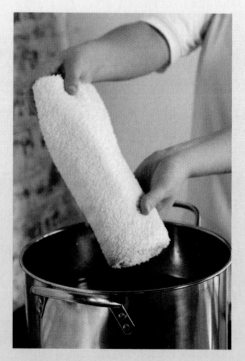

▶ **Figure 4.13**

Procedure

1. Uncover the area of the client's body to be treated.

2. Wearing the insulated gloves, take one towel out of the hot water and wring the towel out quickly and completely; if the towel is too wet, it will cool too quickly. Unroll the towel, but keep it folded in thirds.

TREATMENT 4.2 CONTINUED

Wave the towel to cool it a bit (▶Figure 4.14), and then test the heat by touching the hot compress to the inside of your forearm. If the heat is tolerable, place the hot compress lightly on the client's focus area (▶Figure 4.15).

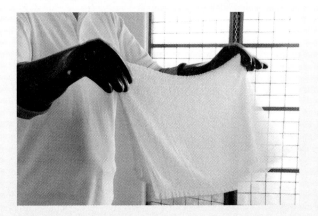

▶ **Figure 4.14**

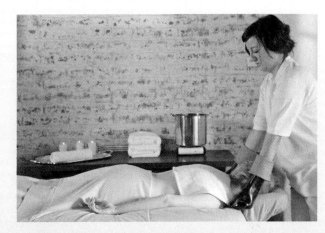

▶ **Figure 4.15**

CLINICAL ALERT !

Check immediately with the client about temperature. If the towel is too hot, remove it immediately and wave it again to cool it more. Place the compress on the client again and recheck about temperature. If it is still too hot, remove it again and cool it until the temperature is comfortable for the client. The first application should be comfortably warm to the client with the temperature gradually increasing with each application, depending on the client's vitality and tolerance to heat.

Cover with a towel to insulate (▶Figure 4.16).

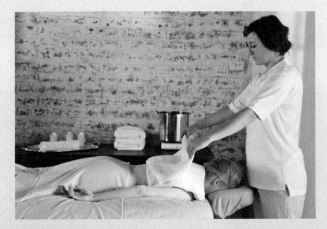

▶ **Figure 4.16**

CLINICAL ALERT !

Do not press down on the insulating towel. This could burn the client.

TREATMENT 4.2 CONTINUED

5. The compress should be replaced as the heat decreases, which should be in 1 to 3 minutes. Before the compress cools completely, prepare the next one for application. Wring out the new hot towel thoroughly, and fan it to cool it a bit. To change compresses, place the new compress on top of the insulating towel (and the old compress), then flip the stack over (▶Figures 4.17 a, b, and c). The insulating towel will now be on top of the new hot compress. This will help retain heat.

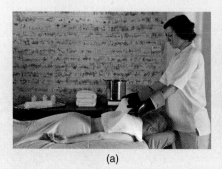 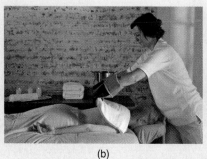 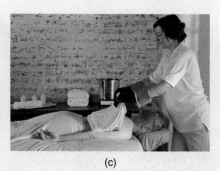

(a)   (b)   (c)

▶ **Figure 4.17**

6. Before removing the towel on top and placing it in the pot to reheat, check to see if the temperature is comfortable for the client. The compress should be a little warmer than the previous hot towel. If it still too hot, remove it immediately and allow it to cool a bit; then replace it when the temperature is tolerable to the client.

7. Keep exchanging the compresses as necessary for 30 to 60 minutes. In the time between towel exchanges, a short scalp and facial massage can be given. The client's feet can be unwrapped for a short foot massage, or other areas of the client's body can be massaged. It is important to stay near the client; the heat may become suddenly unbearable for some clients and the compress will need to be removed immediately.

8. Dry the area with a towel after the last application.

After the Treatment
The client's skin will be reddened, and the tissue should be warm and soft. Massage the area if warranted and appropriate, for example, if the treatment was applied for tight back muscles, and encourage the client to rest and to drink plenty of water afterward.

Hygiene
Launder the sheets and towels with hot water and detergent after each use. Wipe the insulating gloves with alcohol or other disinfectant after each use. Wash the stock pot in warm, soapy water and rinse after each use.

The cooling stage works well for low-grade fever reduction and strengthening immune responses.

Neutral Stage. In the neutral stage, the body reacts to the cold stimulus by dilating blood vessels near the surface in an attempt to create heat. This induces a sedative effect.

The neutral stage has healing benefits for many emotional disorders, including depression, nervousness, restlessness, and anxiety. It is also recommended for insomnia and indigestion and to reduce a low-grade fever.

Heating Stage. In the heating stage, the cold sheet begins to heat up and radiate heat back to the body, stimulating more vasodilation and heating. This causes an increase in metabolism and produces a derivative effect that draws blood and lymph from one part of the body to another.

The heating stage of the cold sheet wrap is good for reducing muscle tension and chest congestion and easing the symptoms of colds and flu.

Sweating Stage. The final stage occurs when the body begins to perspire. The blood vessels near the surface of the skin further dilate, and there is a powerful detoxifying and cleansing effect. This stage can be beneficial for anyone needing to detoxify, such as to eliminate nicotine from the system.

TREATMENT 4.3

Ginger Fomentation

Like the hot compress previously described, a ginger compress is left on the body for approximately 1 to 3 minutes, or until the client feels the compress cooling, then another hot compress is applied. Because the body gets used to the heat, each successive compress can be somewhat hotter than the previous one. There are typically five to ten exchanges, which makes the treatment last about 45 to 60 minutes, including massage of the area after the applications are completed. For weak or frail clients, be sure to decrease the water temperature, decrease the length of time the compress stays on the body, and decrease the number of exchanges.

An amount of fresh ginger root (see ▶Figure 4.18) large enough to yield one cup grated should be purchased for the treatment. Ginger root can be found at grocery stores, especially ones that carry natural, organic food. All the other supplies can also be found at local stores or online.

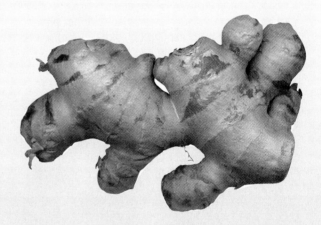

▶ **Figure 4.18 Ginger Root** *(Ilkka Kukko/istockphoto.com)*

CLINICAL ALERT !

Practitioners and clients can be allergic to ginger. It is important for the practitioner to find out from clients any allergies they may have, and note them on an intake form, so there is written documentation. Practitioners allergic to ginger should never use it on clients even when requested to do so, either by clients or employers.

People can develop allergies throughout their lives; therefore, every time a client arrives for a treatment, the practitioner should do a quick allergy update.

Ginger placed on the skin is irritating to all skin types, so a patch test will not show whether clients are allergic to ginger. If clients do not know they are allergic to ginger and a ginger fomentation is performed, the client's body can respond with anything from a few localized hives and itching to a full-blown anaphylactic reaction, which interferes with the client's ability to breathe.

If a client has an allergic reaction, the most important thing the practitioner should do is stay calm and stop the treatment immediately. The ginger should be removed and the client thoroughly rinsed off. If the client's condition worsens, for example, numerous hives, impaired breathing, and/or widespread inflammation occur, emergency care, such as calling 911, should be initiated immediately.

DID YOU KNOW?

Ginger is commonly referred to as a root but it is actually a rhizome. A rhizome is an underground, horizontal stem of a plant, such as a potato.

TREATMENT 4.3 CONTINUED

Rationale

A ginger fomentation can be performed for any and all of the following physiological effects:

- Counterirritant: relieves a deeper inflammation
- Fluxion: brings blood to the area
- Sedative: induces a state of deep relaxation
- Vasodilator: increases local blood flow

Equipment and Supplies (see ▶Figure 4.19)

- Stock pot, 12 quarts or larger
- Heating source, such as an electrical hot plate
- fresh ginger root, enough to yield 1 cup of grated ginger
- Drawstring fomentation bag (made of a loose weave cotton such as muslin), approximately 6″ × 8″, or a square of cheesecloth approximately 8″ × 8″ tied with string
- Four thick soft cloths or towels, approximately 18″ × 30″ (two to moisten, one to insulate, one to dry the client's body area after treatment)
- Insulated gloves

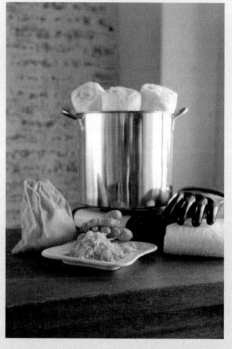

▶ **Figure 4.19**

Indications

- chronic muscle tension
- tight joints (from noninflammatory conditions)
- muscle spasms
- pain from old sprains and strains
- pain from noninflammatory stages of arthritis and bursitis
- insomnia
- congestion in the sinuses and chest from colds, flu, and chronic bronchitis
- congestive headache
- abdominal cramping from premenstrual syndrome and menstruation
- preparation of tissue for massage or other bodywork

Contraindications

- allergy to ginger
- heart conditions
- vascular disorder in area
- numbness or loss of sensation in area
- inflammation in the area
- intolerance to heat
- broken or irritated skin
- high body temperature (fever)

TREATMENT 4.3 CONTINUED

Preparation

1. Fill the stock pot with water to about 3″ below the rim approximately 15 to 30 minutes before the scheduled treatment. Heat water to boiling, and then turn the heat down to medium; the water should not be boiling when the ginger is added to it because boiling destroys the therapeutic properties of ginger. Be ready to turn the heat up or down according to the client's tolerance of the hot compresses.
2. Grate 1 cup of ginger.
3. Place the grated ginger in the fomentation bag or square of cheesecloth. Tie it securely so that the ginger pieces will not leak out.

> **CLINICAL ALERT** !
>
> Ginger can be irritating if the pieces come in direct contact with the skin.

4. Making sure that the water is not boiling, place the bag of ginger in the pot of hot water (▶Figure 4.20).

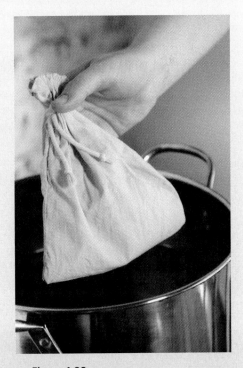

▶ **Figure 4.20**

5. Wearing the insulated gloves, squeeze the bag of ginger to expel juices, and allow it to steep for 10 to 15 minutes.

TREATMENT 4.3 CONTINUED

6. Fold three towels in thirds (or to fit the size of the area being treated) widthwise and then roll two of them up (▶Figures 4.21 a, b, and c).

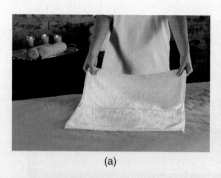
(a)

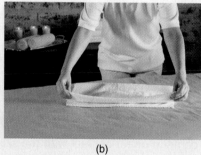
(b)

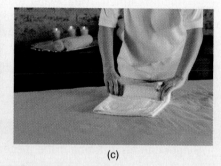
(c)

▶ **Figure 4.21**

Place the two folded, rolled towels in the hot water (▶Figure 4.22). The other folded towel will be used to insulate the compress while it is on the client's body.

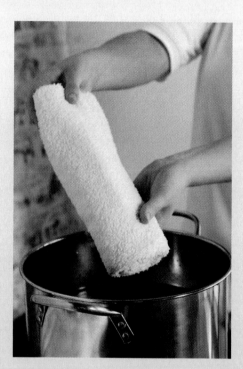

▶ **Figure 4.22**

TREATMENT 4.3 CONTINUED

Procedure

1. Uncover the area of the client to be treated.

2. Wearing the insulated gloves, remove a towel from the pot and wring it out thoroughly (▶Figure 4.23). If the towel is too wet, it will cool too quickly. Unroll the towel, but keep it folded in thirds.

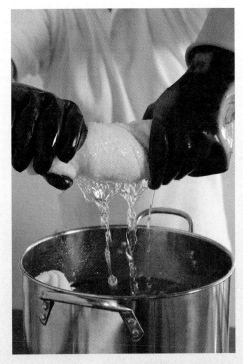

▶ **Figure 4.23**

3. Fan the towel to cool it a bit (▶Figure 4.24), and then test the heat by touching the hot compress to the inside of your forearm. If the heat is tolerable, place the hot compress lightly on the client's focus area (▶Figure 4.25).

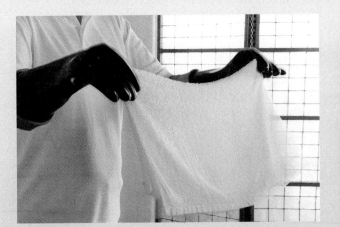

▶ **Figure 4.24**

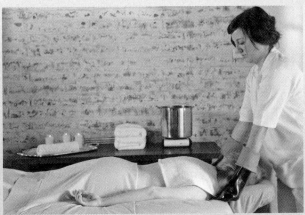

▶ **Figure 4.25**

TREATMENT 4.3 CONTINUED

CLINICAL ALERT !

Check immediately with client about temperature. If the towel is too hot, remove it immediately and wave it again to cool it more. Place the compress on the client again and recheck about temperature. If it still too hot, remove it again and cool it more until the temperature is comfortable for the client. The first application should be comfortably warm to the client with the temperature gradually increasing with each application, depending on the client's vitality and tolerance to heat.

4. Cover with a towel to insulate (▶Figure 4.26).

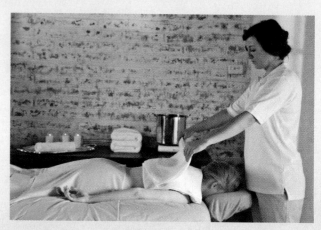

▶ **Figure 4.26**

CLINICAL ALERT !

Do not press down on the insulating towel. This could burn the client.

5. The compress should be replaced as the heat decreases, which should be in 1 to 3 minutes. Before the compress cools completely, prepare the next one for application. Wring out the new hot towel thoroughly, and fan it to cool it a bit. To change compresses, place the new compress on top of the insulating towel (and the old compress), then flip the stack over (▶Figures 4.27 a, b, and c). The insulating towel will now be on top of the new hot compress. This will help retain heat.

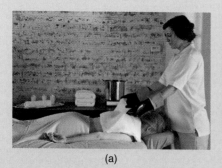

(a)

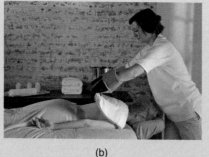

(b)

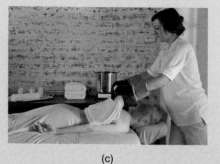

(c)

▶ **Figure 4.27**

TREATMENT 4.3 CONTINUED

6. Before removing the towel on top and placing it in the pot to reheat, check to see if the temperature is comfortable for the client. The compress should be a little warmer than the previous hot towel. If it still too hot, remove it immediately and allow it to cool a bit, and then replace it when the temperature is tolerable to the client.

7. Keep exchanging the compresses as necessary. In the time between towel exchanges, a short scalp and facial massage can be given. The client's feet can be unwrapped for a short foot massage, or other areas of the client's body can be massaged. It is important to stay near the client; the heat may become suddenly unbearable for some clients and the compresses will need to be removed immediately.

8. Dry the area with a towel after the last application.

After the Treatment

The client's skin will be reddened, and the tissue should be warm and soft. Massage the area if warranted and appropriate, such as if the ginger fomentation was applied to tight back muscles, and encourage the client to rest and to drink plenty of water afterwards.

Hygiene

The grated ginger should be used only once and discarded in the waste can after the treatment. The ginger liquid in the stockpot should be drained out and the stockpot washed in warm, soapy water and rinsed after each use. Launder the sheets and towels with hot water and detergent after each use. Wipe the insulating gloves with alcohol or another disinfectant after each use.

Before the treatment, the client should be warmed in some way. This can be done by:

- having the client exercise
- giving the client a modified hot foot bath by placing the client's feet in a basin of comfortably hot water for 5 to 10 minutes
- having the client take a hot shower
- having the client drink a cup of hot tea, or other warming, nonalcoholic beverage

Since everyone is different, clients may go through all four stages in anywhere from 45 minutes to 2 hours; an average time for the entire cold sheet wrap treatment is about 90 minutes.

The supplies can be purchased at your local stores or online.

ALTERNATING OR CONTRAST APPLICATIONS

Alternating or contrast applications use both heat and cold. The treatment begins with the hot application and ends with the cold application, which makes these treatments revulsive. The effects can be dramatic depending on how great the temperature difference is. The major ef-

fect of a contrast application, whether it is local or systemic, is the movement of blood and lymph. Blood and lymph are driven away from the cold (through vasoconstriction) and driven toward the warmth (through vasodilation), resulting in a pumping action. Nutrients and blood cells are brought to an area of tissue; wastes and cell debris are taken away. All the other effects of local and systemic heat applications, and local and systemic cold applications, occur with contrast applications as well.

Indications for alternating applications include:

- chronic muscle tension
- tight joints from noninflammatory conditions
- congestion in the sinuses or the chest
- insomnia
- abdominal cramping from premenstrual syndrome and menstruation
- headache

Contraindications and Considerations for Alternating or Contrast Application Treatments

Because of how powerfully heat and cold can affect the body, certain conditions are contraindicated for the application of alternating treatments, and considerations about certain types of clients need to be kept in mind.

TREATMENT 4.4

Hot Foot Bath

Hot foot baths are typically performed for 20 to 30 minutes. The temperature of the foot bath water starts at 98 to 100°F and can increase up to 115°F. However, it is important that the temperature always be within the client's tolerance. For weak or frail clients, be sure to adjust the water temperature to their tolerance and decrease the duration of the treatment.

The equipment and supplies can be purchased at local stores or online.

Rationale
A hot foot bath can be performed for any or all of the following physiological effects:

- Counterirritant: relieves a deeper inflammation
- Derivative: draws blood and lymph from one part of the body to another
- Sedative: induces a state of deep relaxation

Equipment and Supplies (see ▶Figure 4.28)

- chair
- foot tub or basin, at least 10″ to 12″ inches deep
- stock pot, 12 quarts or larger
- heating source, such as an electrical hot plate
- one flat sheet
- one wool blanket
- three to four towels, approximately 18″ × 30″
- washcloth
- pitcher
- ice water
- pool thermometer
- dry mustard powder (optional)

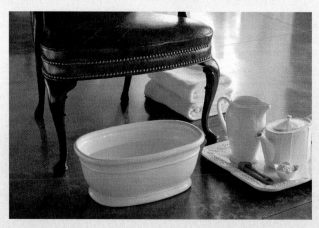

▶ **Figure 4.28**

Indications

- congestion in the sinuses and chest, sinus from colds, flu, and chronic bronchitis
- headache
- onset or ending of a cold or flu
- relief of nosebleeds
- need to detoxify
- need for relaxation and stress relief
- insomnia
- warming the body for a cold treatment or a body wrap
- abdominal cramping from premenstrual syndrome and menstruation

TREATMENT 4.4 CONTINUED

Contraindications

- heart conditions
- untreated hypertension
- numbness or loss of sensation
- neuropathy
- vascular disorders
- any disorders that can accompanying vascular issues or neuropathy, such as diabetes
- high body temperature (fever)
- intolerance to heat
- broken or irritated skin on the feet

Preparation

1. Fill the stock pot to within 3″ of the rim and heat it to just under boiling approximately 15 to 30 minutes before the scheduled treatment.
2. Place ice water in the pitcher and position it within easy reach.
3. Place the washcloth in the ice water
4. Cover the chair with a towel.

Procedure

1. Have the client undress and wrap in the sheet, with the opening at the back, and then sit on the chair. The client's bare feet are on the floor (▶Figure 4.29). Tent the sheet around the client and the chair (▶Figure 4.30).

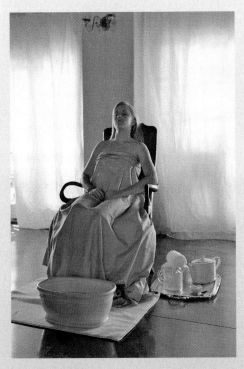

▶ **Figure 4.29**

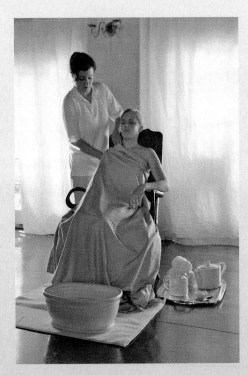

▶ **Figure 4.30**

TREATMENT 4.4 CONTINUED

2. Place a towel around the client's neck to prevent itching (▶Figure 4.31).

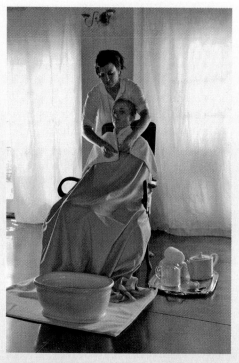

▶ **Figure 4.31**

Wrap the client snugly in the wool blanket. Loosen the blanket around the client's neck to prevent itching if necessary (▶Figures 4.32 a and b).

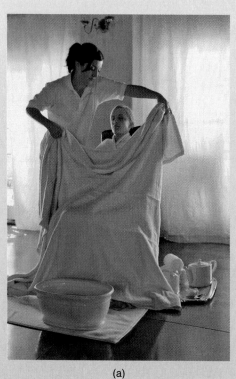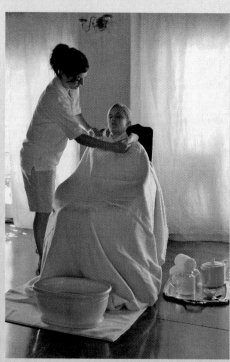

(a)   (b)

▶ **Figure 4.32**

3. Fill the foot tub or basin with about 3″ of water that is comfortably warm to the client, 98 to 100°F. (Use a combination of the hot and ice water, checking with the pool thermometer for the desired temperature (▶Figure 4.33). A teaspoon or two of dry mustard can be added to enhance the heating effect (▶Figure 4.34).

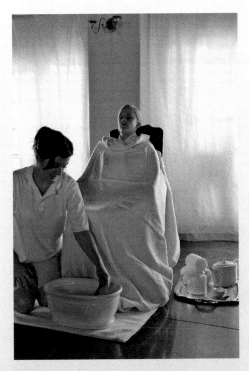

▶ **Figure 4.33**

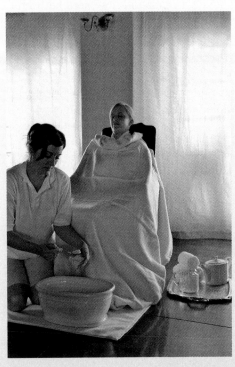

▶ **Figure 4.34**

4. Place the client's feet in the foot tub (▶Figure 4.35). Tent the sheet and blanket over the foot bath.

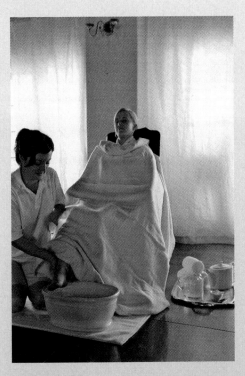

▶ **Figure 4.35**

TREATMENT 4.4 CONTINUED

> **CLINICAL ALERT** !
>
> Check with the client about the temperature—it should be comfortably warm. If the temperature needs adjusting, remove the client's feet *before* adding more hot water or ice water to the basin so the client is not shocked by the rapid change in temperature. Mix the water before returning the client's feet to the tub.

5. Stand behind the chair and massage the client's shoulders, neck, scalp, and face while the feet are soaking (▶Figure 4.36).

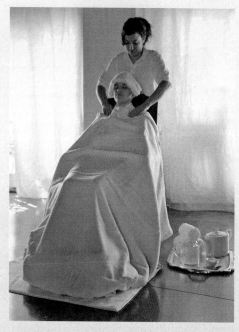

▶ **Figure 4.36**

6. Apply a cool washcloth to the client's forehead as the client begins to heat up (▶Figure 4.37). This will feel cool and refreshing and will stimulate the retrostasis action, pushing congestion toward the client's feet.

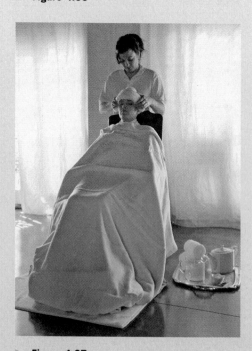

▶ **Figure 4.37**

TREATMENT 4.4 CONTINUED

7. Continue to add hot water to the foot tub, gradually increasing the temperature to 105 to 115°F, or to a temperature that is comfortable for the client (▶Figure 4.38), bringing the water level to at least 2″ above the client's ankles. This ensures that the larger blood vessels in the legs will be affected, increasing the effects of the treatment.

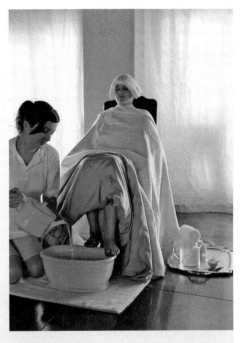

▶ **Figure 4.38**

8. Continue the treatment for approximately 20 to 30 minutes total (massaging the client's neck and shoulders, changing the cool washcloth, and adding hot water periodically to the foot basin).

9. At the end of the treatment, lift one of the client's feet out of the tub and splash with ice water; be sure to cover the entire foot (▶Figure 4.39). Thoroughly dry the foot with a towel (▶Figure 4.40). Repeat the cold splash on the client's other foot. The feet should be reddened from hyperemia.

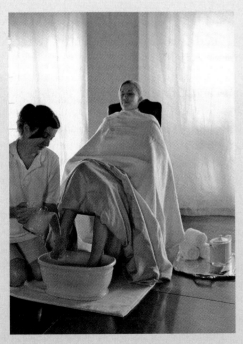

▶ **Figure 4.39**

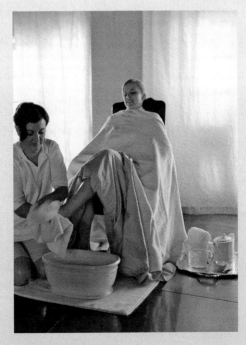

▶ **Figure 4.40**

TREATMENT 4.4 CONTINUED

After the Treatment
Encourage the client to rest and to drink plenty of water.

Hygiene
Launder the sheets, towels, and washcloth with hot water and detergent after each use. The foot tub or basin and pitcher should be used only once; they should be washed in warm, soapy water and rinsed between each use. Wipe the thermometer down with alcohol or another disinfectant after each use. The wool blanket should not have come in contact with the client's skin, so dry cleaning it every two weeks (or after six uses) should be sufficient. If the wool blanket did come in contact with the client's skin, it needs to be cleaned before being used on another client. An easier solution is to buy washable wool blankets and launder them in hot water and detergent after each use.

These contraindications and considerations apply for both local and systemic alternating application treatments.

Contraindications to alternating applications include:

▶ heart conditions
▶ untreated hypertension or hypotension
▶ respiratory conditions
▶ numbness or loss of sensation in area
▶ neuropathy
▶ vascular disorders
▶ acute inflammation
▶ burns
▶ flare-up stages of autoimmune disorders such as lupus, rheumatoid arthritis, and multiple sclerosis (there is generally a great deal of pain and accompanying widespread inflammation with flare-up stages of autoimmune disorders; a heat and cold application would only be more painful and debilitating)
▶ any disorders that can accompanying vascular issues or neuropathy, such as diabetes
▶ cancer
▶ high body temperature (fever)
▶ broken or irritated skin
▶ any condition in which the person is not able to communicate or give accurate feedback about temperature such as treatments on infants, those under the influence of drugs or alcohol, or those who are unconscious

Considerations are needed for clients who are fragile physically or emotionally, such as from aging or chronic disease. They may be able to receive hydrotherapy treatments, but the treatments must be modified for their particular conditions. Generally, more moderate temperatures and decrease in duration of alternating treatments are warranted. The same is true for people with intolerance to heat and cold.

Revisit Table 4.5 to see the indication, contraindications, and considerations for contrast applications.

Treatments

Local alternating or contrast treatments can take the form of showers applied to certain parts of the body, compresses, and partial baths (baths in which only part of the body is bathed such as the feet or hands). Systemic alternating or contrast treatments can take the form of heating such as in a sauna, steam room, or sweat lodge, then a cold plunge into cold water or the snow, or contrast full immersion baths. Alternating compresses are discussed next, and alternating full immersion and partial baths are covered later in this chapter.

SHOWERS

A shower is defined as controlled streams of water. Single or multiple shower heads are generally used and are applied either to the entire body or localized areas. Different pressures and temperatures (hot, cold, tepid, or alternating) for different durations can be used, depending on the desired outcome. ▶Table 4.6 shows the temperature range, duration, and therapeutic benefits of hot, warm, tepid, and cold showers. Resting comfortably for at least 20 minutes after the shower and drinking plenty of water will continue the therapeutic benefits.

Showers can be a useful supplement to hydrotherapy treatments and can be used to:

▶ warm clients before a cold treatment, such as a cold sheet wrap
▶ give clients a chance to rest and relax before or after a treatment
▶ cleanse clients before they receive other spa, massage, and bodywork treatments
▶ energize and rejuvenate before or after receiving a treatment

TABLE 4.6

Therapeutic Benefits of Showers

Type of Shower	Temperature Range	Duration	Therapeutic Benefits
Hot (should not be taken by those who have areas intolerant to heat)	100–105°F	1–6 minutes	Relief from muscle tension, pain, and spasms
			Relief from noninflammatory joint pain
			Relief from congestion in the sinuses and chest from colds, flu, and bronchitis
			Relaxation and stress relief
			Headache relief
			Help with insomnia
Warm	92–100°F	5–10 minutes	Relief from muscle tension, pain, and spasms
			Relief from noninflammatory joint pain
			Relaxation and stress relief
			Help with insomnia
			Soothing to the skin
Tepid	86–92°F	4–6 minutes	Relaxation and stress relief
			Help with insomnia
			Soothing to the skin
Cold (should not be taken by those who are physically frail, have heart conditions, have untreated high blood pressure, or are intolerant to cold)	50–60°F	30 seconds–2 minutes	Increase muscle tone
			Invigorate the body
			Warm the body (the body responds to the cold stimulus by heating up)

Therapeutic benefits of showers vary by temperature. Notice that hot and cold showers have some strong contraindications.

Showers can offer other benefits as well. By manipulating the temperature and duration of the shower, heating or cooling of the body can be enhanced through derivation. A hot shower on a hot day will actually cool the body. The heat of the water draws blood to the superficial blood vessels of the skin, so heat radiates away and the body cools. On a cold day, a cold shower will do the opposite. Blood is driven to the body's core, thereby conserving the warmth and preventing its escape from the body. An alternating shower starting with increasing heat and decreasing cold will produce vascular gymnastics; blood vessels vasodilate and vasoconstrict. This action invigorates and tonifies the body and stimulates the immune system.

Spa Showers

Resort and hotel spas, destination spas, medical and medispas, and certain day spas may have specialized showers

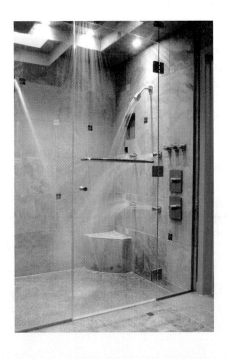

TREATMENT 4.5

Heating (Cold Sheet) Wrap

Rationale
A heating wrap can be performed for any and all of the following physiological effects:

- Tonifier: increases vitality and strengthens the immune system
- Sedative: induces a state of deep relaxation and stress relief
- Stimulant: invigorates
- Detoxifier: eliminates toxins
- Derivative: draws blood and lymph from one part of the body to another

Equipment and Supplies (see ▶Figure 4.41)

- one or more wool blankets (washable wool is the easiest to clean)
- four sheets (one fitted and three flat; 100% cotton such as muslin works the best for this treatment)
- two bath towels, approximately 30″ × 60″
- one washcloth
- Large basin (enough to hold about 2 gallons of water)
- Ice; may be necessary to keep water cold
- Insulating sheet (rubber, plastic, Mylar, etc.)

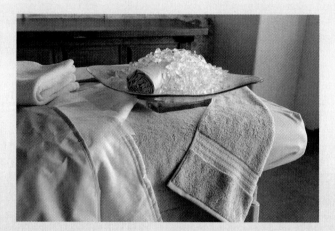

▶ **Figure 4.41**

Indications
The indications for performing a heating wrap are

- need for stress relief
- fever
- insomnia
- muscle tension
- congestion in the sinuses and chest from colds, flu, and chronic bronchitis
- congestive headache
- anxiety and restlessness
- depression
- detoxification
- need to stimulate the immune system to ward off a cold or flu

Contraindications

- heart conditions
- skin conditions made worse by heat
- claustrophobia
- intolerance to cold

TREATMENT 4.5 CONTINUED

Preparation

1. Fill the basin with water and ice. Position the ice within easy reach to refresh the cool water in the basin as it warms.
2. Fold the sheet in half widthwise, then in thirds lengthwise, and then roll it up (see ▶Figure 4.42). Place the sheet in the ice water; make sure it becomes thoroughly soaked and chilled. The washcloth can also be placed in the ice water.

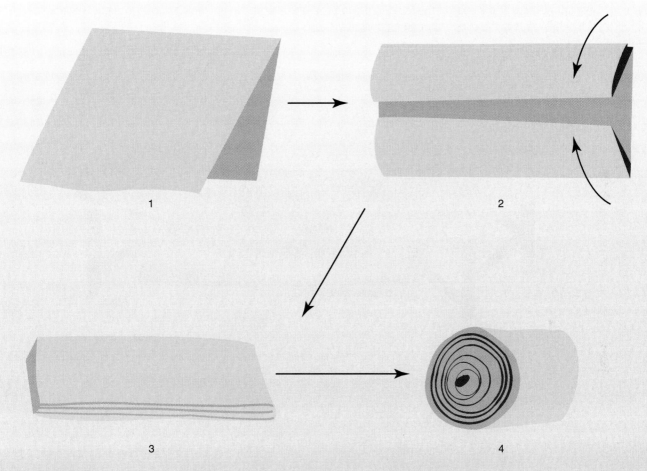

1

2

3

4

▶ **Figure 4.42**

3. Layer the table in the following order (see ▸Figures 4.43 a and b):
   - fitted sheet to protect table
   - large towel placed horizontally across the head of the table, leaving enough room for the head
   - wool blanket placed horizontally across the table, on top of the towel
   - flat sheet placed horizontally on top of the wool blanket
   - insulating sheet on top of the cloth sheet
   - one flat sheet on top of the insulating sheet (extend the cloth sheet at least 1″ beyond the wool blanket and insulating sheet at the head of the table so it can be folded over the wool blanket once the client is wrapped; this helps protect the client from being in contact with the wool, which may be itchy).

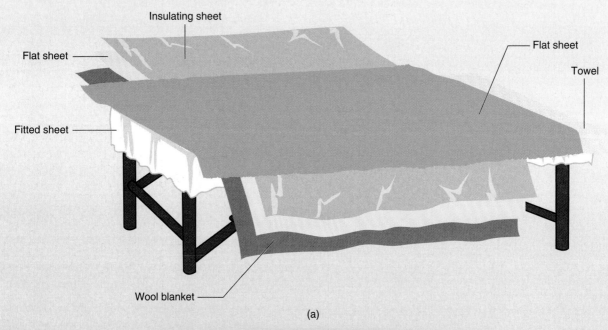

(a)

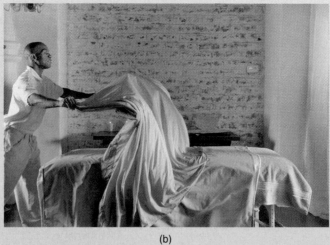

(b)

▸ **Figure 4.43**

TREATMENT 4.5 CONTINUED

4. Have the client warm up, for example, through a hot foot bath (▶Figure 4.44).

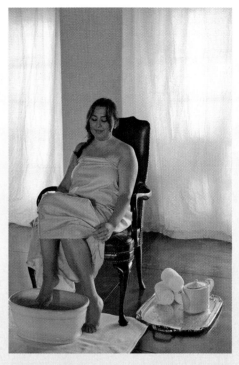

▶ **Figure 4.44**

5. Make sure the client is draped with a sheet or towel that opens at the back (▶Figure 4.45).

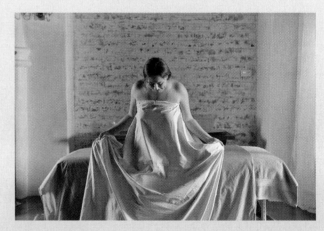

▶ **Figure 4.45**

Procedure

1. Take the sheet out of the basin of cold water and thoroughly wring it out (▶Figure 4.46). If the sheet is not wrung out tightly, it will be harder for the client's body to warm up in the heating stage.

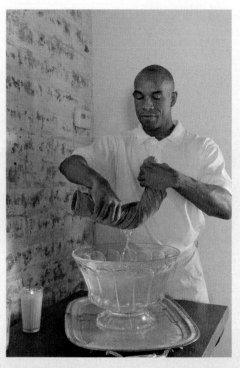

▶ **Figure 4.46**

2. Quickly spread the cold sheet on the table horizontally and help the client lie supine on top of it, spreading the sheet or towel drape out on both sides so the client is lying directly on the cold wet sheet (▶Figure 4.47).

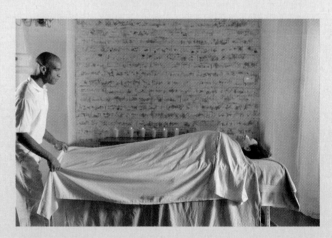

▶ **Figure 4.47**

TREATMENT 4.5 CONTINUED

3. Starting at the client's feet, quickly wrap the wet sheet around the body, pulling the towel or draping sheet out as the client is wrapped. The wet sheet should come in contact with the client's skin in all areas, leaving no air pockets (▶Figures 4.48 a and b). The client's arms can be at the sides or crossed over the chest. For best results, the client's arms should be inside the wrap. However, if the client is more comfortable, the arms can be left outside the wrap.

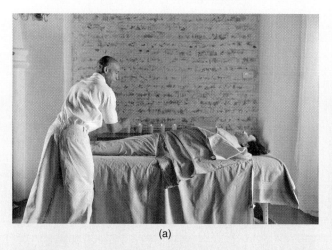
(a)

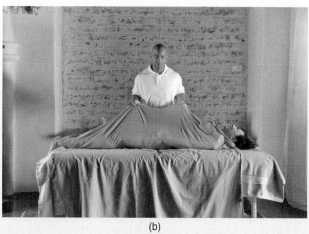
(b)

▶ **Figure 4.48**

4. Next, starting at the client's feet, wrap (individually) the dry sheet, the insulating sheet, and the wool blanket around the client (▶Figures 4.49 a, b, c, and d).

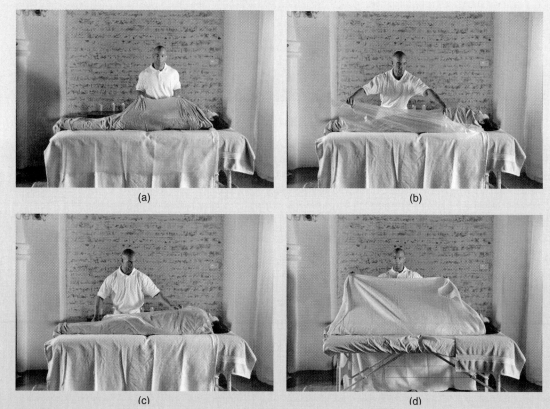
(a)

(b)

(c)

(d)

▶ **Figure 4.49**

TREATMENT 4.5 CONTINUED

5. Secure the towel at the head of the table around the client's neck and shoulders (▶Figures 4.50 a and b).

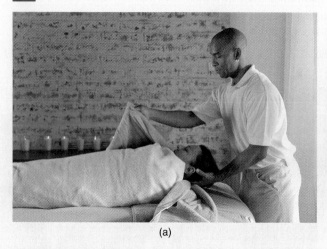

(a)

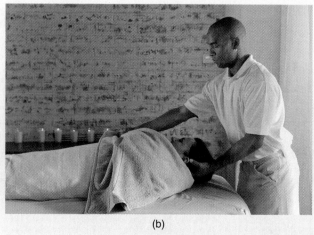

(b)

▶ **Figure 4.50**

Each layer of the wrap, as well as the towel, should be tucked snugly under the client's body, creating a mummy-like effect (▶Figure 4.51).

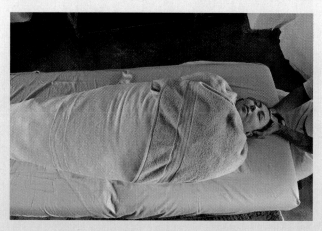

▶ **Figure 4.51**

6. Make sure the client is comfortable, using bolsters, pillows, or other props as needed. If the client experiences any discomfort from the tight wrapping, loosen the upper chest layers and ask the client to take some deep breaths. The wrap at the feet can also be loosened. It is important for the practitioner to be present and attentive. The client may need anything from having an itch on the nose scratched to additional blankets to feel an increase in the heating process. It can make one feel very vulnerable to be wrapped and immobile; the practitioner's presence can be reassuring.

TREATMENT 4.5 CONTINUED

7. The client should remain wrapped for 45 to 90 minutes. During this time, a scalp and facial massage can be given or the client's feet can be unwrapped for a foot massage. Another option is to sit quietly at the head or foot of the table (▶Figure 4.52). It is helpful to synchronize breathing with the client's breathing. Sometimes it is possible to see signs that the client is moving from stage to stage: cooling to neutral to heating to sweating.

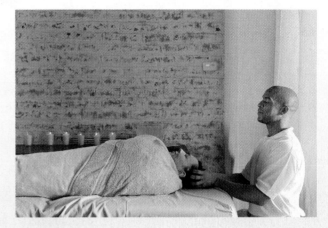

▶ **Figure 4.52**

CLINICAL ALERT !

It is important to stay near the client; some clients may become claustrophobic and need to have the wrappings removed as soon as they start feeling uncomfortable.

---

8. When the client begins to sweat, wring out the washcloth and place it on the client's forehead.

9. When the client is ready to be unwrapped, there will usually be signs such as opening the eyes, twitching, and stirring. Clients tend to want to be unwrapped right away so make sure you are ready to do so immediately.

10. Unwrap quickly, draping the client with the sheet or towel drape as layers are removed. The air will feel chilly to the client so it is important to redrape as quickly as possible.

After the Treatment
Have the client rest quietly approximately 20 minutes, and encourage drinking of plenty of water afterward.

Hygiene
Launder the sheets, towels, and washcloth with hot water and detergent after each use. Clean the insulating sheet by spraying it with alcohol or another disinfectant. It can also be washed with soap and water, but it should still be sprayed with alcohol after that. The wool blanket should not have come in contact with the client's skin so dry cleaning it every two weeks (or after six uses) should be sufficient. If the wool blanket did come in contact with the client's skin, it needs to be cleaned before being used on another client. An easier solution is to buy washable wool blankets and launder them in hot water and detergent after each use.

---

available for clients to receive specific hydrotherapy treatments. Specially trained practitioners in these spas use the thermal and mechanical effects of water to stimulate or relax the body. These showers include jet or percussion sprays, also called Scotch douche, Blitzguss, and Vichy showers.

These showers involve a certain amount of nudity for the client. Even though practitioners may be comfortable with this, first-time clients are usually not prepared for the level of undress necessary for these treatments. Since most client dissatisfaction comes from communication issues,

it is important that practitioners who perform these showers explain clearly to the client how the procedure is performed and what the client can expect.

Each spa has its own protocol on how to perform the treatments involved with these showers and trains its practitioners accordingly. Additionally, each spa has its own protocols for cleaning and disinfecting the showers and trains its personnel in these methods. Generally, each shower is cleaned with a disinfectant after every individual client use. To prevent the spread of fungal infections,

TREATMENT 4.6

Alternating or Contrast Compress

An alternating or contrast compress application involves alternating hot and cold compresses. These are sometimes called circulatory whips because of their effect on circulation. The hot compresses cause vasodilation of blood vessels, and cold compresses cause vasoconstriction of blood vessels, so there is a pumping action of blood into and out of the area, sometimes referred to as "vascular gymnastics" or "vasogymnastics." The purpose is to bring blood and nutrition to the area with heat, and then to decrease blood flow, which give tissues time for toxins to diffuse into blood. Additional applications of heat then help move toxins out of the area. The end result is that congestion is flushed out and local healing is promoted.

A heated compress starts the treatment and is followed by the brief application of a cold compress. The first hot compress starts at a temperature that is comfortably warm for the client and gets successively hotter, within the client's tolerance. The cold compress starts at a temperature that is comfortably warm for the client and gets successively colder, within the client's tolerance. Contrast compresses are typically performed for 20 to 30 minutes. For clients who are weak, frail, or sensitive to hot and cold, use milder temperatures and decrease the duration of the treatment.

The supplies for alternating compresses can be purchased in local stores or online. These treatments can also be performed by clients at home with proper instruction from practitioners.

Rationale

Alternating compresses can be performed for any and all of the following physiological effects:

- Analgesic: relieves pain
- Antispasmodic: relieves muscle spasms
- Vasoconstrictor: decreases local blood flow
- Vasodilator and vasoconstrictor: increases and decreases local blood flow; performs a pumping action of blood in and out of the tissues

Equipment and Supplies

- stock pot, 12 quarts or larger
- heating source, such as an electrical hot plate
- basin of cold or ice water
- ice (as needed to keep water at the level of coolness)
- four thick soft cloths or towels, approximately 18″ × 30″; the thicker the compress, the longer it stays cold
- insulated gloves

Indications

- chronic muscle tension
- tight joints (from noninflammatory conditions)
- muscle spasms
- pain from old sprains and strains
- abdominal cramping from premenstrual syndrome and menstruation
- congestion in the sinuses and chest from colds, flu, and chronic bronchitis
- headache
- preparation of tissue for massage or other bodywork

Contraindications

- heart conditions
- numbness or loss of sensation in area
- vascular disorders in area
- inflammation in the area
- broken or irritated skin
- high body temperature (fever)
- intolerance to cold
- intolerance to heat

TREATMENT 4.6 CONTINUED

Preparation

1. Fill the stock pot with water to about 3″ below the rim approximately 15 to 30 minutes before the scheduled treatment. Heat water to just under boiling, and then turn the heat down to medium. Be ready to turn the heat up or down according to the client's tolerance of the hot compresses.
2. Cool water and place it in the basin. Position ice within easy reach for adding during the treatment.
3. Fold four towels in thirds (or to fit the size of the area being treated) widthwise, and then roll up three of them. Wearing the insulated gloves, place two folded, rolled towels in the hot water. Place one folded rolled towel in the ice water. The other folded towel will be used to insulate the compress while it is on the client's body.

Procedure

CLINICAL ALERT !

Always start with a hot compress, and end with a cold compress.

1. Uncover the area to be treated.

2. Wearing the insulated gloves, take one towel out of the hot water and wring out the towel quickly and completely; if the towel is too wet it will cool too quickly. Unroll the towel, but keep it folded in thirds.

3. Wave the towel to cool it a bit; then test the heat by touching the hot compress to the inside of your forearm. If the heat is tolerable, place the hot compress lightly on the client's focus area.

CLINICAL ALERT !

Check immediately with the client about temperature. If the towel is too hot, remove it immediately and wave it again to cool it more. Place the compress on the client again and recheck about temperature. If it still too hot, remove it again and cool it until the temperature is comfortable for the client. The first application should be comfortably warm to the client with the temperature gradually increasing with each application, depending on the client's vitality and tolerance to heat.

4. Cover with a towel to insulate.

CLINICAL ALERT !

Do not press down. This could burn the client.

5. Leave the hot compress on for about 1 to 3 minutes or until heat decreases. Wring out the cold towel and place it on top of both the hot and insulating towels. Have the client take a deep breath, and then flip the stack of towels so the cold compress is now on the client's body, and have the client exhale (having the client take a deep breath keeps the client focused on the breath rather than the cold application and also helps the client relax). Remove the hot towel; the insulating towel will now be on top of the cold compress.

6. Place the hot towel in the basin of hot water to reheat.

7. Leave the cold compress on for only about 30 to 60 seconds. During this time, while wearing the insulated gloves, wring out the second hot towel (the first hot towel will not be reheated enough yet to reapply).

TREATMENT 4.6 CONTINUED

8. Put the new hot towel on top of both cold and insulating towels, and flip the stack of towels so that the hot compress is in place.

CLINICAL ALERT ❗

Check to see if the temperature is comfortable for the client. The compress should be a little warmer than the previous hot compress. If it is still too hot, remove it immediately and wave it to cool it more, and then replace it when the temperature is tolerable to the client.

---

9. Remove the cold compress, leaving the insulating towel on top of the hot towel. Place the cold towel back in the basin of cold water.

10. Continue exchanging the compresses. For optimum benefit, the treatment should include approximately three to five hot/cold exchanges lasting for 20 to 30 minutes, but this is always determined by the client's vitality and needs.

11. Dry the area with a towel after the last application.

After the treatment
Massage the area if warranted and appropriate, such as tight back muscles treated with the hot compress. Encourage the client to rest and to drink plenty of water afterward.

Hygiene
Launder the sheets and towels with hot water and detergent after each use. Wipe the insulating gloves with alcohol or other disinfectant after each use. Wash the stock pot and basin in warm, soapy water and rinse after each use.

---

clients are given shower footwear to use, which they can either keep or discard when the spa visit is over.

Jet or Percussion Shower (Scotch Douche)
A jet or percussion shower takes place in a large shower or wet room with a wall bar for the client to hold. A special high-pressure showerhead, which is the Scotch douche (*douche* is French for "shower"), produces a highly pressurized stream of water of varying temperature, beginning at 94°F and increasing from there. Either fresh water or seawater can be used. The routine starts at the feet and works up the body and lasts about 20 minutes. The focus is on the client's muscles; bony landmarks and sensitive areas of the body are avoided. The treatment is highly tonifying and stimulating and increases systemic blood flow by causing vasodilation of blood vessels. Afterward, the client should rest for about 20 minutes.

A jet or percussion shower is contraindicated for use with clients who have:

▶ become pregnant (first trimester)
▶ heart conditions
▶ untreated hypertension or hypotension
▶ severe asthma
▶ uncontrolled epilepsy

▶ severe varicose veins (the stream of water should avoid area)
▶ broken or irritated skin
▶ tendency to bruise easily

The Blitzguss (Jet Blitz)
Jet Blitz, or Blitzguss, is a therapeutic cold shower treatment using a high-pressure stream of water directed at different parts of the body, focusing on muscular areas. This is stimulating and intense and is done for strengthening the body's vitality and immune response by decreasing superficial circulation, driving blood to the core of the body. The temperature and duration of the treatment vary depending on its goals.

A Jet Blitz is contraindicated for use with clients who have:

▶ heart conditions
▶ untreated hypertension or hypotension
▶ frailty or weakness
▶ become pregnant (all stages of pregnancy)
▶ severe asthma
▶ uncontrolled epilepsy
▶ severe varicose veins (stream of water should avoid area)

▶ broken or irritated skin

▶ tendency to bruise easily

▶ intolerance to cold

Vichy shower

A Vichy shower consists of multiple showerheads spraying water of varying temperatures and pressures, suspended over a wet table (see ▶Figure 4.53). The sprays can be used to relax the body, as in a gentle rain application, or the pressure can be increased to stimulate the body, which also increases blood and lymphatic flow. A Vichy shower can be used to rinse the body after a body scrub or mud or seaweed application. The temperature and duration of the treatment vary depending on its goals.

Practitioners can also recommend showers for clients to perform at home. For example, if the client was just starting to relax and wanted to continue the relaxation at home, a warm or hot shower could be suggested. Or perhaps a cooling shower in the heat of the summer is needed. Other reasons could be detoxification, to alleviate insomnia, or to relieve congestion.

Showers and Baths in Private Practice

A shower or bath can be used as a way to heat the client's body before doing a treatment in which it is important the client be warmed up, such as a cold sheet or herbal wrap. Showers and baths can also be used by the client to cool down if overheated, such as from a ginger fomentation or mud wrap. Even if a client is not receiving a spa or hydrotherapy treatment, access to a shower or bath can be inviting. For example, clients may feel more comfortable showering before receiving a massage if they have done a vigorous workout, or it may be a way of starting to relax after a long and grueling day. It could also be

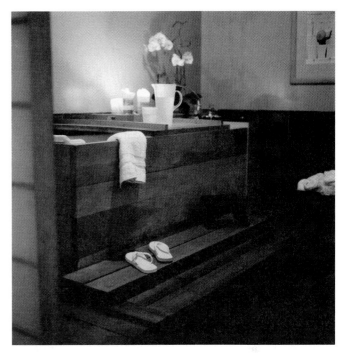

(Angela Wyant/Getty Images Inc.—Stone Allstock)

used by the client to wash off the lubricant used during massage.

It is important that the shower and bath area is clean and inviting. There should be a rubber mat in the shower stall and the bathtub to prevent falls. Provide soap, shower gel, shampoo, and hair conditioner, and have bath towels and washcloths easy to reach. A robe and bath footwear should be provided, especially if the shower or bath is outside the treatment room.

Practitioners who are considering installing a shower or bath should check their local regulations to see if it is allowed. If showers are permitted, practitioners should keep in mind that they will also need to meet requirements of the Americans with Disabilities Act, as well as health and hygiene codes. Those with home practices who want to have clients use their home showers or baths would need to check local regulations to see if this is allowed and which municipal codes need to be met.

As with all showers and baths, no matter what the setting, hygiene is a major factor. Practitioners would need to ensure that their sanitation methods are of the highest caliber to prevent the spread of any possible infection. Footwear would need to be provided and clients would be required to wear them in the shower or bath. After use, clients can take the footwear with them or dispose of them. The shower or bath would need to be thoroughly disinfected using commercial grade disinfectants between each and every client. There are some environmentally safe products available and worth researching.

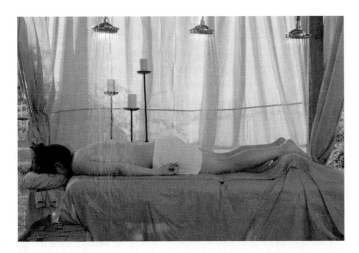

▶ **Figure 4.53** A Vichy shower can be used to relax or stimulate the body or rinse the body after a treatment.

BALNEOLOGY

Balneology is the science of baths and bathing. The warmth and gentle pressure of water surrounding the body both stimulates and soothes. Blood vessels dilate, heart rate slows, and relaxation occurs. Cold baths, on the other hand, stimulate and invigorate, driving blood to the core of the body, resulting in a secondary warming action. There are also contrast baths, which involve hot then cold water and are sometimes referred to as hot and cold plunges. Baths can be taken in fresh water, in seawater, and with restorative substances added.

The many types of restorative substances include skin-soothing agents such as muds, salts, and peat (discussed in Chapter 6), seaweed and sea salt (discussed in Chapter 7), and essential oils and herbs (discussed in Chapter 8). The following are some examples of how substances can be used to enhance a bath:

▶ Essential oils can be added: Five to six drops for a full bath, one to two drops for a partial bath. Pour the essential oil under the running water as the bath is filling and mix well. See ▶Table 4.7 for a list of essential oils and their effects.

▶ An herbal infusion can be made by using one to two cups of dried herbs (double the amount if the herbs are fresh) and placing them in a 10″ × 12″ muslin drawstring back or a 20″ × 20″ square of cheesecloth tied with a string. Bring one quart of water to a boil and then remove from heat. Add the bag of herbs and let it steep in the hot water for 15 to 30 minutes, depending on the strength of the infusion desired. Remove the bag of herbs and add the infused water to the bath, mixing well. See Table 4.7 for a list of herbs and their effects. Herbs can usually be purchased at local stores or online.

▶ Skin softening and soothing agents, such as baking soda and oats, can be added by pouring one to two cups under the running water as the bath is filling and mixing well. See Table 4.7 for a list of skin softening and smoothing agents.

Spa Baths

Resort and hotel spas, destination spas, medical and medispas, and certain day spas may have specialized baths available for clients to receive specific spa and hydrotherapy treatments, such as a mud bath. Each spa has its own protocol on how to perform the treatments involved with these baths and trains its practitioners accordingly. Additionally, each spa has its own protocols for cleaning and disinfecting the baths and trains staff in these methods. Generally, each tub is cleaned with a disinfectant after each individual client use. To prevent the spread of fungal infections, clients are given bath footwear to use, which they either keep or discard when the spa visit is over.

Baths generally involve nudity for the client, that is, in front of the practitioner. Even though practitioners may be comfortable with this, first-time clients are usually not prepared for the level of undress necessary for these treatments. Since most client dissatisfaction comes from communication issues, it is important that practitioners in spas who perform these baths explain clearly to the client how the procedure is performed and what the client can expect.

Baths are generally either full-immersion baths, which involve being submerged up to the neck, or partial, which are performed on body parts that need specific attention. Hot, warm, neutral, and cold temperatures can be used, as well as alternating between temperatures. Each temperature has specific benefits for the body. ▶Table 4.8

> **CLINICAL ALERT** ❗
>
> Practitioners and clients can be allergic to any or all restorative substances. It is important for the practitioner to find out from clients any allergies they may have, and note them on an intake form, so there is written documentation. Practitioners allergic to any or all restorative substances should never use them on clients even when requested to do so, either by clients or employers.
>
> People can develop allergies throughout their lives; therefore, so every time a client arrives for a treatment, the practitioner should do a quick allergy update. Before any treatment is performed, the substance should be applied to a small area on the client's skin and on the practitioner's skin, usually the forearm, to see if there is an allergic reaction.

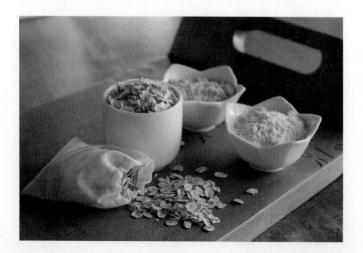

TABLE 4.7

Restorative Substances to Add to Baths

	Herbs	Essential oils
Calming and relaxing	Chamomile	Marjoram
	Lavender	Lavender
	Linden flowers	Geranium
	Hops	Bergamot
	Valerian	
	Lemon Balm	
	Clary sage	
	Jasmine	
	Marjoram	
Energizing and Balancing	Chamomile	Rosemary
	Clary sage	Juniper berry
	Rosemary	Peppermint
	Geranium	Geranium
	Lemongrass	Eucalyptus
	Orange	Bergamot
	Ylang-ylang	
Detoxifying	Hayflower	Eucalyptus
	Oatstraw	Sage
	Ginger	Grapefruit
	Juniper	Juniper berry
	Grapefruit	Cypress
	Eucalyptus	
	Clove	
	Fennel	
	Nettle	
Skin Softening and Smoothing	Bran	
	Oats	
	Cornstarch	
	Baking soda	
	Organic apple cider vinegar	
Other		
Epsom salts		
Mineral salts		
Sea Salt		
Apple Cider Vinegar		

TABLE 4.8

Therapeutic Benefits of Full Immersion Baths

Type of Bath	Temperature Range	Duration	Therapeutic Benefits
Hot (should not be taken by those who have areas of inflammation or intolerance to heat or who are physically frail or pregnant)	98–105°F	2–45 minutes	Short bath (2 minutes) is stimulating Prolonged bath (30–45 minutes) is sedating Relief from muscle tension, pain, and spasms Relief from noninflammatory joint pain Relief from congestion in the sinuses and chest from inflammation or colds, flu, and bronchitis Relaxation and stress relief Headache relief Help with insomnia
Warm	92–100°F	2–45 minutes	Relief from muscle tension, pain, and spasms Relief from noninflammatory joint pain Relaxation and stress relief Help with insomnia Soothing for the skin
Tepid	86–92°F	2–45 minutes	Relaxation and stress relief Help with insomnia Soothing for the skin
Cold* (should not be taken by those who are physically frail, have heart conditions, have untreated high blood pressure, or are intolerant to cold)	50–80°F	10 seconds–3 minutes	Increase muscle tone Invigorate the body Stimulate the immune system Warm the body (the body responds to the cold stimulus by heating up)

* First warm the body with a hot cup of tea, hot full bath, or shower.

Therapeutic benefits of full-immersion baths vary by temperature. Notice that hot and cold baths have some strong contraindications.

shows the temperature range, duration, and therapeutic benefits of hot, warm, tepid, and cold full-immersion baths. Resting comfortably for at least 20 minutes after the bath and drinking plenty of water will continue the therapeutic benefits.

Alternating or Contrast Full-Immersion Baths

Alternating or contrast full-immersion baths can be done at home but may be more effective in a spa, health resort, or fitness center where a heated pool and cold plunge are available. The temperature of the heated water is 100 to 110°F, and the cold water is 40 to 55°F. The duration of time in the heated water is 3 to 5 minutes and in the cold water 30 to 60 seconds. Immersion in the heated water should always be done first. For optimal results, alternating temperature immersions should be done in rapid succession three times.

Because clients who are taking alternating baths will have wet bath footwear, and the floor will most likely be wet as well, practitioners should assist the clients as they go back and forth between the baths to ensure that they do not slip and fall.

The benefits of alternating full-immersion baths are:

▶ relief from muscle tension, pain, and spasms
▶ relief from noninflammatory joint pain
▶ relief from congestion in the sinuses and chest from colds, flu, and bronchitis
▶ relaxation and stress relief
▶ invigoration of the body
▶ stimulation of the immune system

Alternating full-immersion baths should not be taken by those who have:

▶ heart conditions
▶ untreated hypertension or hypotension
▶ numbness or loss of sensation
▶ neuropathy
▶ vascular disorders
▶ burns
▶ flare-up stages of autoimmune disorders such as lupus, rheumatoid arthritis, and multiple sclerosis (there is generally a great deal of pain with flare-up stages; heat and cold would only be more painful and debilitating)
▶ any disorders with accompanying vascular issues or neuropathy, such as diabetes
▶ high body temperature (fever)
▶ broken or irritated skin
▶ frail physical health
▶ become pregnant
▶ intolerance to heat
▶ intolerance to cold

Partial Baths

Partial baths is the term for immersing only a part of the body in water and is generally performed for areas that need specific attention. For example, foot baths submerge the feet up to mid-calf, leg baths submerge the leg up to the knee, and hand baths submerge the hands up to the mid-upper arm. These baths are performed at the same temperatures as the hot, warm, tepid, and cold immersion baths. Either a bathtub or a basin can be used for the water.

Alternating Partial Bath

Partial baths of the feet/legs and hands result in both local and consensual responses. In other words, applications can affect issues that are local as well as elsewhere in the body. A basin of heated water at 100 to 110°F and a basin of cold water at 40 to 55°F are needed. The duration of the body part in the basin of heated water is 3 to 5 minutes and in the basin of cold water is 30 to 60 seconds. The body part should always be placed in the heated water first and the treatment ended with the body part placed in the cold water. For optimal results, alternating temperature placement should be done in rapid succession five times.

Alternating partial baths can be taken for local benefits that include:

▶ warming chilled feet
▶ invigorating tired feet
▶ relieving swollen ankles or feet
▶ pain relief from carpal tunnel syndrome
▶ relieving noninflammatory joint pain

Alternating partial baths can be taken for reflexive benefits that include:

▶ relief from congestive headache
▶ relief from congestion in the sinuses and chest from colds, flu, and bronchitis
▶ relief from pelvic congestion
▶ stoppage of nosebleeds
▶ stimulation of circulation in the opposite extremity
▶ relaxation and stress relief
▶ help with insomnia

Alternating partial baths should not be taken by those who have:

▶ heart conditions
▶ untreated hypertension or hypotension
▶ numbness or loss of sensation in area
▶ neuropathy
▶ vascular disorders in area
▶ burns
▶ flare-up stages of autoimmune disorders such as lupus, rheumatoid arthritis, and multiple sclerosis (there is generally a great deal of pain with flare-up stages; heat and cold would only be more painful and debilitating)
▶ any disorders with accompanying vascular issues or neuropathy, such as diabetes
▶ high body temperature (fever)
▶ broken or irritated skin
▶ frail physical health
▶ become pregnant
▶ intolerance to heat
▶ intolerance to cold

The basins should be washed in warm, soapy water and rinsed after each use.

Sitz Bath

The sitz bath is sometimes referred to as a shallow, hip, or half bath. *Sitz* means "sit" in German. It is a partial bath that addresses the lower back, abdomen, pelvis, and lower extremities. Specially designed tubs are often found in hospitals and physical rehabilitation centers. In these facilities, a sitz bath is used most commonly after childbirth or to encourage postsurgical healing. Although sitz baths are not usually done in a spa, massage, or bodywork setting, a sitz bath can easily be performed by clients at home using single or multiple tubs. The person sits in a bathtub or large basin filled with water up to the navel and, in some types of sitz baths, puts the feet in a second smaller tub of water of contrasting temperature.

Hot Sitz Bath   Hot sitz baths relieve the pain from sciatica, pelvic inflammatory disease, and anal fissures; decrease lower lumbar muscle spasms; soothe anal and vaginal irritation and hemorrhoids; and alleviates uterine cramping. It is important to use a cold compress on the head during a hot sitz to prevent overheating of the body. A hot sitz bath should not be received by those who have:

- ▶ heart conditions
- ▶ untreated hypertension or hypotension
- ▶ intolerance to heat

A bathtub is filled with hot water at a temperature of 100 to 110°F. For weak or frail clients, the bathtub water temperature should be decreased to 92 to 100°F. The water should come to the level of the hips and cover the abdomen. A smaller foot tub is placed in the bath and filled with hotter water at a temperature of 110 to 112°F, which can be decreased to 100 to 110°F for weak or frail clients. The person sits in the bathtub and places the feet in the smaller foot tub. The duration should be 10 to 20 minutes, or shorter for weak or frail clients. A cold compress can be placed on the person's head. A short cold shower or rinse may be done at the end of the treatment. The person should dry thoroughly and rest for at least 20 minutes afterward.

Cold Sitz Baths   Cold sitz baths increase muscle tone in the uterus, bladder, and colon. They can stop bleeding; increase blood circulation to the core; increase overall muscle tone; and help relieve constipation, incontinence, and hemorrhoids.

A bathtub is filled with cold water at a temperature of 50 to 75°F. Water should come to the level of the hips and cover the abdomen. The person soaks in water for 2 to 5 minutes, then dries thoroughly and rests for at least 20 minutes.

Contrast Sitz Baths   Contrast sitz baths use separate tubs of hot and cold water. They improve circulation in the pelvic area, soothe anal and vaginal irritation and hemorrhoids, reduce pelvic pain, and relieve uterine cramping and constipation.

One bathtub is filled with hot water at 100 to 110°F or a temperature that is comfortable. Water should come to the level of the hips and cover the abdomen. The other bathtub is filled with cold water at 50 to 75°F. Water should come to the level of the hips and cover the abdomen. The person soaks in hot water tub for 3 to 4 minutes and then soaks in the cold water for 30 to 60 seconds. This should be repeated two to four times, ending with the cold bath. The person should dry thoroughly and rest for at least 20 minutes.

VAPOR TREATMENTS

A vapor treatment can be as simple as inhaling the steam from a pot of hot water or as elaborate as steam baths and saunas that have been augmented with, for example, eucalyptus for decongestion or lavender for relaxation.

Simple Inhalation Treatment

Simple inhalation treatments are used to clear congestion from colds, flu, or other respiratory conditions because the steam liquifies mucus so that it moves out of the nose and mouth easily. Steam inhalations also warm and moisturize the sinuses and respiratory passageways. One quart of water is brought to a boil and then removed from heat. The hot water can remain in the pot or be poured into a bowl. The person tents the head with a towel and stands or sits over the pot and breathes deeply (see ▶Figure 4.54). This procedure can also be used to moisturize the

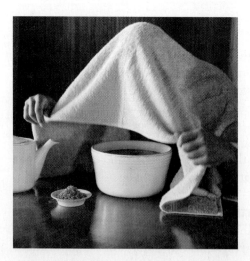

▶ **Figure 4.54** Boiling water is poured into a bowl, from which the client inhales the vapor for a variety of ailments.

skin of the face; when it is used this way, it is called a facial sauna.

Five to eight drops of essential oil can be added to the hot water for added therapeutic effect. Revisit Table 4.7 for a list of some essential oils and their benefits; more information about essential oils is found in Chapter 8.

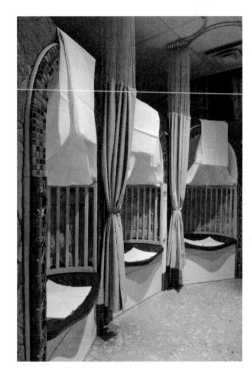

► **Figure 4.55** Treatment in an alpine steam room can stimulate blood flow, soothe the skin, and relieve chest and sinus congestion.

An herbal infusion, described in Chapter 8, can also be used. After the herbs are removed, the remaining water can be used for the simple inhalation treatment. Again revisit Table 4.7 for a list of some herbs and their benefits, and more information about herbs is found in Chapter 8.

Steam Bath

A steam bath is just what it sounds like: being immersed (like a bath) in steam. It is done in a room where the whole body is enveloped in steam, and the steam can be enhanced with, for example hayflower. ►Figure 4.55 shows an alpine steam room. Behind the wooden slats surrounding the seats are coarse fabric bags filled with hayflower blossoms, seeds, and small leaves. The steam brings out the therapeutic effects of the hayflower, which include stimulating blood flow, soothing the skin, and relieving chest and sinus congestion.

A steam bath can also be taken in an enclosed cabinet, with the head exposed (see ►Figure 4.56 a) or in a room where the whole body is enveloped in steam. A steam bath is good for detoxification; warming the body before a wrap or cold plunge; relieving the effects of cold or flu, arthritis, general congestion, or congestive headache; or general relaxation. Steam canopies that fit over the top of a wet table or massage table are also available (see ►Figure 4.56 b). These can be used in place of the blanket and insulating sheet for wraps, or as an enhancement to a massage treatment.

Resort or hotel spas, destination spas, medical and medispas, and certain day spas may have steam baths available for clients. Each spa has its own protocol on how the

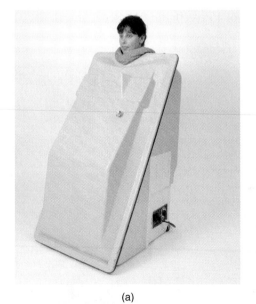

(a)

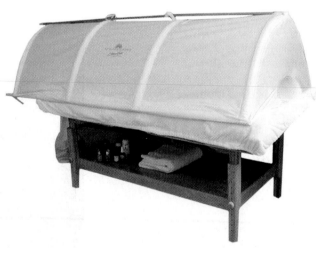

(b)

► **Figure 4.56** A steam bath can be taken in an enclosed cabinet with the head exposed or on a wet table or massage table fitted with a steam canopy. A steam bath is good for detoxification, warming the body, relieving various ailments, or general relaxation. *(Image (a) Andy Crawford © Dorling Kindersley and image (b) courtesy of Universal Companies, Inc.)*

CLINICAL ALERT ❗

Since the heat from the steam bath can be intense, it may be best to acclimate to it in stages. For example, stay in for 3 to 4 minutes at first, then leave to cool down. Go back in for 5 to 6 minutes, if it is tolerable, and then leave to cool down. Continue this process of being in the steam room and leaving to cool down, within tolerance levels, for up to a maximum of 20 minutes total in the steam room. It is very important to not overheat. Be sure to remain hydrated by drinking plenty of water.

---

steam baths are to be used and trains its practitioners accordingly. Additionally, each spa has its own protocols for cleaning and disinfecting the steam baths and trains its staff in these methods. To prevent the spread of fungal infections, clients are given shower footwear to use, which they either keep or discard when the spa visit is over.

The temperature of steam baths is 110 to 114°F, with humidity at or near 100%. The time spent in the steam bath should gradually increase from 3 to 4 minutes up to a maximum of 15 to 20 minutes (see Clinical Alert). At the end of the steam bath, the client should apply a cool cloth to the head and end with a cold rinse or cold plunge.

Generally, steam baths are used for:

- detoxification
- relief from muscle tension, pain, and spasms
- relief from noninflammatory joint pain
- relief from congestion in the sinuses and chest from colds and flu
- relieve from congestive headache
- relaxation and stress relief
- energizing
- preparation for massage or body wrap

Steam baths should not be used by those who have:

- heart conditions
- untreated hypertension or hypotension
- numbness or loss of sensation
- neuropathy
- vascular disorders
- burns
- flare-up stages of autoimmune disorders such as lupus, rheumatoid arthritis, and multiple sclerosis (there is generally a great deal of pain and accompanying widespread inflammation with flare-up stages; the heat would only be more painful and debilitating)
- any disorders with accompanying vascular issues or neuropathy, such as diabetes

- high body temperature (fever)
- broken or irritated skin
- physical frailty
- become pregnant
- intolerance to heat

SAUNA

The sauna is a dry heat treatment done in a small room or cabinet lined with either cedar or redwood (see ▶Figure 4.57). Saunas with electric heaters are popular because of convenience. Traditional saunas were heated with wood-burning stoves. The *savusauna*, or smoke sauna, has a large wood-burning heater with 200- to 300-pound rocks and no stovepipe. The smoke is allowed to remain in the sauna while it is heating up to the desired temperature and then is released through a small vent before the sauna is used (Roy, 2004).

Resort or hotel spas, destination spas, medical and medispas, and certain day spas may have saunas available for clients. Each spa has its own protocol on how the saunas are to be used and trains its practitioners accordingly. Additionally, each spa has its own protocols for cleaning and disinfecting the sauna and trains its staff in these methods. To prevent the spread of fungal infections, clients are given shower footwear to use and either keep or discard when the spa visit is over.

With temperatures nearing 180 to 190°F, sauna treatments are dry-heat treatments that induce sweating and are cleansing, purifying, and detoxifying. The time spent in the sauna should gradually increase from 3 to 4 minutes up to a maximum of 15 to 20 minutes (see Clinical Alert).

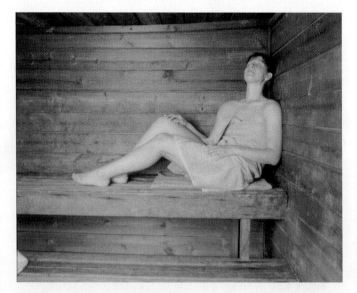

▶ **Figure 4.57** A cedar- or redwood-lined sauna provides dry-heat treatment for cleansing, purifying, and detoxifying. *(Andy Crawford © Dorling Kindersley)*

Since the heat from the sauna can be intense, it may be best to acclimate clients to it in stages. For example, they can stay in for 3 to 4 minutes at first, then leave to cool down. They can then go back in for 5 to 6 minutes, if it is tolerable, and then leave to cool down. Continue this process of being in the sauna and leaving to cool down, within tolerance levels, for up to a maximum of 20 minutes total in the steam room. It is very important to not overheat so make sure clients drink plenty of water.

At the end of the sauna, the client should apply a cool cloth to the head and end with a cold rinse or cold plunge.

Generally saunas are used for:

▶ detoxification
▶ relief from muscle tension, pain, and spasms
▶ relief from noninflammatory joint pain
▶ relaxation
▶ energizing
▶ preparation for massage or body wrap

Saunas should not be used by those who have:

▶ heart conditions
▶ untreated hypertension or hypotension
▶ numbness or loss of sensation
▶ neuropathy
▶ vascular disorders
▶ burns
▶ flare-up stages of autoimmune disorders such as lupus, rheumatoid arthritis, and multiple sclerosis (there is generally a great deal of pain and accompanying widespread inflammation with flare-up stages; the heat would only be more painful and debilitating)
▶ any disorders with accompanying vascular issues or neuropathy, such as diabetes
▶ high body temperature (fever)
▶ broken or irritated skin
▶ physical frailty
▶ become pregnant
▶ intolerance to heat

STEAM BATHS AND SAUNAS IN PRIVATE PRACTICE

Practitioners who are considering installing a steam bath or sauna should check their local regulations to see if it is allowed. If steam baths or saunas are permitted, prac-

titioners should keep in mind that they need to meet the parameters of the Americans with Disabilities Act, as well as health and hygiene codes. If practitioners have steam baths or sauna in a home office and want to have clients use them, they too would need to check local regulations to see if this is allowed, and which municipal codes need to be met.

With all steam baths and saunas, no matter what the setting, hygiene is a major factor. Practitioners would need to ensure that their sanitation methods are of the highest caliber in order to prevent the spread of any possible infection. Shower footwear would need to be provided and clients required to wear them in the steam bath. After use, clients can take the footwear with them or dispose of them. The steam bath would need to be thoroughly disinfected regularly using commercial-grade disinfectants. There are some environmentally safe products available and worth researching.

OTHER HYDROTHERAPY

Hydrotherapy Tub (Hydro Tub)

The hydrotherapy tub is a specially designed tub with jets and an underwater pressure hose that can be used to perform hydrotherapy massage. It is typically found in health spas and rehabilitation clinics (see ▶Figure 4.58). The water temperature is 90 to 100°F. A trained practitioner does a series of massage techniques starting at the client's feet and, working upward, includes stretching and joint mobilization exercises and gentle range-of-motion techniques. The treatment lasts 20 to 40 minutes. Pressure is controlled and can be light as in lymphatic massage or deeper for deep tissue massage and trigger points. The jets can be set for relaxation or stimulation.

Generally, treatments in a hydrotherapy tub are used for:

▶ increasing circulation
▶ relief from muscle tension, pain, and spasms
▶ relief from noninflammatory joint pain
▶ relaxation
▶ energizing
▶ preparation for body wrap

Hydrotherapy tub treatments should not be performed on those who have:

▶ heart conditions
▶ untreated hypertension or hypotension
▶ numbness or loss of sensation
▶ neuropathy
▶ vascular disorders

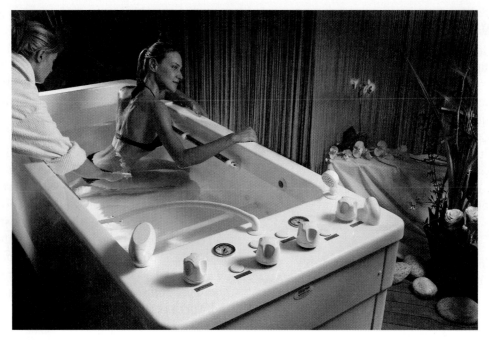

▶ **Figure 4.58** A specially designed hydrotherapy tub can be used to perform hydrotherapy massage. *(Image courtesy Stas Doyer Hydrotherapy)*

- ▶ burns
- ▶ flare-up stages of autoimmune disorders such as lupus, rheumatoid arthritis, and multiple sclerosis (there is generally a great deal of pain and accompanying widespread inflammation with flare-up stages; the heat would only be more painful and debilitating)
- ▶ any disorders with accompanying vascular issues or neuropathy, such as diabetes
- ▶ high body temperature (fever)
- ▶ broken or irritated skin
- ▶ physical frailty
- ▶ become pregnant
- ▶ intolerance to heat

Whirlpool (Jacuzzi®)

A whirlpool (also known by the trade name Jacuzzi®) is a tub with high-pressure jets that circulate heated water. The temperature of the water is between 100 and 108°F, and a session usually lasts 20 to 30 minutes. The motion of the water relaxes the body; relieves pain; eases muscular tightness, arthritis, joint, ligament, and tendon problems; and alleviates insomnia. The mechanical effect of the water's movement against the body can be both relaxing and stimulating at the same time.

Whirlpools should not be used by those who have:

- ▶ heart conditions
- ▶ untreated hypertension or hypotension

- ▶ numbness or loss of sensation
- ▶ neuropathy
- ▶ vascular disorders
- ▶ burns
- ▶ flare-up stages of autoimmune disorders such as lupus, rheumatoid arthritis, and multiple sclerosis (there is generally a great deal of pain and accompanying widespread inflammation with flare-up stages; the heat would only be more painful and debilitating)
- ▶ any disorders with accompanying vascular issues or neuropathy, such as diabetes
- ▶ high body temperature (fever)
- ▶ broken or irritated skin
- ▶ physical frailty
- ▶ become pregnant
- ▶ intolerance to heat

Flotation Tank or Sensory Deprivation Tank/Room

A flotation tank or sensory deprivation tank (see ▶Figure 4.59 a) or room (see ▶Figure 4.59 b) is a tank or small tiled room that is filled with body-temperature water (94 to 98°F) to a depth of approximately 10 inches. Enough Epsom salt is dissolved in the water to allow the body to float. The tank or room can be closed to all exposure to sound and light so the client can experience true sensory deprivation for a session that lasts 20 to 60 minutes. Visits to a flotation tank or sensory deprivation tank/room

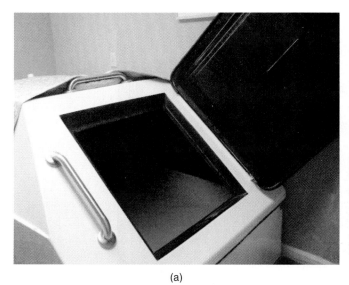

(a)

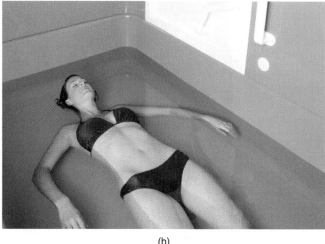

(b)

▶ **Figure 4.59** A flotation or sensory deprivation tank or room is closed to all sound and light so the client can experience true sensory deprivation. *Photos courtesy of (a) Harmony Learning Center, Decatur, GA Now Harmony Learning org. and (b) Ocean Float Rooms Ltd. Photos by Adrian Nettleship.*

aim to release muscle tension, stress, and anxiety but are not recommended for those with claustrophobia.

Hubbard Tank

A Hubbard tank is a specially constructed full-immersion tank. It is equipped with a hoist for lifting and supporting patients who are injured or immobile. It has support bars for doing water exercise and jets for hydrotherapy massage (see ▶Figure 4.60). Therapists assist patients with stretching and joint mobilization exercises and gentle range of motion. Treatments generally last 20 to 40 minutes. Neutral-temperature water can be mixed with a brine solution to soothe and cleanse burn victims or those

with decubitis ulcers. Warm or hot water, 90 to 100°F, is used to relax muscles and warm joints for increased range of motion for those, for example, with sports injuries, rheumatoid arthritis, Parkinson's disease, cerebral palsy, multiple sclerosis, polio and postpolio syndrome, and spinal cord injuries, as well as for rehabilitation for postoperative conditions.

Watsu® and Aquatic Massage

Watsu® is a flowing treatment that is done by floating the client in body-temperature water (98°F) and doing a series of stretches and pressure-point massage that strengthen muscles and increase flexibility (see ▶Figure 4.61). It was developed in 1980 by Harold Dull of Harbin Springs, CA, who combined the principles of zen shiatsu with the buoyancy of water (water + shiatsu = Watsu®). As the client effortlessly floats, the practitioner is able to address the body completely. It is known as an intimate and nurturing water therapy and is being offered by an increasing number of spas as well as private practitioners (Sinclair, 2008. WABA, 2008a). Aquatic massage grew out of Watsu® and was developed by Elaine Marie, the foremost teacher of this modality. It involves the same principles and techniques as Watsu® but has a shorter training program (Marie, 2008).

Water Dance (Wassertanzen)

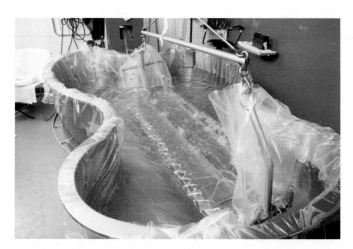

▶ **Figure 4.60** A Hubbard tank is a full-immersion tank for patients who are injured or immobile. It has support bars for doing water exercise and jets for hydrotherapy massage.

Water Dance (WasserTanzen®) is a form of underwater aquatic bodywork that was developed by a Swiss couple, Arjana Brunschwiler and Aman Schroter, in 1987. It is

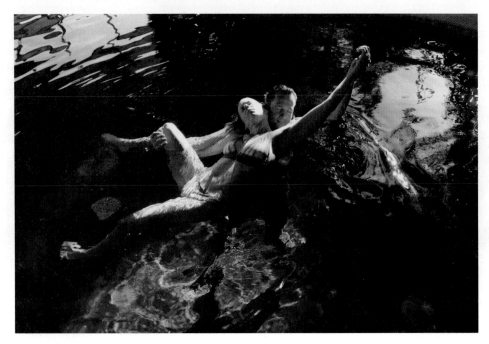

▶ **Figure 4.61** Watsu combines the principles of zen shiatsu with the buoyancy of water to strengthen muscles and increase flexibility. The practitioner is able to do a series of stretches and pressure-point massage as the client floats effortlessly in the water.

similar to Watsu® except that both the practitioner and client are completely underwater. The client is given nose clips and holds the breath while beneath the water's surface. The practitioner then takes the client through a series of gentle gyrations and stretches (see ▶Figure 4.62). It is truly an underwater dance. Free from the bounds of gravity, clients can experience a deep state of relaxation and perhaps release emotions. Like Watsu® Water Dance is being offered by an increasing number of spas as well as private practitioners (WABA, 2008b).

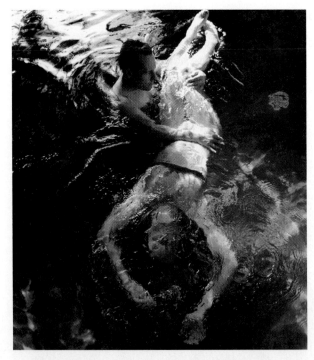

▶ **Figure 4.62** Water Dance is similar to Watsu® except that both the practitioner and client are completely underwater.

Summary

Hydrotherapy is one of the oldest treatment methods known to humankind, and because of its versatility, it has been in continual use up to the present day. Understanding the components of hydrotherapy gives practitioners tools they need to help their clients choose the best treatment options. One of these components is the properties of water. Water exists in three states: solid, liquid, and gas; hydrotherapy treatments in the form of ice, water, and steam use water in all three states. Water affects the body mechanically, chemically, and thermally. Being an effective solvent; participating in chemical reactions; acting as a lubricant; being readily available and easy to use; and having buoyancy, hydrostatic pressure, and a high heat capacity all make water an ideal medium for treatments.

The other components of hydrotherapy are its four main variables. These include temperature of the treatment, duration of the treatment, the client's health and vitality, and location (on which part of the client's body the treatment is applied or if application is to the client's entire body). Also important are indications, contraindications, and considerations for local and systemic heat, cold, and contrast applications.

Generally, cold applications penetrate more deeply than heat applications do. The effects of cold applications on the body include vasoconstriction of skin blood vessels and vasodilation of core blood vessels; decreased lymphatic flow in the application area; decrease in metabolic reaction rates in the tissue area; and slowing of nerve impulse conduction, resulting in an analgesic effect. In addition, muscle tone increases, connective tissue becomes less pliable and more rigid, and leukocyte activity increase. Examples of cold applications are cold compresses, cryotherapy, cold showers, and cold baths.

Heat from applications that use water penetrate more deeply into tissues than applications that use dry heat do. Effects of heat applications include detoxification (through diaphoresis) and vasodilation of skin blood vessels, which helps tissues heal and facilitates the transportation of heat to other parts of the body. Heat applied to one part of the body can draw blood from another part of the body, relieving congestion and inflammation in the untreated area. Other effects include increasing cellular metabolism, stimulating the activities of leukocytes, warming and increasing the pliability of muscle and connective tissue, and relieving pain. Examples of heat applications include hot compress, ginger fomentation, hot foot bath, heating wraps, hot showers, hot baths, steam inhalation treatments, steam baths, and saunas.

Alternating treatments make use of both cold and heat; the effects on the body are the same as for both cold and heat treatments. Alternating treatments include compresses, showers, and baths.

Other types of hydrotherapy include the use of hydrotherapy tubs, flotation tanks/sensory deprivation tanks or rooms, Hubbard tanks, whirlpools/Jacuzzis®, and the modalities of Watsu® and Water Dance.

Activities

1. List three benefits of local cold application.

_____

_____

_____

2. List five indications of local cold application.

_____

_____

_____

_____

3. List three benefits of systemic cold application.

_____

_____

_____

4. List five indications of systemic cold application.

_____

_____

_____

_____

5. List three benefits of local heat application.

_____

_____

_____

6. List five indications of local heat application.

_____

_____

_____

_____

_____

7. List three benefits of systemic heat application.

_____

_____

_____

8. List five indications of systemic heat application.

_____

_____

_____

_____

_____

9. List three benefits of alternating applications.

_____

_____

_____

10. List five indications of alternating applications.

_____

_____

_____

_____

_____

11. List ten contraindications or considerations for cold, heat, and alternating applications.

_____

_____

_____

_____

_____

_____

_____

_____

_____

_____

12. Receive a single cold compress treatment. What did you like about it? What did you not like about it? How did you feel 24 hours after the treatment? 48 hours after the treatment?

_____

_____

_____

_____

_____

13. Receive a cryotherapy treatment. What did you like about it? What did you not like about it? How did you feel 24 hours after the treatment? 48 hours after the treatment?

_____

_____

_____

_____

_____

14. Receive a hot compress treatment. What did you like about it? What did you not like about it? How did you feel 24 hours after the treatment? 48 hours after the treatment?

_____

_____

_____

_____

15. Receive a hot ginger fomentation treatment. What did you like about it? What did you not like about it? How did you feel 24 hours after the treatment? 48 hours after the treatment?

_____

_____

_____

_____

16. Receive a hot foot bath treatment. What did you like about it? What did you not like about it? How did you feel 24 hours after the treatment? 48 hours after the treatment?

_____

_____

_____

_____

_____

17. Receive a heating (cold sheet) wrap treatment. What did you like about it? What did you not like about it? How did you feel 24 hours after the treatment? 48 hours after the treatment?

_____

_____

_____

_____

_____

_____

_____

_____

18. Receive an alternating compress treatment. What did you like about it? What did you not like about it? How did you feel 24 hours after the treatment? 48 hours after the treatment?

_____

_____

_____

_____

_____

19. Try taking a cool shower on a cool day. How did you feel the rest of the day?

_____

_____

_____

20. Try taking a hot shower on a warm day. How did you feel the rest of the day?

_____

_____

_____

21. For a week, try ending each bath or shower you take with cold water. How did you feel throughout the week?

_____

_____

_____

_____

_____

_____

22. Try taking a steam bath. What did you like about it? What did you not like about it? How did you feel 24 hours after the treatment? 48 hours after the treatment?

_____

_____

_____

_____

_____

_____

23. Try taking a sauna. What did you like about it? What did you not like about it? How did you feel 24 hours after the treatment? 48 hours after the treatment?

_____

_____

_____

_____

_____

_____

24. Receive a Watsu®, aquatic massage, or water dance treatment. What did you like about it? What did you not like about it? How did you feel 24 hours after the treatment? 48 hours after the treatment?

_____

_____

_____

_____

_____

_____

Study Questions

1. Transferring heat away from the body as a result of water currents is the definition of
   a. convection
   b. conduction
   c. radiation
   d. buoyancy

2. Which temperature is considered painfully hot?
   a. 92–100°F
   b. 100–104°F
   c. 105–110°F
   d. 110–124°F

3. A reaction that occurs in one area of the body is called
   a. consensual
   b. local
   c. systemic
   d. diaphoretic

4. Using heat to draw blood and lymph from one area of the body to another is called
   a. hyperemia
   b. convection
   c. derivation
   d. hypotension

5. Hypotension is the term for
   a. high blood pressure
   b. excessive sweating
   c. lowered body temperature
   d. low blood pressure

6. A fomentation is defined as a
   a. layer of towels
   b. cold application
   c. hot moist compress
   d. a body wrap

7. The temperature range of a hot foot bath is
   a. 85–90°F
   b. 92–99°F
   c. 98–115°F
   d. 110–112°F

8. The "pumping action" of blood into and out of an area is referred to as
   a. fluxion
   b. vascular gymnastics
   c. derivation
   d. reflexion

9. Vasoconstriction of blood vessels will have which of the following effects?
   a. increase of local blood flow
   b. revulsive action
   c. stimulation of muscle tissue
   d. flushing of toxins out of the area

10. A revulsive treatment is defined as one that involves
    a. the use of tepid temperatures
    b. addressing one area of the body to have an effect on another area
    c. prolonged heat, followed by brief cold
    d. immersion into a cold bath

11. A local cold application of short duration has which effect on the body?
    a. sedation
    b. stimulation
    c. warming
    d. numbing

12. Which of the following is a contraindication for a sauna?
    a. tight muscles
    b. pregnancy
    c. noninflammatory joint pain
    d. toxin buildup

13. Which of the following treatments would best help relieve chest congestion?
    a. sauna
    b. cold compress
    c. tepid bath
    d. cold shower

14. The power of a fluid to exert an upward force on a body placed in it is the definition of
    a. hydrostatic pressure
    b. balneology
    c. buoyancy
    d. heat capacity

15. In which of the following ways does water affect the body?
    a. chemically
    b. thermally
    c. mechanically
    d. all of the above

16. A great difference between body temperature and treatment temperature will cause the treatment to
    a. be ineffective
    b. intensify
    c. lessen
    d. remain constant

17. The loss of fluids and electrolytes during a systemic heat application can lead to which of the following?
    a. heat stroke
    b. heat cramps
    c. heat exhaustion
    d. all of the above

18. An accurate description of a stage the body goes through when stimulated by cold is that in the
    a. third stage, there is an immediate cardiovascular response
    b. first stage, hormones increase metabolism to generate more heat
    c. second stage, blood vessels in the skin vasconstrict
    d. third stage, muscle tone increases

19. Clients are generally not good candidates to receive cold or heat therapies if they have
    a. chest congestion
    b. heart disease
    c. joint tightness
    d. chronic pain

20. A combination of shiatsu and water describes
    a. Blitzguss
    b. Vichy shower
    c. Watsu®
    d. sensory deprivation

Case Samples

A. Leona Chen is a 36-year-old stock trader who works 70 hours a week. Lately, the stock market has taken a downturn, which is concerning Leona greatly. She has been getting sick a lot in the last couple months with bothersome colds and stomach upset. This is adding to her stress, and as a result, she has been experiencing insomnia. Her regular massage therapist, Maribel Grijalva, suggests to Leona that during her next appointment, she might benefit from a hydrotherapy treatment.

1. Which hydrotherapy treatments would be best for Leona to receive?
2. What are the rationale, equipment and supplies, indications, contraindications, preparation, after-treatment care, and hygiene for these treatments?
3. Which questions should Maribel ask Leona to determine which treatment would be most beneficial?

B. Lina Safar is a busy graduate student who is spending long hours on the computer, working on her master's degree. She has chronic tightness in her mid- and upper back.

1. Which hydrotherapy treatment could be recommended?
2. What are the rationale, equipment and supplies, indications, contraindications, preparation, after-treatment care, and hygiene for this treatment?

C. Ralph Evans is a pharmacist who spends long hours on his feet filling prescriptions and consulting with sick customers. His resistance is worn down and he feels like he is coming down with a cold or, worse yet, the flu. His daughter has recommended that Ralph receive a hydrotherapy treatment from her massage therapist, Imani.

1. What are the rationale, equipment and supplies, indications, contraindications, preparation, after-treatment care, and hygiene for this treatment?
2. Which questions should Imani ask Ralph to determine which treatment would be most beneficial?

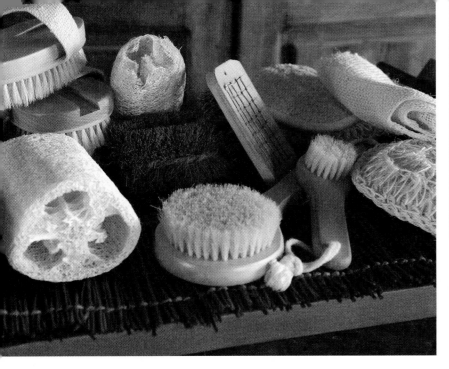

LEARNING OBJECTIVES

After studying this chapter, the reader will have the information to

1. Explain what exfoliation is and list the benefits it has for the body.

2. Distinguish between manual exfoliation and chemical (enzyme, dissolving) exfoliation.

3. Discuss the structure of the skin in relation to exfoliation.

4. Outline the tools and substances used for dry brushing, scrubs (frictions), body polishes, and chemical exfoliation.

5. Delineate the supplies needed, rationale, indications, contraindications, treatment procedure, hygiene, and after-treatment care for full-body dry brushing and quick-prep dry brushing.

6. Delineate the supplies needed, rationale, indications, contraindications, treatment procedure, hygiene, and after-treatment care for manual exfoliations using natural substances.

7. Delineate the supplies needed, rationale, indications, contraindications, treatment procedure, hygiene, and after-treatment care for salt and sugar glows.

Think of your skin as a rose—sometimes petals must be removed to reveal a more beautiful bloom.
— Author unknown

KEY TERMS

Body polishes	Dry brushing (body brushing)	Keratin	Scrubs (frictions, glows)
Chemical (enzyme or dissolving) exfoliation	Emollient	Manual exfoliation	

WHAT IS EXFOLIATION?

Exfoliation is the removal of dead skin cells from the surface of the body. An overabundance of dead skin cells can cause skin pores to clog with natural body oils, dirt, and debris, which can lead to the formation of pustules. Dryness and flakiness can also occur. Removal of the dead cells brightens skin color and clarity by encouraging the body to produce new skin cells. It also unclogs the follicles and pores; improves skin texture by making it smoother; and allows moisturizers, lotions, serums, and other preparations to better hydrate and nourish the skin. Exfoliation leaves the skin invigorated and increases vasodilation of skin blood vessels so that blood is brought to the surface of the body. It also energizes superficial lymphatic flow and stimulates nerve endings.

A full-body exfoliation is a powerful therapy in and of itself that can have a positive impact on the entire body. The removal of dead skin cells, the vasodilation of skin blood vessels, and the stimulation of nerve endings make it an invigorating treatment. Exfoliation can also be a prelude to another treatment, such as a mud or herbal wrap. It not only prepares the skin for the wrap, it also gives clients the benefit of receiving more than one treatment, enhancing their spa experience (Williams, 2007).

TYPES OF EXFOLIANTS

The term *exfoliant* refers to both the substances and the tools used to remove dead skin cells. There are two main types of exfoliation treatments. The physical process of applying friction with abrasives is called **manual exfoliation.** Manual exfoliants include dry brushes, mitts, loofahs, and abrasive cloths (for applying friction), and natural substances such as salt, sugar, cornmeal, and coffee that are abrasive. These substances are typically mixed with water, oils, or crèmes before being rubbed over the surface of the skin.

The other type is **chemical, enzyme,** or **dissolving exfoliation.** These exfoliants consist of chemicals or enzymes that work by dissolving dead skin cells, but they do not overstimulate the skin like manual abrasives can. After application, the enzymes are washed or rubbed off. Natural substances such as yogurt, milk, and papaya contain acids and enzymes that act as natural exfoliants. Cleopatra, renowned in history for her beauty, was famous for taking regular milk baths. In ancient Turkish palaces, entire harems bathed in large pools filled with milk. There are many different commercial preparations, and the manufacturer's instructions need to be followed carefully if they are used.

It is also important to note that practitioners should never go beyond their scope of practice. They need to check their local or state regulations regarding the use of exfoliants in their practice. It is possible that practitioners need to be licensed as estheticians or cosmetologists to perform exfoliations. It is recommended that practitioners check with all pertinent regulatory bodies to make sure they are in compliance with the laws that govern them and their practice.

A CLOSER LOOK AT THE SKIN

As discussed in Chapter 2, the skin is one of the body's major protections. Its functions include:

▶ physically shielding the body from bacteria; ultraviolet radiation; and cuts, scratches, and scrapes
▶ playing a considerable role in regulating body temperature
▶ providing information about the external environment via stimulation of its nerve endings
▶ excreting toxins and excess salts in perspiration
▶ playing a role in the complicated process of vitamin D synthesis

Layers of the Skin

Skin is composed of three layers:

▶ **epidermis**—the thinnest, outermost layer of skin
▶ **dermis**—the inner, thicker layer composed of connective tissue; contains blood and lymph vessels, nerves, and glands that open onto the surface of the skin. The sudoriferous (sweat) glands excrete perspiration. The sebaceous (oil) glands excrete oil that keeps skin and hair soft and supple.
▶ **hypodermis or superficial fascia**—the layer that connects the skin to underlying muscle and bone

The epidermis is the layer affected by exfoliation. It has five layers (see ▶Figure 5.1):

▶ **Stratum basale**—the deepest layer. This is a single layer of cells that continually divide. The newly formed cells, called *keratinocytes*, gradually travel upward through the rest of the layers of the epidermis. Keratinocytes produce the protein **keratin,** which makes skin waterproof. However, as the keratinocytes fill with keratin, they die.
▶ **Stratum spinosum**—superficial to the stratum basale. This layer has eight to ten layers of keratinocytes that are beginning to produce keratin.

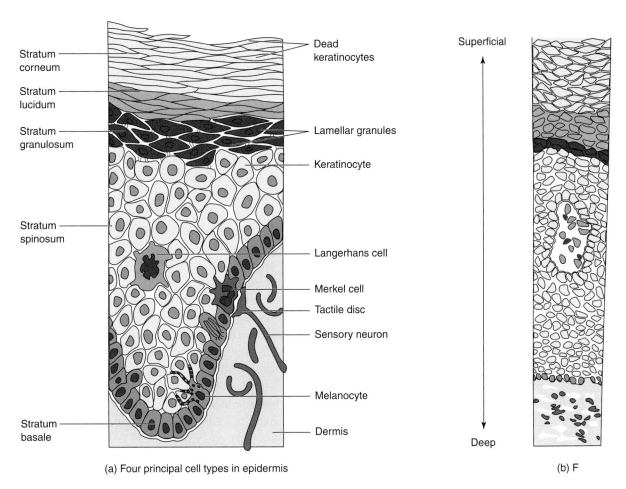

Stratum corneum

Stratum lucidum

Stratum granulosum

Stratum spinosum

Stratum basale

Dead keratinocytes

Lamellar granules

Keratinocyte

Langerhans cell

Merkel cell

Tactile disc

Sensory neuron

Melanocyte

Dermis

Superficial

Deep

(a) Four principal cell types in epidermis

(b) F

▷ **Figure 5.1** The layer of skin affected by exfoliation is the epidermis, which has five layers

▷ **Stratum granulosum**—superficial to the stratum spinosum. The keratinocytes are in three to five layers of flattened cells and continue to produce keratin. At this point, the keratinocytes are beginning to die.

▷ **Stratum lucidum**—found only in the thick skin of the fingertips, palms, and soles. It is three to five layers of flattened, clear, dead keratinocytes.

▷ **Stratum corneum**—the most superficial. Consists of twenty-five to thirty rows of flat, dead skin cells filled with keratin. These cells are continuously sloughed off and replaced by others traveling upward from the deeper layers. This layer is susceptible to cellular buildup, which may lead to dry, flaky skin.

It takes approximately 28 to 30 days for the keratinocytes to travel from the stratum basale up to the stratum corneum, so the skin completely renews itself about every month (Tortora and Derrickson, 2006).

It is a myth that the skin's pores open and close. The pores are actually openings in the skin that allow sebum (oil) to travel to the surface and keep it soft and supple. Pores that appear larger than usual could result from dead skin cells that have accumulated in the pore. Exfoliation helps remove the dead skin cells and helps keep the pores clean, which makes them look smaller.

DID YOU KNOW?

Approximately 30,000 to 40,000 skin cells are shed each day. That adds up to almost nine pounds per year!

MANUAL EXFOLIATION

Manual exfoliation can be done using many different tools and substances, depending on the level of abrasion needed. Exfoliation using brushes or fiber tools is known as **dry brushing** or **body brushing.** Other manual exfoliation tools that can be used for dry brushing include loofahs,

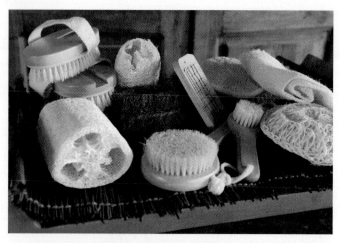

▶ **Figure 5.2** Examples of manual exfoliation tools: lower left—loofah; top and center—various brushes; top right—ayate cloth; bottom right—sisal scrub

nylon mitts, sisal mitts (sisal is a coarse fiber), ayate cloths (ayate is a woven fiber that is less coarse than sisal), and other abrasive cloths depending on the level of abrasion desired. See ▶Figure 5.2 for examples of manual exfoliation tools. Dry brushing can be performed anywhere from mild to moderate to vigorous.

Clients can also do this exfoliation for themselves at home. They can purchase any of the manual exfoliation tools and perform dry brushing with proper instruction from practitioners. The equipment and supplies can be purchased at local stores, online, or from spa supply stores.

Scrubs or **frictions** are manual exfoliation methods using salts or coarser organic substances. These tend to be brisk treatments that leave the client energized. The exfoliant substance is mixed with a fluid such as water, oil, crème, milk, yogurt, water, or a body wash, and essential oils can be added to the mixture to enhance the treatment. Since these treatments both remove the top layers of the skin and cause vasodilation of skin blood vessels, the person is left with pink skin and a characteristic "glow." Because of this, scrubs using salt and sugar are often referred to as salt and sugar **glows.**

The salt glow exfoliation is thought to have originated in Scandinavian countries. The long winter months of inactivity and little bathing would result in dry, flaky skin that built up on people's bodies. When springtime arrived, they needed to cleanse and refresh themselves. Making use of the nearby ocean, they used sea salt rubs to tonify and exfoliate themselves (Nikola, 1997). Salt is a natural detoxifier; it draws toxins from the body.

More recently, sugar has been adapted for use in glows as well. There are glows made of table sugar, brown sugar, and raw sugar. Unlike salt, sugar has moisturizing properties; like salt, it leaves the skin soft and smooth. The salt or sugar is usually mixed with a little water to make it the consistency of snow. The amount of water needed to make the mixture is minimal enough that it does not dissolve the salt and sugar crystals. The salt or sugar can be mixed completely with oil for the exfoliation but this makes for a messier treatment. The oil is difficult to remove from the client's body and to launder from the sheets. It is easier to use an oil-based scrub in the shower.

Body polishes are a gentler form of exfoliation using softer granules such as those found in fine blue cornmeal or finely ground natural substances such as crushed almonds or grape seed meal. A skin **emollient** such as oil, lotion, or crème can be used as part of the mixture. A skin emollient is a substance that makes the skin soft and supple. For more coarse grains, the emollient should be thicker; for smaller grains, the emollient can be thinner.

Many different substances can be used for scrubs and body polishes. In addition to salt, sugar, and the other previously mentioned materials, just about anything that occurs in granular form, or that can be ground into granules, can be used as long as it is natural. ▶Table 5.1 lists suggested substances to use in scrubs and body polishes. ▶Figure 5.3 shows some examples of substances used in scrubs and body polishes.

Additionally practitioners can explore the use of materials found in their geographic areas. For example, grape seeds, wine, and grape seed oil are used for scrubs at spa and bodywork practices in Napa Valley, CA, and the Spa at the Hotel Hershey in Hershey, PA, offers a chocolate sugar scrub.

As discussed, practitioners can use many different tools and substances to perform manual exfoliation treat-

TABLE 5.1
Suggested substances to use in scrubs and body polishes

Barley
Coffee grounds
Cornmeal—blue, white, yellow
Crushed pearls
Ground nuts—almonds, peanuts, hazel nuts, and so on
Oatmeal
Pulverized pumice
Salt—sea salt, Epsom salt, Dead Sea salt, desert mineral salt
Seeds—grape, poppy, sunflower, sesame
Sugar—table sugar, raw sugar, brown sugar

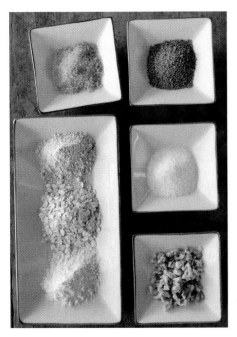

▶ **Figure 5.3** Common substances for scrubs and/or body polishes: top left—flax seeds; top right—poppy seeds; middle left (top to bottom)—blue cornmeal, oatmeal, yellow cornmeal; middle right—sea salt; bottom right—grape seeds

ments. What follows are some basic methods and materials. Once these can be performed skillfully, practitioners can develop more creative treatments and build their treatment menus. Practitioners who work in spas should note that each spa has its own treatment protocols, often called signature treatments, and practitioners are trained

CLINICAL ALERT

Practitioners and clients can be allergic to any or all exfoliation substances and fluids. One of the more well-known allergies is to nuts. It is important for the practitioner to find out from clients any allergies they may have, and note them on an intake form, so there is written documentation. Practitioners allergic to any or all exfoliation substances and fluids should never use them on clients, even when requested to do so either by clients or employers.

People can develop allergies throughout their lives; therefore, every time a client arrives for a treatment, the practitioner should do a quick allergy update. Before any treatment is performed, the substance should be applied to a small area on the client's skin and on the practitioner's skin, usually the forearm, to see if there is an allergic reaction.

accordingly. The items used in these signature treatments can vary widely, depending on the spa's menu. What is presented in this chapter may or may not be consistent with how individual spas perform their treatments; however, the following presentation will help practitioners acquire basic exfoliation skills, become comfortable handling supplies and equipment, and become able to discuss exfoliation treatment options with clients in a knowledgeable manner.

A full-body dry brushing takes about 30 minutes and can be offered as an individual treatment or in conjunction with other therapies. For example, body brushing can be done before a body wrap. When the dead skin cells are removed, the substances used in body wraps, such as mud or crèmes, can have a much better effect on the skin.

Lymphatic Flow and Manual Exfoliations

As discussed in Chapter 2, the lymphatic system flows one way; it is not circular like the cardiovascular system. Interstitial fluid flows into lymphatic capillaries and becomes lymph. The lymphatic capillaries drain into lymphatic vessels, which have lymph nodes situated on them. There are superficial lymphatic vessels, which are close to the surface of the skin, and there are deep lymphatic vessels buried within tissues along with arteries, deep veins, and nerves.

Lymph nodes filter pathogens and cellular debris out of the lymph. There are many lymph nodes along both the superficial and deep lymphatic vessels—some singular, some in clusters. Superficial clusters of lymph nodes are found in the inguinal, cervical, and axillary regions. Deep clusters of lymph nodes are found in the iliac, thoracic, and intestinal regions.

All the lymphatic vessels drain into one of nine larger lymphatic trunks. By the time lymph reaches a trunk, it is completely filtered. All the lymphatic trunks drain into one of two lymphatic ducts.

The left lymphatic duct (also called the thoracic duct) is about 15 to 18 inches long and begins just anterior to the second lumbar vertebra. The thoracic duct is the main collecting duct of the lymphatic system. It receives lymph from the entire body inferior to the ribs, the left upper extremity, the left side of thorax, and the left side of the head and neck.

The right lymphatic trunk is about one-half-inch long and receives lymph from the right side of the thorax, head, and neck.

Both lymphatic trunks empty the freshly filtered lymph into the bloodstream. The thoracic duct connects with the left subclavian vein; the right lymphatic duct connects with the right subclavian vein. As discussed in Chapter 2, as soon as lymph enters the bloodstream, it is

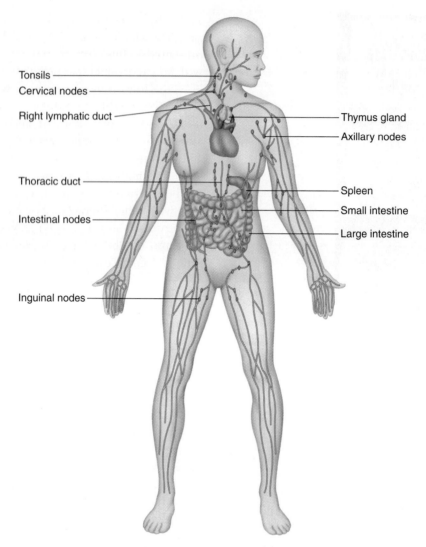

Tonsils
Cervical nodes
Right lymphatic duct
Thoracic duct
Intestinal nodes
Inguinal nodes

Thymus gland
Axillary nodes
Spleen
Small intestine
Large intestine

▶ **Figure 5.4** All the lymphatic vessels drain into one of nine larger lymphatic trunks. All the lymphatic trunks drain into one of two lymphatic ducts.

considered plasma, the liquid portion of blood (see ▶Figure 5.4).

Lymphatic flow is slow. It does not move quickly like blood, which has the force of the heart pumping it into arteries. In fact, sometimes lymph moves so slowly that not enough interstitial fluid can enter the lymphatic capillaries, and it accumulates in the tissues. This is called edema (Tortora and Derrickson, 2006).

Dry brushing and all manual exfoliation methods actually help stimulate the flow of lymph in the superficial vessels by physically encouraging the movement of lymph forward through the lymphatic vessels. This clears the way for more interstitial fluid to enter the lymphatic capillaries.

As discussed in Chapter 2, superficial lymphatic vessels are close to the surface of the body. Therefore, dry-brushing strokes applied to the extremities, face, neck, and upper chest are done lightly. However, strokes on the abdomen and back can be applied with more depth to help stimulate the deeper flow of lymph.

Because the lymphatic system flows in one direction, the strokes performed in dry brushing and other manual exfoliation techniques travel along the pathway of lymph flow:

▶ In the extremities, the strokes are performed toward the client's heart.
▶ Strokes on the face, neck, and upper chest are performed downward.
▶ The abdominal and back strokes are designed to help stimulate the deeper flow of lymph forward: abdominal strokes are performed in a clockwise direction, then up each side to the center of the abdomen; back strokes are performed downward from the neck and shoulders to the mid-back, then from the lumbar area up to the mid-back.

The steps outlined for full-body dry brushing, quick-prep dry brushing, and manual exfoliations using natural substances are designed specifically to assist the flow of lymph in the proper direction. As with massage, it is important that the strokes on the extremities be performed toward the client's heart (Benjamin and Tappan, 2005).

For clients who have mild edema not resulting from medical conditions, such as from standing for long periods of time, these methods may be useful. Practitioners, however, should never go beyond their scope of practice. Specific courses of study in lymphatic drainage, including accreditation courses, give practitioners the skills and tools needed to address more serious medical conditions that have edema as a symptom.

Dry brushing can be performed as an individual treatment or as part of a body wrap or other treatment. Although the dry-brushing techniques for either case are the same, the equipment, supplies, and setup are somewhat different. Because of that, dry brushing that is part of a body wrap or other treatment is shown as part of those treatments in subsequent chapters.

When using the body brush or exfoliation tool, the most efficient stroke is a brisk half-moon stroke, using a flick of the wrist. These brisk movements remove the maximum amount of dead skin cells with each stroke (see ▶ Figures 5.5 a and b).

Manual Exfoliation Using Natural Substances

Many different natural substances can be used for manual exfoliations. Salts and sugars are particularly useful because in addition to being abrasive, they contain glycolic acid that dissolves away dead skin cells. Therefore, they can be considered chemical or enzymatic exfoliants as well; sugar is also hydrating to the skin (Williams, 2007). Other popular substances include oatmeal, barley, poppy seeds, ground coffee, cornmeal (yellow or blue), ground grape seeds, ground almonds, ground sunflower seeds, and even pulverized pumice (crushed volcanic rock).

There are several factors to consider when helping clients choose which exfoliation substance would work best for them. If they have delicate or sensitive skin, milder abrasive such as those used in body polishes would be more appropriate. Clients with dry skin may benefit more from the hydrating aspects of a sugar scrub. Salt scrubs may be more useful for a client with oily skin. Since pumice tends to be more abrasive than many other exfoliation substances, pumice scrubs are excellent for the feet.

Since an exfoliation can be very invigorating, practitioners should keep communicating with the client about pressure of application. Sometimes deeper pressure and more time are needed to exfoliate the soles of the feet, palms of the hands, elbows, and knees.

When using natural substances, it is best to grind them to a desired consistency and make them into a paste or slurry using water, oil, crème, milk, yogurt, a body wash, or any other liquid of choice. When using salt or sugar, enough liquid should be added to make the salt or sugar the consistency of snow. Essential oils can be added to the mixtures to enhance the treatment. Generally, two drops of a carrier oil should be added first; then the essential oil can be added drop by drop and mixed in with the fingers or a spatula.

Since natural exfoliation substances leave residue on the body, it may be best to use them where there is access to a shower. Certain spa settings will have a wet table or Vichy shower available for rinsing the client thoroughly. However, this may involve the client wearing little or being completely nude while the practitioner rinses off the exfoliation substance. Even though practitioners may be comfortable with this, first-time clients are usually not prepared for the level of undress necessary.

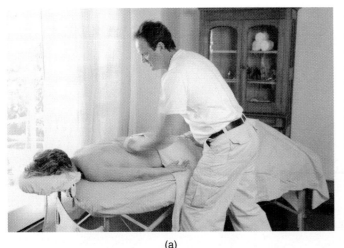
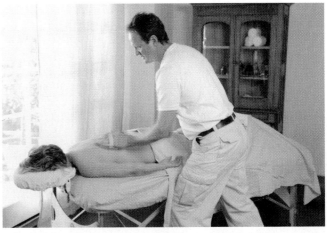

(a)　　　　　　　　　　　　　　　　(b)

▶ **Figure 5.5** A brisk half-moon stroke is the most efficient stroke to use with the body brush or exfoliation tool because it removes the maximum amount of dead skin cells with each stroke.

TREATMENT 5.1

Full-Body Dry Brushing

Rationale
A full-body dry brushing can be done for any or all of the following physiological effects:

- Exfoliant: removes dead skin cells
- Vasodilator: increases local blood flow
- Stimulant: invigorates the whole body and promotes movement of the digestive tract; stimulates lymphatic flow
- Tonifier: strengthens vitality and the immune system

Equipment and Supplies
(see ▶Figure 5.6)

- Two cloth sheets (one fitted and one flat)
- One large towel, approximately 30″ × 60″
- Choice of dry brush, loofah, ayate fiber cloth, sisal fiber gloves or cloth, or nylon mitts. A softer version of the dry-brushing tool will be needed for the client's face.

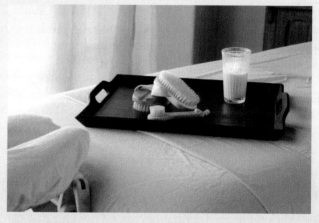

▶ **Figure 5.6**

Indications

- need for exfoliation
- low vitality
- fatigue
- constipation

Contraindications

- skin irritation
- rash
- sunburn (clients should be made aware that there is a higher chance of getting sunburned after having an exfoliation treatment)
- contagious skin condition
- athlete's foot—only the feet would be contraindicated; the rest of the body could be dry brushed
- recent tattoo
- area shaved 24 hours prior to treatment

Preparation

- Have dry-brushing tools within easy reach.
- If performing full-body dry brushing as an individual treatment, drape the massage table with the fitted sheet and then the flat sheet. Leave the room while the client gets on the table under the top sheet. The treatment can be performed starting with the client lying either prone or supine. In the following steps, the procedure is shown starting with the client lying prone.

TREATMENT 5.1 CONTINUED

Procedure

> **CLINICAL ALERT** !
>
> It is important to check with the client about the pressure of the brush or tool on the skin, and adjust the pressure as necessary. More pressure can be used and more time can be spent on the bottom of the feet, the knees, and the elbows, where the skin is a bit thicker than it is on the rest of the body, and where there tends to be more of a buildup of dead skin cells.

1. Standing at the foot of the table, undrape the client's left leg and gluteal region. Brush the sole of the foot (▶ Figure 5.7). Since the skin is thicker on the bottom of the foot, brushing can take longer here than elsewhere on the body.

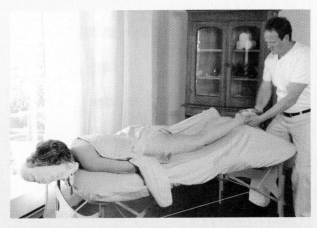

▶ **Figure 5.7**

2. Visually divide the rest of the client's leg into three sections: lateral, posterior, and medial. Beginning at the client's ankle, brush up each section three times, stroking from the ankle toward the client's heart (▶ Figure 5.8). Be sure to include the client's gluteal region. Redrape the client's left leg.

3. Move to the client's right leg. Undrape and brush the foot, leg, and gluteal region the same as for the left leg. Redrape the client's right leg.

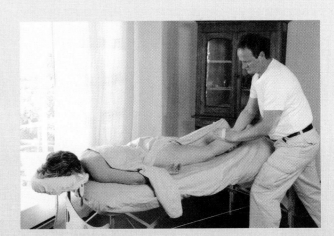

▶ **Figure 5.8**

TREATMENT 5.1 CONTINUED

4. Move to the client's left arm and undrape it. Brush the palm of the client's hand and fingers (▶Figure 5.9).

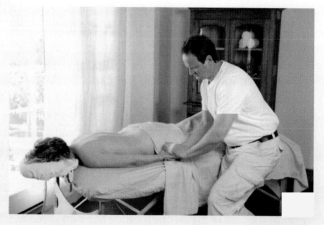

▶ **Figure 5.9**

5. Beginning at the client's wrist, brush up the arm, stroking from the wrist toward the client's heart (▶Figure 5.10). Redrape the client's left arm.

6. Move to the client's right arm. Undrape and brush the hand and arm the same as for the left arm. Redrape the client's right arm.

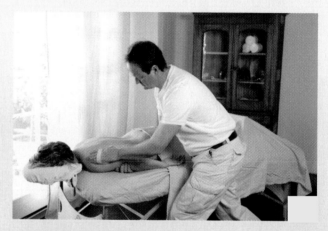

▶ **Figure 5.10**

7. Move to the head of the table and undrape the back. Starting at the neck (▶Figure 5.11 a) and shoulders (Figure 5.11 b), brush down to the client's mid-back. Brush the area three times.

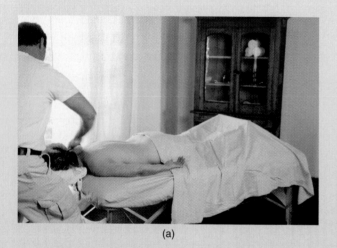

(a)

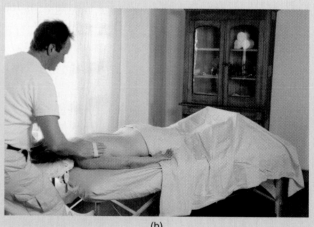

(b)

▶ **Figure 5.11**

TREATMENT 5.1 CONTINUED

8. Move to the right side of the table. Reaching across the client's back, brush the client's left lumbar to mid-back area, using angling and upward strokes toward the client's heart (▶Figure 5.12). Brush the area three times.

9. Move to the left side of the table. Brush the client's right lumbar to mid-back area the same as for the left side.

10. Move to the head of the table and do some light feather strokes with your fingertips from the client's low back to the shoulders. Redrape the back.

11. Help the client turn over.

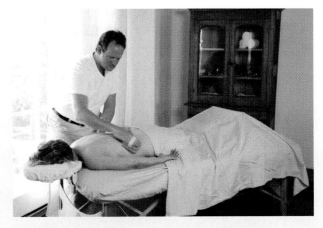

▶ **Figure 5.12**

12. Standing at the foot of the table, undrape the client's right foot. Brush the dorsal surface of the foot (▶Figure 5.13).

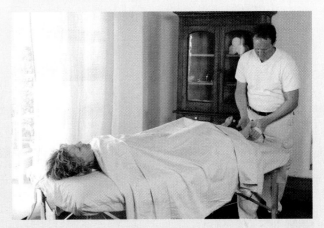

▶ **Figure 5.13**

13. Undrape the client's right leg. Visually divide the rest of the client's leg into three sections: lateral, anterior, and medial. Beginning at the client's ankle, brush up each section three times, stroking from the ankle toward the client's heart (▶Figure 5.14). Redrape the client's right leg.

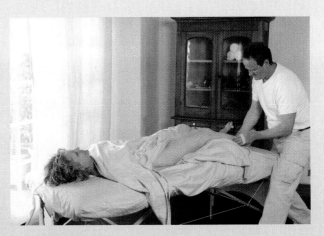

▶ **Figure 5.14**

TREATMENT 5.1 CONTINUED

14. Move to the client's left leg. Undrape and brush the foot and leg same as for the right leg. Redrape the client's left leg.

15. Move to the client's abdomen and drape the large towel across the client's chest area. Have the client hold it firmly as you pull the sheet inferiorly until the client's abdomen is undraped.

16. Using smaller strokes, brush the client's abdomen in a clockwise direction (▶Figure 5.15 a). Finish the abdomen by brushing up each side and coming to the center of the abdomen (Figure 5.15 b).

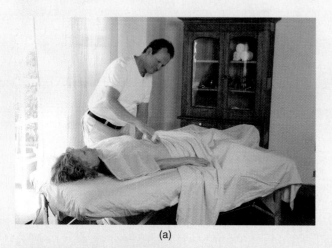 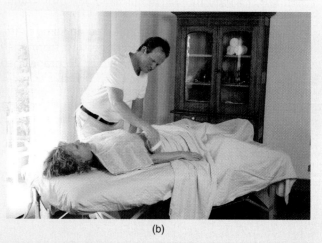

(a)   (b)

▶ **Figure 5.15**

17. Redrape the client's abdomen by pulling the sheet up over the abdomen and the draping towel on the client's chest area. Move to one side of the client, and while the client holds the sheet firmly, gently pull the draping towel out from under the sheet.

18. Move to the client's right arm and undrape it. Brush the back of the client's hand and fingers (▶Figure 5.16).

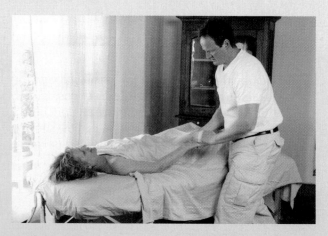

▶ **Figure 5.16**

TREATMENT 5.1 CONTINUED

19. Visually divide the rest of the client's arm into three sections: lateral, anterior, and medial. Beginning at the client's wrist, brush up each section three times, stroking from the wrist toward the client's heart (▶Figure 5.17). Redrape the client's right arm.

20. Move to the client's left arm. Undrape and brush the hand and arm the same as for the right arm. Redrape the client's left arm.

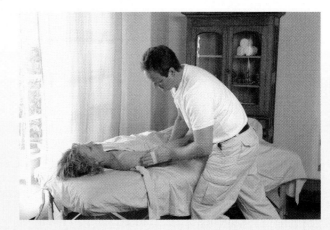
▶ **Figure 5.17**

21. Move to the head of the table. To brush the client's upper chest area, start at the right clavicle and brush downward three times, then brush downward three times from the left clavicle (▶Figure 5.18).

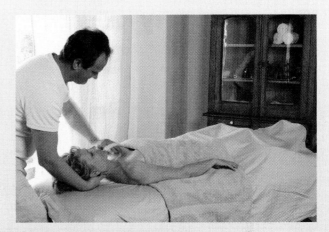
▶ **Figure 5.18**

22. If the client wants the face included, use a softer brush. With small, gentle strokes, brush from the client's chin to the forehead (▶Figure 5.19).

After the Treatment

An emollient can be applied to the client's skin, either by the practitioner or the client. The client should be made aware that there is a higher chance of getting sunburned after having an exfoliation treatment.

Hygiene

The exfoliation tools, sheets, and towels should be washed after each use. Wash the brushes in warm, soapy water and rinse. After rinsing, place them in rubbing alcohol for at least 20 minutes, then let them air dry. The tools can also be placed in a dishwasher and washed that way. Store them in an airtight container. Brushes will need to be replaced often since alcohol will cause them to deteriorate over time. Launder the sheets and towel in hot water and detergent between uses.

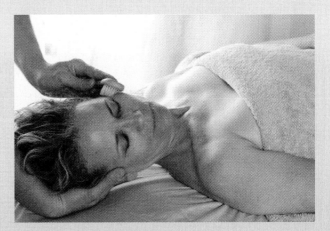
▶ **Figure 5.19**

TREATMENT 5.2

Quick-Prep Dry Brushing

The "quick-prep" dry brushing technique is basically the same as the full-body dry brushing except that it is an abbreviated version. It can be performed as an individual treatment or in preparation for other treatments, such as a body wrap. It is especially useful when the treatment time is limited. It usually only takes a total of 10 minutes—5 minutes with the client prone and 5 minutes with the client supine.

The rationale, equipment and supplies, indications, contraindications, preparation, after-treatment care, and hygiene are the same for the quick-prep dry brushing technique as they are for the full-body dry-brushing technique.

Procedure

1. Standing at the foot of the table, undrape the client's left leg and gluteal region. Working toward the client's heart, start brushing at the feet, move up the leg, and include the gluteals (▶Figure 5.20). Redrape the client's left leg.
2. Move to the client's right leg. Undrape and brush the foot, leg, and gluteal region the same as for the left leg. Redrape the client's right leg.

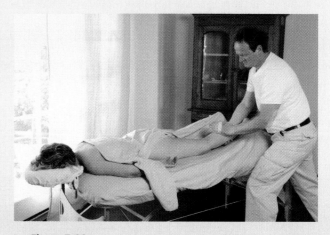

▶ Figure 5.20

CLINICAL ALERT !

Check with the client about pressure and adjust as necessary.

---

3. Move to the client's left arm and undrape it. Brush the palm of the client's hand and fingers. Beginning at the client's wrist, brush up the arm, stroking from the wrist toward the client's heart (▶Figure 5.21). Redrape the client's left arm.
4. Move to the client's right arm. Undrape and brush the hand and arm the same as for the left arm. Redrape the client's right arm.

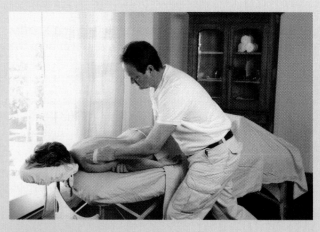

▶ Figure 5.21

TREATMENT 5.2 CONTINUED

5. Move to the head of the table and undrape the back. Starting at the neck and shoulders (▶Figure 5.22), brush down to the client's mid-back. Move to the right side of the table.

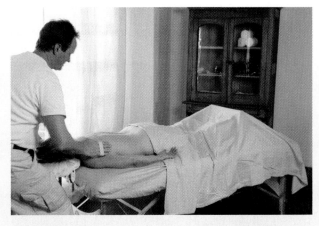

▶ **Figure 5.22**

6. Reaching across the client's back, brush the client's left lumbar to mid-back area, using angling upward strokes toward the client's heart (▶Figure 5.23). Move to the left side of the table. Brush the client's right lumbar to mid-back area the same as for the left side. Redrape the back. Help the client turn over.

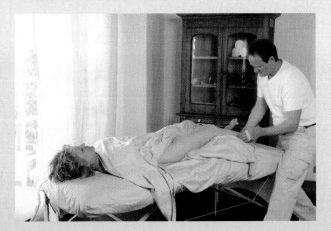

▶ **Figure 5.23**

7. Standing at the foot of the table, undrape the client's right leg. Working toward the client's heart, start brushing at the feet and move up the leg (▶Figure 5.24). Redrape the client's right leg.

8. Move to the client's left leg. Undrape and brush the foot and leg the same as for the right leg. Redrape the client's left leg.

9. Move to the client's abdomen and drape the large towel across the client's chest area. Have the client hold it firmly as you pull the sheet inferiorly until the client's abdomen is undraped.

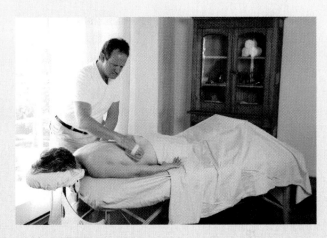

▶ **Figure 5.24**

TREATMENT 5.2 CONTINUED

10. Using smaller strokes, brush the client's abdomen in a clockwise direction (▶Figure 5.25 a). Finish the abdomen by brushing up each side and coming to the center of the abdomen (Figure 5.25 b).

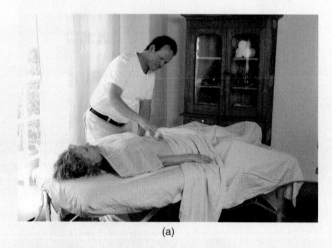

(a)   (b)

▶ **Figure 5.25**

11. Redrape the client's abdomen by pulling the sheet up over the client's abdomen and the draping towel over the client's chest area. Move to one side of the client, and while the client holds the sheet firmly, gently pull the draping towel out from under the sheet.

12. Move to the client's right arm and undrape it. Brush the back of the client's hand and fingers. Beginning at the client's wrist, brush up the arm, stroking from the wrist toward the client's heart (▶Figure 5.26). Redrape the client's right arm.

13. Move to the client's left arm. Undrape and brush the hand and arm the same as for the right arm. Redrape the client's left arm.

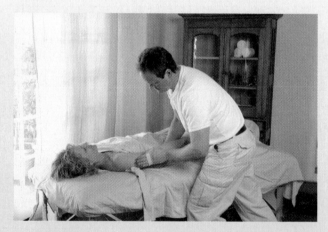

▶ **Figure 5.26**

14. Move to the head of the table. To brush the client's upper chest area, start at the right clavicle and brush downward three times, then brush downward three times from the left clavicle (▶Figure 5.27).

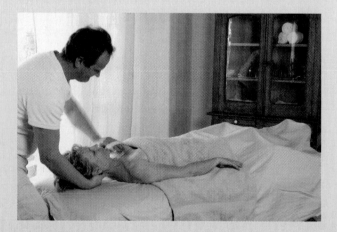

▶ **Figure 5.27**

Since most client dissatisfaction comes from communication issues, it is important that practitioners in spas who perform these showers explain clearly to the client how the procedure is performed and what the client can expect.

There is a method for removal of the residue when working in a dry room, and it is included in the description of Treatment 5.3.

Clients can do manual exfoliations using natural substances at home with proper instruction from practitioners. For example, exfoliations in the shower are easy to do. A container of oatmeal, seeds, or salts can be kept in the bathroom. When clients want to exfoliate, they simply mix the exfoliation substance with a bit of liquid such as oil or yogurt and then rub the exfoliant on their skin before or in the shower and rinse it off. After the shower, they can apply a soothing skin lotion. All of the equipment and supplies can be purchased at local stores, online, and from spa supply stores.

CHEMICAL, ENZYME, OR DISSOLVING EXFOLIATION

The other type of exfoliant is a chemical, enzyme, or dissolving exfoliant. Enzymes and alphahydroxy acids (AHA) or betahydroxy acids (BHA) are found in commercial products. They are also found in nature as:

► citric acid in citrus fruits
► malic acid in apples
► tartaric acid in grapes
► lactic acid in dairy products such as milk, cream, and yogurt
► glycolic acid in sugar and sugar cane

When these acids are applied to the skin, they loosen the keratin that holds skin cells together, allowing the cells to be easily sloughed off. Papaya (papain) and pineapple (bromelain) also contain enzymes that are effective exfoliants. Because they are nonacid enzymes, they are considered the safest for sensitive skin, unless there is an allergy to papaya or pineapple (Latona, 2000).

A chemical exfoliation can be gentle on the skin or aggressive like a medical facial peel. It is recommended that a reputable esthetician be consulted regarding any over-the-counter chemical, enzyme, or dissolving exfoliation products. It is also very likely that spas will carry chemical, enzyme, or dissolving exfoliation products. Spa staff members who are expected to use these on their clients will receive training on how to apply them properly.

Clients can perform these exfoliations at home with proper instruction from practitioners. For an exfoliating milk bath, one to two cups of milk or cream can be added to bath water, or the entire bath can be filled with milk. Clients should be urged to follow the manufacturers' instructions if using a commercial exfoliation product.

TO GET YOU STARTED

Hydrating Aroma Body Scrub #1

½ cup liquid glycerin
½ cup water
1½ to 3 cups fine sea salt or unrefined sugar
1 tsp solid coconut butter or oil
6 drops of essential oil of choice

Combine glycerin and water. Starting with one cup, add salt or sugar and mix until it is completely dissolved. Add the remaining salt or sugar and mix. Melt the coconut butter or oil in a small container in the microwave on low; do not overheat. Pour the melted coconut oil into the salt or sugar mixture and mix well. Add the essential oil of choice. More coconut oil can be melted and added until the desired consistency is reached. Store in an airtight jar or container.

Hydrating Aroma Body Scrub #2

1 cup fine sea salt or unrefined sugar
3 tsp liquid glycerin
1 tsp pure honey
3–5 drops essential oil
Optional: pinch of lavender flowers or dried herb of choice

Combine ingredients. Mix well and store in airtight jar or container.

Coffee Body Scrub

2 cups ground coffee (as fine or coarse as desired)
½ cup fine sea salt or unrefined sugar
2–3 tbsp carrier oil (such as sweet almond, apricot kernel, jojoba, sesame, grapefruit, etc.)

Combine all ingredients. Store in airtight container or jar.

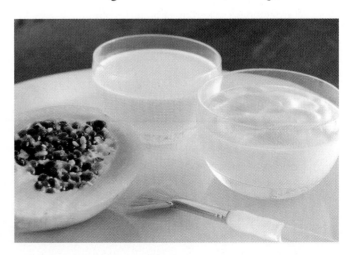

TREATMENT 5.3

Manual Exfoliation Using Natural Substances

Rationale

A manual exfoliation using natural substances can be applied for any or all of the following physiological effects:

- Exfoliant: removes dead skin cells
- Vasodilator: increases local blood flow
- Stimulant: invigorates the whole body, promotes movement of the digestive tract
- Tonifier: strengthens vitality and the immune system

Equipment and Supplies
(see ▶ Figure 5.28)

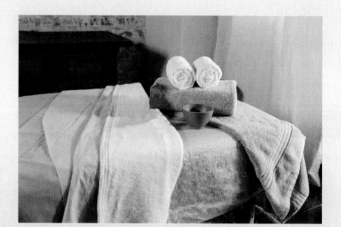

▶ **Figure 5.28**

- small, nonmetal bowl for exfoliation substance—nonmetal because the substance may react chemically with metal, changing the substance's properties
- natural substance of choice (1/4 to 1/2 cup). If performing a salt glow, use 50% fine salt and 50% medium grain salt (sea salt, Epsom salt, Dead Sea salt, desert mineral salt; see Chapters 6 and 7 for more information about these salts). If performing a sugar glow, use table, brown, or raw sugar.
- essential oil(s) of choice—If using an essential oil, a couple drops of a carrier oil will also be needed
- liquid of choice to make paste or slurry (water, milk, yogurt, oil, etc.)
- one cloth sheet and two large towels, approximately 30″ × 60″.
- If there is no access to a shower, a basin of warm water and three to four towels, approximately 18″ × 30″, are needed for substance removal. A towel cabi or crock pot filled with moist towels can also be used. More than three to four towels may be necessary for clients who have a large body size and for clients with a lot of body hair (it may be more difficult to remove the substance from the hair).

Indications

- need for exfoliation
- need for detoxification
- fatigue
- low endurance
- beginning or ending of a cold or flu

Contraindications

- skin irritations
- rashes
- sunburn
- allergy to substances being used
- contagious skin condition
- athlete's foot—only the feet would be contraindicated; the rest of the body could be exfoliated
- recent tattoo
- area shaved 24 hours prior to treatment

TREATMENT 5.3 CONTINUED

Preparation

1. Place the cloth sheet and two large towels lengthwise on top of the table.
2. Place the exfoliation substance, liquid, and small bowl within easy reach.
3. If working in a dry room and using a crock pot or cabi, turn on the warmer to warm the towels for substance removal at the end of the treatment. Moisten the three or four (or more) 18″ × 30″ towels and put them in the crock pot or cabi. If using the basin of warm water and towels, place the basin in a convenient place to fill it with warm water during the treatment.

Procedure

1. Have the client get on the table in supine position underneath the top large towel.

2. In the small bowl, blend the natural substance of choice with the fluid being used until it resembles a slurry (▶Figure 5.29).

If using salt, measure equal parts fine and medium grain salt into the small bowl. If using sugar, place the sugar in the small bowl. Use just enough warm water to make the salt or sugar the consistency of snow; blend the mixture with your fingers (▶Figure 5.30).

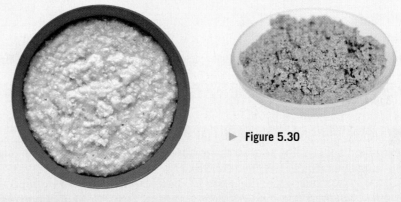

▶ **Figure 5.30**

▶ **Figure 5.29** (© Dorling Kindersley)

If desired, add essential oil to the exfoliation mixture. First, add a couple drops of a carrier oil, then add a drop or two of essential oil; mix well.

3. Take the bowl of mixture to the foot of the table.

4. Undrape the client's right leg.

5. Pour some water in your hands; then, starting at the client's right foot, apply it up the client's leg (▶Figures 5.31 a and b).

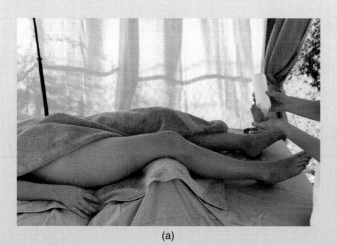

(a)

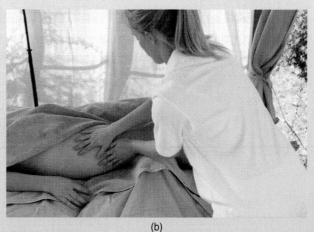

(b)

▶ **Figure 5.31**

TREATMENT 5.3 CONTINUED

6. Take a small amount of the mixture and rub it between your hands. Take more as needed during the treatment (▶Figures 5.32 a and b).

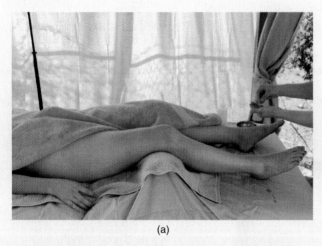
(a)

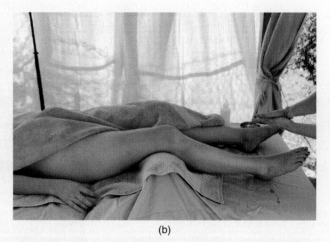
(b)

▶ **Figure 5.32**

7. Apply the mixture to the dorsal surface of the client's foot using small circular strokes to thoroughly exfoliate it (▶Figure 5.33).

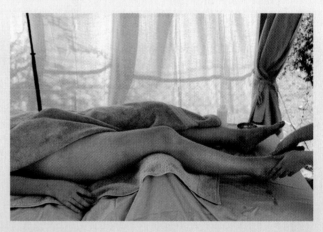

▶ **Figure 5.33**

CLINICAL ALERT !

Check with client about pressure and adjust as necessary.

8. Continue using small circular strokes up the ankle and anterior right leg (▶Figures 5.34 a and b). Redrape the client's right leg.

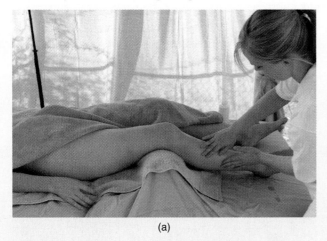 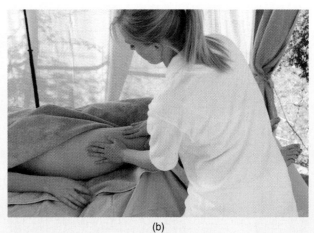

(a)   (b)

▶ **Figure 5.34**

9. Move to the client's left leg. Undrape and exfoliate the foot and leg the same as for the right leg. Redrape the client's left leg.

10. Move to the client's right arm and undrape it. Use small circular strokes to thoroughly exfoliate the client's hand and right arm, up to the shoulder (▶Figures 5.35 a and b). Redrape the client's right arm.

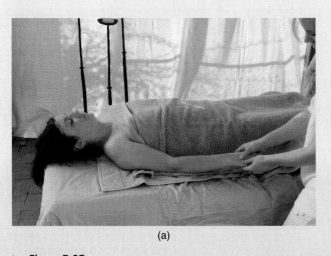 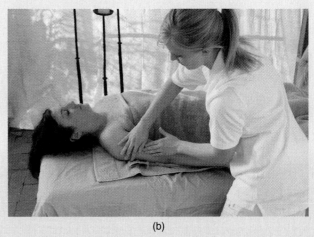

(a)   (b)

▶ **Figure 5.35**

11. Move to the client's left arm. Undrape and exfoliate the hand and arm the same as for the right arm. Redrape the client's left arm.

TREATMENT 5.3 CONTINUED

12. Move to the client's abdomen. Fold the large towel like an accordion cross-wise over the client's chest area and grasp the top of the large, length-wise towel on top of the client. As you unfold the cross-wise towel, fold down the length-wise towel until the client's chest is draped by the cross-wise towel, and the abdomen is undraped (▶Figures 5.36 a, b, c, and d).

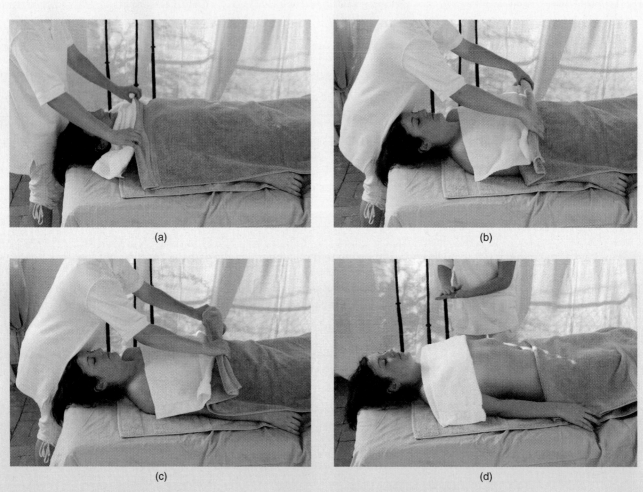

(a)

(b)

(c)

(d)

▶ **Figure 5.36**

13. Stand at the side of the table. Using smaller movements and a lighter touch, stroke in a clockwise direction (▶Figures 5.37 a and b).

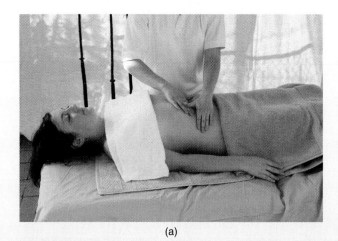

(a)

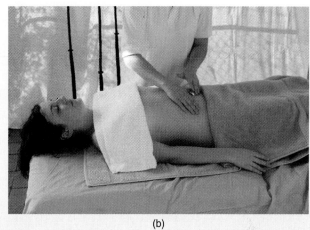

(b)

▶ **Figure 5.37**

Finish by exfoliating each of the client's sides and coming to the center of the abdomen (▶Figure 5.38).

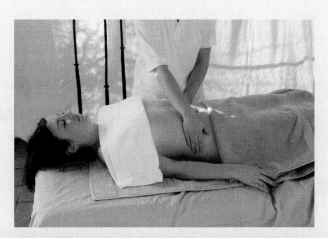

▶ **Figure 5.38**

14. Pull the towel up over the client's abdomen and draping towel on the client's chest area. Gently pull the draping towel out from under the sheet (▶Figure 5.39).

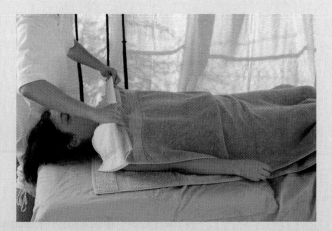

▶ **Figure 5.39**

TREATMENT 5.3 CONTINUED

15. Move to the head of the table. To exfoliate the client's upper chest area, use smaller movements and a lighter touch, working downward from the clavicles (▶Figures 5.40 a and b).

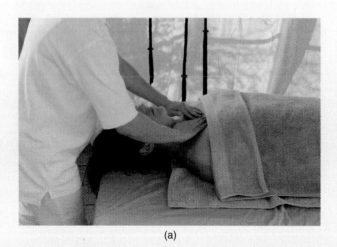
(a)

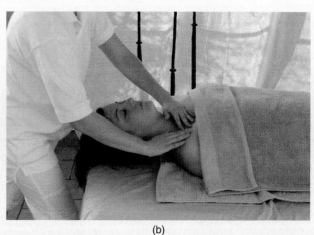
(b)

▶ **Figure 5.40**

16. If the client's face is to be included, use a light touch. With small gentle strokes, exfoliate from the client's chin to forehead.

17. Before the client turns over, the exfoliation substance can be removed. If using a wet table or Vichy shower, rinse the client thoroughly. If working in a dry room, use the dry room removal technique.

DRY ROOM REMOVAL TECHNIQUE

If the exfoliation is being done in a dry room with no access to a shower, the exfoliation substance can be removed by placing a warm, moist towel on the area for a few seconds. Remove a towel from the crock pot, cabi, or basin and wring it out if it is too wet (▶Figure 5.41 a). Apply the towel to the client's body and pat down firmly; then remove the substance with one firm, smooth stroke (▶Figure 5.41 b). Do not scrub or wipe with the towel. Use a new towel from the crock pot, cabi, or basin for each area of the body from which the substance is removed.

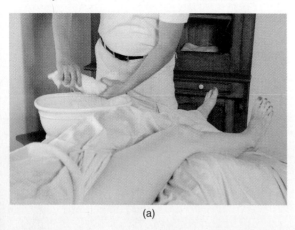
(a)

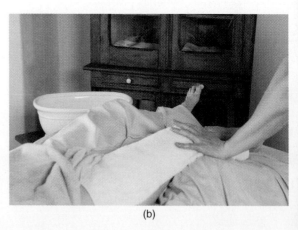
(b)

▶ **Figure 5.41**

TREATMENT 5.3 CONTINUED

18. Help the client turn over.

19. Move to the foot of the table. Standing at the foot of the table, undrape the client's left foot and leg. Exfoliate the sole of the client's foot using small, circular strokes (▶Figure 5.42).

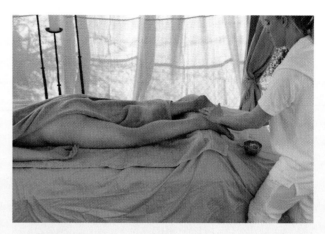

▶ **Figure 5.42**

20. Continue using small circular strokes up the posterior left leg, including the gluteal area (▶Figures 5.43 a and b). Use less pressure on the back of the client's knee. Redrape the client's left leg.

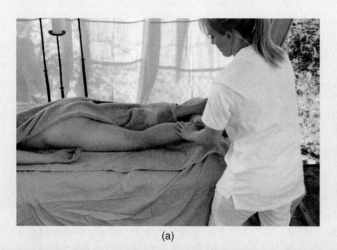

(a)

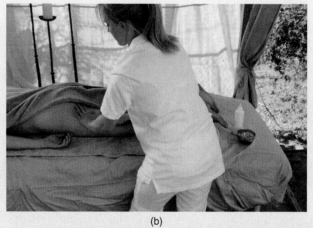

(b)

▶ **Figure 5.43**

21. Move to the client's right leg. Undrape and exfoliate the foot and leg the same as for the left leg. Redrape the client's right leg.

TREATMENT 5.3 CONTINUED

22. Move to the head of the table and undrape the client's back. Using small circular strokes, exfoliate the client's neck and back (▶Figure 5.44 a) and move around to the side of the table to include the lateral sides of the back. (Figure 5.44 b).

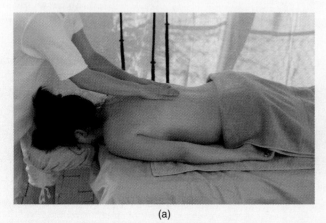
(a)

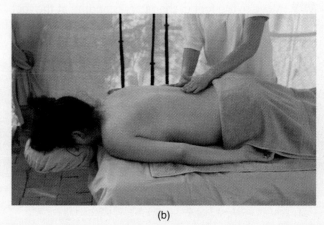
(b)

▶ **Figure 5.44**

23. Once the exfoliation is complete, the exfoliation substance needs to be removed. If using a wet table or Vichy shower, rinse the client thoroughly. If there is a separate shower facility, help the client off the table, draping the top sheet around for modesty. Guide the client to the shower and then back to the massage table after rinsing off. If the exfoliation is being done in a dry room with no access to a shower, use the dry room removal technique and skip to step 26.

24. While the client is in the shower, remove the top remaining sheet on the massage table, uncovering the fresh sheet underneath.

25. When the client returns, apply a moisturizing oil or lotion to the body.

26. If the exfoliation is being done in a dry room, remove the top remaining towel from underneath the client using the dry room sheet removal technique.

DRY ROOM SHEET REMOVAL TECHNIQUE

Ask the client to lift the head slightly. Reach across the client and grasp the sheet on both sides; gently pull down (▶Figure 5.45 a). Have the client lay the head back down and lift the shoulders; then lay the shoulders down and lift the hips (▶Figure 5.45 b); then lay the hips down as you continue to pull the sheet toward the foot of the table (▶Figure 5.45 c).

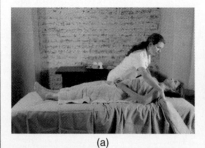
(a)

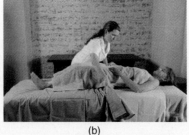
(b)

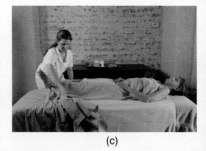
(c)

▶ **Figure 5.45**

27. When the exfoliation substance is removed, apply a moisturizing oil or lotion to the body.

TREATMENT 5.3 CONTINUED

After the Treatment
Once the exfoliation is complete, another treatment can be performed, such as a massage or body wrap. Otherwise, assist the client off the table, provide plenty of water to drink, and encourage rest.

Hygiene
The exfoliation mixture should be used on only one client; any leftover mixture should be immediately discarded. The sheets and towels should be laundered with hot water and detergent after each use. The bowls should be washed in warm, soapy water and rinsed between each use. Since a towel cabi holds multiple towels, it should be washed out daily and sprayed with disinfectant. Used towels should *never* be placed back in a towel cabi. If a crock pot is used, it should be used for only one treatment. It should be washed in warm, soapy water; rinsed; and sprayed with disinfectant between each use.

A full-body chemical, enzyme, or dissolving exfoliation treatment can be done in much the same way as Treatment 5.3, with a few modifications:

▶ Under equipment and supplies, approximately ½ cup of the exfoliation substance is needed and no additional liquid should be needed.

▶ The rationale, indications, and contraindications are all the same.

▶ Preparation is the same except to place the large towel horizontally at the head of the table

▶ The procedure is the same, with the exfoliation substance being applied either by hand or by painting it on the client's body. Once the exfoliation substance has been applied to both the front and back of the client, instead of being immediately removed, wrap the two top sheets around the client securely

(▶Figure 5.46 a), then wrap the towel around the client securely (▶Figure 5.46 b). The client should stay wrapped for about 20 minutes. After 20 minutes, the exfoliation substance should either be rinsed off or removed using the dry room removal technique.

▶ Once the exfoliation is complete, another treatment can be performed, such as a massage or body wrap. Otherwise, assist the client off the table, provide plenty of water to drink, and encourage rest.

▶ Hygiene is the same.

CLINICAL ALERT !

Practitioners and clients can be allergic to any or all of the chemical, enzyme, or dissolving exfoliation substances, including natural products such as milk and papaya. It is important for the practitioner to find out from clients any allergies they may have, and note them on an intake form, so there is written documentation. Practitioners allergic to any or all of the chemical, enzyme, or dissolving exfoliation substances should never use them on clients even when requested to do so, either by clients or employers.

People can develop allergies throughout their lives; therefore, every time a client arrives for a treatment, the practitioner should do a quick allergy update. Before any treatment is performed, the substance should be applied to a small area on the client's skin and on the practitioner's skin, usually the forearm, to see if there is an allergic reaction.

TO GET YOU STARTED

Papaya exfoliation for the face
Put the pulp of one papaya in a food processor or a blender and blend. Coat face with fresh papaya. Leave on 10 to 15 minutes. Rinse face with warm water and pat dry.

Enhanced papaya exfoliation for the body
½ ripe papaya, peeled and mashed
3 tbsp kaolin clay (green or white clay may be used)
3 drops essential oil (cooling oils such as peppermint or rosemary are recommended)
1 tsp lime juice

Combine all ingredients. Brush skin with a dry brush or loofah to prepare for absorption of the papaya mixture. Apply to skin and wait 20 minutes. Since this is a cooling mask, covering with towels before rinsing off may be necessary to keep warm.

Sweetened Yogurt Scrub for the face
1 tsp unrefined sugar
1 tbsp plain yogurt
½ tsp honey

Combine ingredients and apply to the face. Leave on 10 to 15 minutes. Rinse with warm water and gently pat skin dry.

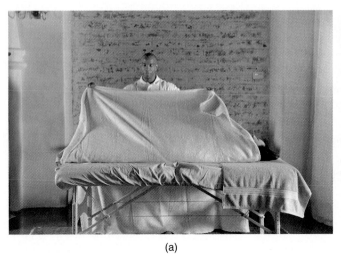

(a)

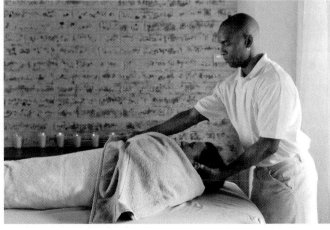

(b)

▶ **Figure 5.46**

Summary

Exfoliation is the removal of dead skin cells from the surface of the body. Benefits include brightening the skin, encouraging the production of new skin cells, making the skin smoother, allowing other preparations to hydrate and nourish the skin, and stimulating superficial blood and lymph flow. Exfoliation can be performed as a stand-alone treatment or as a preparation for other treatments, such as body wraps. Manual exfoliation is the physical process of applying friction with abrasives. Chemical, enzyme, or dissolving exfoliants are chemicals or enzymes that work by dissolving dead skin cells.

Manual exfoliation methods include dry brushing, in which natural bristle brushes, loofahs, nylon mitts, sisal mitts, and ayate cloths are used with mild, moderate, or vigorous pressure and speed. Scrubs or frictions use salts or coarser organic substances mixed with a fluid that allows them to glide onto the body. This tends to be a brisk treatment that leaves the client energized. Scrubs using salt or sugar are often referred to as salt glows or sugar glows. Body polishes are a gentler form of exfoliation using soft granules mixed with a skin emollient. Treatments that can be performed are full-body dry brushing, quick-prep dry brushing, manual exfoliations using natural substances, salt glows, sugar glows, and chemical (enzyme or dissolving) exfoliations using natural substances or commercial exfoliants.

Activities

1. List three benefits of skin exfoliation.

   _____

   _____

   _____

2. Name three different ways, using tools or substances, to exfoliate the body as a stand-alone treatment or in preparation for a wrap.

   _____

   _____

   _____

3. List three indications for dry-brushing treatment.

_____

_____

_____

4. On the figure, draw arrows indicating the appropriate direction of the application of strokes in a dry-brushing treatment.

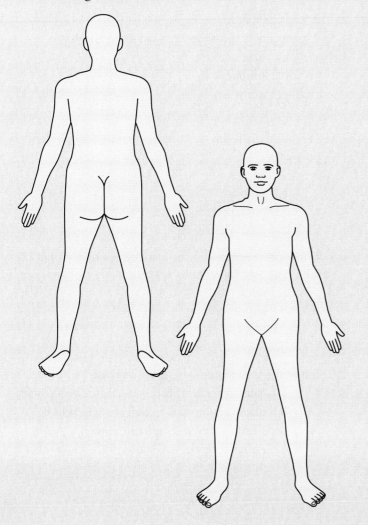

5. List three natural substances that can be used to exfoliate the skin.

_____

_____

_____

6. Receive an exfoliation treatment. Describe what type of exfoliation you received, including methods and materials used. What did you like about it? What did you not like about it? What would you have done differently?

_____

_____

_____

_____

_____

_____

_____

_____

_____

_____

Study Questions

1. Which of the following is an example of a chemical exfoliation treatment?
   a. dry brushing
   b. milk bath
   c. salt glow
   d. cornmeal scrub

2. The layer of the epidermis that is the most superficial is the stratum
   a. corneum
   b. spinosum
   c. basale
   d. granulosum

3. Which of the following treatments is the most vigorous?
   a. chemical exfoliation using papaya
   b. body polish using cornmeal
   c. salt glow using sea salt
   d. scrub using poppy seeds

4. Which of the following is an indication for an exfoliation treatment?
   a. high blood pressure
   b. fatigue
   c. sunburn
   d. inflammation

5. What should the practitioner do with the sugar mixture that is left over from performing a sugar glow?
   a. save it
   b. use it on another client
   c. discard it
   d. microwave it to kill any pathogens

6. To assist in the flow of lymph, dry-brush techniques are performed in the direction of the client's
   a. heart
   b. fingers
   c. toes
   d. back

7. A contraindication for exfoliation is skin that is
   a. dry
   b. sunburned
   c. itchy
   d. scaly

8. Which of the following can be used for its exfoliating properties?
   a. apples
   b. grapes
   c. pineapple
   d. all of the above

9. More pressure and time can be spent exfoliating which part of the client's body?
   a. neck
   b. abdomen
   c. feet
   d. upper chest

10. Exfoliation treatments benefit the body by
    a. causing surface blood vessels to vasoconstrict
    b. discouraging the growth of new skin cells
    c. slowing down lymphatic flow
    d. enhancing the hydrating effects of other preparations

Case Sample

Padma Chopak is a 45-year-old physician. She relaxes and stays fit by taking long hikes on the weekends. She has seen Antonio Mascarone regularly for massage for 6 months. Antonio has noticed that now that it is summer, Padma's skin is more dry and scaly, especially when she comes in for treatments after her hikes. He suggests to Padma that she try one of his exfoliation treatments.

1. Which exfoliation treatments would be best for Padma to receive?
2. What are the rationale, equipment and supplies, indications, contraindications, preparation, after-treatment care, and hygiene for these treatments?
3. Which questions should Antonio ask Padma to determine which treatment would be most beneficial?

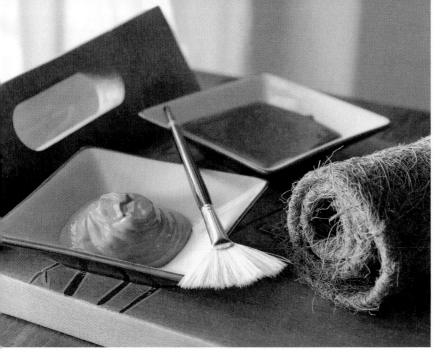

Pelotherapy

LEARNING OBJECTIVES

After studying this chapter, the reader will have the information to

1. Distinguish among the different types of pelotherapy.

2. Explain the therapeutic properties of muds, clays, peats, earth salts, paraffin, and geothermal therapy.

3. Describe different types of muds, clays, peats, and salts.

4. Delineate the supplies needed, rationale, indications, contraindications, treatment procedure, hygiene, and after-treatment care for a mud or peat body wrap.

5. Delineate the supplies needed, rationale, indications, contraindications, treatment procedure, hygiene, and after-treatment care for a mud, peat, or clay mask.

6. Delineate the supplies needed, rationale, indications, contraindications, treatment procedure, hygiene, and after-treatment care for a salt glow.

7. Delineate the supplies needed, rationale, indications, contraindications, treatment procedure, hygiene, and after-treatment care for paraffin applications.

8. Delineate the supplies needed, rationale, indications, contraindications, treatment procedure, hygiene, and after-treatment care for hot and cold stone therapy.

Nature has generously provided for us everything that we need to remain in good health.
—Father Sebastian Kneipp

KEY TERMS

Clays	Geothermal	Parafango	Peloids (pelos)
Emulsifier	Illite	Paraffin	Pelotherapy
Emulsion	Kaolinate	Peat	Smectite
Fuller's earth	Muds		

TYPES OF PELOTHERAPY

Pelotherapy is the therapeutic use of **muds, clays, peat**, earth salts, **paraffin**, and stones. *Pelo-* is Greek for "mud." Throughout time, civilizations have discovered therapeutic uses for the multitude of substances that make up the Earth's crust and are dissolved in the Earth's waters. Muds, peats, and clays have been integrated into cultural healing traditions. Stones were discovered to have curative powers through their ability to absorb heat and cold; these thermal aspects were then applied to the body. Salts have always been important to the health of the body, as discussed in Chapter 2. Early on, sources of salt were highly prized, both for flavoring food and for external application to the body.

Native Americans used many different types of soil for healing, purification, and spiritual ceremonies. Tribal warriors painted their faces with earthen clays tinted with the juice of roots and berries. Clays were, and still are, used in sweat lodge ceremonies and taken internally for medicinal reasons. The Egyptians used clay in their embalming process. The Greek physician Galen touted the properties of muds and clays. The Dead Sea, located in the Judean desert between Israel and Jordan, is the lowest point on Earth. The ancient world knew of the curative properties of its water, salts, and mud. For centuries, people have traveled there to heal their aching muscles and joints and to treat their skin disorders. Cultures in Mexico and South America used clays for ceremonial and health reasons (Eyton's Earth, 2007b; Knishinsky, 1998).

Many different types of soils and waters are found around the Earth, and they have varying compositions and therapeutic properties. For example, the Neydharting Moor near Salzburg, Austria, is the home of Austrian Moor Mud, a famous mud that is used as a therapeutic treatment for skin conditions, sports injuries, aching muscles and joints, arthritis, and rheumatism. In addition to minerals and trace minerals, it contains the beneficial remnants of plants. Canadian, German, and Hungarian Moor mud, also long known for their restorative properties, have different ratios of soil, minerals, and plants. Karlsbad, Czechoslovakia, is rich with hot springs and mud high in minerals salts, CO_2, calcite, and trace iron deposits. Argiletz clay, well known for its use in health and beauty treatments, is mined from the bedrock quarries in

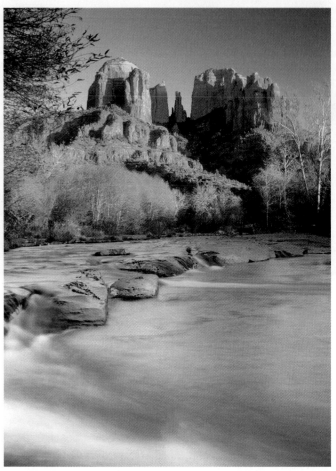

(Chad Ehlers/Stock Connection)

Argiletz, France. Natural red clay from Corona, CA, is known for its purifying effects, and volcanic mud from Calistoga, CA, may differ in its ash and mineral content from volcanic mud from Costa Rica, but they are both useful for therapeutic treatments (Crebbin-Baily, Harcup, and Harrington, 2005; Minton, 2008b; Williams, 2007).

Paraffin is a substance used in pelotherapy that is derived from petroleum, wood, coal, or shale. It is a waxy by-product from the processing of these materials (Merriam-Webster Dictionary, 2004). Discovered to be a good insulator, it is used in spa and hydrotherapy treatments to increase heat penetration into the body. Similar to paraffin is **parafango,** which also provides the slow release of healing warmth. It is a mixture of dehydrated volcanic mud and paraffin with talcum and magnesium oxide added.

Geothermal comes from the Greek words *geo,* meaning "earth" and *thermal* meaning "heat." Smooth river stones that were warmed in the sun were used by early humans to soothe their aches and pains, and stones chilled in the snow were applied to reduce swelling and relieve pain. Stones were used instinctively by many populations for many generations before modern science established the physiological reasons for their therapeutic effects (Nelson and Scrivner, 2004).

DID YOU KNOW?

Peloids, or **pelos,** are the fine grains making up muds, clays, and peat. They are highly absorbent and possess unique heat-retention abilities. They can be thought of as the "pulp" that holds the heat.

It is important to note that practitioners should never go beyond their scope of practice. They need to check their local and/or state regulations regarding the performance in their practice of the treatments presented in this chapter. Some areas require that anyone who performs body wraps and masks on another person be an esthetician or cosmetologist. It is recommended that practitioners check with all pertinent regulatory bodies to make sure they are in compliance with the laws that govern them and their practice.

MUDS

Sometimes the terms *mud* and *clay* are used interchangeably because they can resemble each other. However, they have different constituents and different properties and need to be considered separately.

Muds are differentiated based on the soils and marine sediments from which they are derived. Muds are composed mostly of silica, alumina, water, iron, alkalis, and trace minerals—Ca^{++}, Mg^{++}, Na^+, K^+, SO_4^{2-} (sulfur oxide), Cu, and Zn. Inorganic muds contain mostly minerals that result from lake and river sedimentation and have little organic material. Volcanic muds can be found near hot mineral springs; some spas specialize in hot mud baths for clients. Organic muds are formed from algae, plant, and animal matter that has mixed with lime, clay, and sand in the soil. The colors of the muds depend on the amounts of various minerals in them. For instance, muds that are red have a high amount of iron (Ashworth and Little, 2001b; Mitchell, 1993).

Therapeutic Properties of Muds

One of several properties of muds that can make them therapeutic is their mineral content. The minerals in muds are in ionic form, which means they are either cations or anions (recall from Chapter 2 that cations are positively charged ions, and anions are negatively charged ions). The minerals (ions) in muds help with deep skin cleansing and aid in the removal of waste products by their drawing action, which also can stimulate local blood and lymphatic flow. Some of the small ions in the muds can pass into the body through the skin, although the structure and properties of the skin do not allow many to do so.

Muds easily suspend in water or other liquid, forming an emulsion. An **emulsion** is basically a fluid that has particles suspended in it because the particles do not dissolve. There is a lot of room for water molecules in and among the particles of the muds (Mitchell, 1993). When applied, the combination of mud particles and water forms a covering that acts as an insulator on the body,

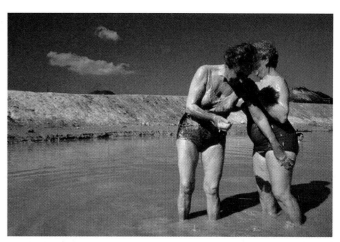

(Catrina Genovese/Omni-Photo Communications, Inc.)

trapping heat and keeping it from radiating away while also keeping water from evaporating from the body. Thus, muds are excellent warming and hydrating treatments. The trapped heat also serves to increase local blood circulation. The suspended particles of mud are of various sizes and textures, and they can have an abrasive quality. This makes them useful for exfoliation, which also stimulates superficial blood circulation.

Overall, muds are used therapeutically to help relieve pain in muscles and joints and pain from tendonitis, muscle strain, joint injuries such as sprains, and noninflammatory stages of arthritis and bursitis and to soothe certain skin conditions (Abel, 2005; Barron, 2003; Crebbin-Bailey, Harcup, and Harrington, 2005; O'Rourke, 1995; Williams, 2007).

Types of Muds

Muds are categorized based on their region of origin and composition. New ones are continually being discovered, and new treatments are developed that are location specific. ▶Table 6.1 shows representative examples of muds from the United States and around the world.

CLAYS

Because they are so plentiful and because they have so many uses, clays are employed in industry and agriculture, as well as therapeutically. Clays are found throughout the world, and many regional clays have become well known. For example, one of the largest clay deposits in the world is located in Bavaria, Germany. The most recognized clay comes from a large deposit in France, which is why it is sometimes argued that the French have the most experience in the modern use of clays. The term *Indian Clay* refers to a product from India, where some of the highest-quality clays deposits in the world are found (Eyton's Earth, 2007b).

TABLE 6.1		
Examples of muds from the United States and around the world		
Mud	**Location**	**Comments**
Calistoga Mud	Calistoga, CA	Volcanic mud and hot springs known for their healing properties; Native Americans first made use of the mud baths, and later the Spaniards; today, many spas are located in the area
Natural red clay	Glen Ivy Hot Springs Corona, CA	Clay known for healing and purifying; Native Americans designated the area as sacred; later, the Spaniards took advantage of the healing benefits; today, a spa on the site offers treatments from local mud (http://www.glenivy.com)
Dead Sea Mud	Dead Sea, Israel	Mineral-rich, highly saline mud that draws impurities and retains heat (see ▶Figure 6.1); used for a wide range of skin disorders such as psoriasis and eczema; especially beneficial for muscle pain and stiffness, arthritis, and other joint pain
Rotorua Thermal	New Zealand	Silky volcanic mud; rich in minerals and trace elements; QE Health (formerly known as the Queen Elizabeth Hospital) in Rotorua uses the mud (see ▶Figure 6.2) as part of its standard care in the treatment of arthritis and other joint conditions (http://www.rotoruanz.com/attractions/spa_wellness.php, http://www.qe-health.co.nz)
Muds and Clays	Australia	Found near mineral-rich, natural springs; harvested from undeveloped areas so are essentially free from chemical pollutants; sun dried after being harvested; used for more than 60,000 years by Aboriginal tribes for healing, sacred, and ceremonial purposes; muds and clays have only recently become available outside Aboriginal culture (http://www.aeocaustralia.com/)
Rasul (Rhassoul)	Morocco	Lava clay (see ▶Figure 6.3) mined in the Atlas Mountains of Eastern Morocco; used alone or in a combination mud and steam treatment originating in the Middle East; a description of a Rasul (Rhassoul) spa treatment is included on page 197–198.

(Calistoga Spas, 2008; Glen Ivy Hot Springs Spa, 2008; Minton, 2008b; Williams, 2007).

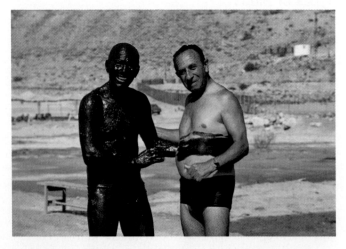

▶ **Figure 6.1** Mineral-rich mud from Israel's Dead Sea draws impurities and retains heat, is used to treat a range of skin disorders, and can be beneficial for muscle pain and stiffness, arthritis, and other joint pain. *(Linda Troeller/Phototake NYC)*

Therapeutic Properties of Clays

Clays are composed mostly of silica, alumina, water, iron, alkalis, and trace minerals—Ca^{++}, Mg^{++}, Na^+ and K^+. Marine-based clays have a higher mineral content than soil-based ones do. It is the mineral content of clays and their ability to suspend easily in an emulsion with water or other liquid that give them their therapeutic properties. As with muds, the minerals in clays are in ionic form, which means they are either cations or anions (positively or negatively charged ions). Clays draw impurities from the body to do deep skin cleansing and aid in the removal of waste products. As with muds, this drawing action stimulates local blood circulation and lymphatic flow. The ionic composition is also how clays tighten and tone the skin: water from the skin is drawn to the high concentration of ions in the clays and, as it leaves, the skin tightens. Some of the small ions in the clays may pass into the body through the skin, although the structure and properties of the skin do not allow many to do so.

Clays form emulsions with water or other liquids because clays are very porous; there is a lot of room for water

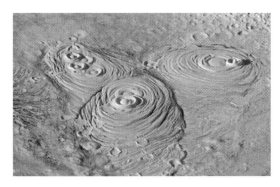

▶ **Figure 6.2** New Zealand's Rotorua thermal is a silky volcanic mud that is rich in minerals and trace elements. *(Rob Francis/Robert Harding World Imagery)*

molecules in and among the particles of the clays. Because of the water, clays readily react to temperature and hold heat especially well (Knishinsky, 1998; Mitchell, 1993; Williams, 2007). They are excellent for heat applications, such as to warm the body or provide local heat penetration into tight muscles and aching, noninflamed joints.

Clays can be taken internally as well. Before the advent of nutritional supplements, people would eat small bits of clay or "medicinal earth" to replenish their minerals and absorb toxins from their digestive tracts. Today, bentonite is the clay that provides trace minerals for most commercially prepared mineral nutrition supplements. Clays are also still taken internally to absorb toxins (Abehsera, 2001; Knishinsky, 1998).

Types of Clays

Even though clays may be similar in composition, no two clays are completely alike; even clays found in the same location but in different veins can vary somewhat. There are many different ways to categorize clays: by their physical properties, the location in which they are found, or their color. As will be seen, individual clays can fit into more than one category.

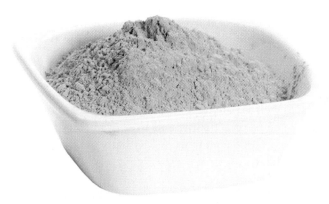

▶ **Figure 6.3** Moroccan Rasul can be used alone or in a combination mud and steam treatment originating in the Middle East. *(Photo courtesy of Universal Companies, Inc.)*

Classification by Physical Properties

Smectite clays are made of mineral crystals that absorb water and swell considerably. Most smectite was created through the chemical reaction of seawater or rain water on volcanic ash as the ash settled from volcanic eruptions early in the Earth's history. Over time, deposits of smectite clays were covered by other layers of earth and rock. Smectite absorbs moisture and toxins present in or on skin it. Examples of smectite clays are bentonites and Fuller's earth.

Kaolinate is made of mineral crystals that have a low capacity to swell when in contact with water. It is mined in China, Brazil, France, the United Kingdom, Germany, India, Australia, Korea, and, in the United States, in Georgia, Florida, and South Carolina. The commercial names for it are kaolin, China white, and China clay.

Illite is made of mineral crystals but is a nonexpanding clay. In other words, it does not swell when in contact with water. Illite is common in sediments and soils throughout the world. An example of illite clay is French green (Knishinsky, 1998; Mitchell, 1993. U.S. Geological Survey, 1999).

Classification by Color

Mineral content determines the color of clay. The color classification was created to distinguish particular properties among clays, including the ability to draw impurities and balance the skin's natural pH. These clays, in addition to other properties, are highly absorbent, drying, detoxifying, and toning and are used in face masks, back masks, and full-body masks (although oil is sometimes applied first to alleviate the drying effect):

- ▶ **green**—intensely drawing, exfoliating, and purifying
- ▶ **red**—best for dry and sensitive skin types
- ▶ **yellow**—gentle and revitalizing; good for sensitive, sun-damaged skin
- ▶ **white**—excellent for body powder and hand masks; gentle for mature skin
- ▶ **pink**—good for daily use; gentle and softening

Classification by Location

French Argiletz clay, bentonite, Coso green clay, montmorillonite, and pascalite are all named for the area of the world in which they were initially discovered. Since initial discovery and naming of these clays, sources have been found in places other than the original location, which is why, for example, there are different types of bentonite.

Montmorillonite—discovered in Montmorillon, France, in 1847. Found in many locations worldwide, it is a green clay and a smectite.

Bentonite—named for the Benton Formation in eastern Wyoming; discovered around 1890. Closely resembling montmorillonite, it is usually found as green clay with a high pH. The quality of these clays varies according to the location of the deposit, and the mineral content varies quite a bit among different sources. Sodium bentonite, calcium bentonite, and magnesium bentonite are all found in various places around the world. Bentonite is a smectite.

French Argiletz Clay—mined in Argiletz, France. After it is mined, it is sun dried. A versatile clay, it comes in all five clay colors and is used quite often for face, hand, and body masks. Sometimes this clay is referred to as French clay, as in French green or French white. French Argiletz clay is an illite (Eyton's Earth, 2007b; Knishinsky, 1998; Mitchell, 1993; Williams, 2007).

Pascalite—unearthed in Wyoming by French Canadian fur trapper Emile Pascale in 1830. It is a white clay that closely resembles montmorillonite and bentonite, but it is a nonswelling clay or illite (Eyton's Earth, 2007a). See ▶Figure 6.4 for examples of different clays.

Fuller's Earth

A name commonly recognized in the clay realm is **Fuller's earth,** a smectite derived from a different geological layer of the earth than other smectites so it has a different chemical composition from typical smectite clays. Its name comes from how it was used in the past as a cleaner. In powder form, this clay has the ability to absorb lanolin (oil that naturally occurs in wool) and other oils. It was kneaded into

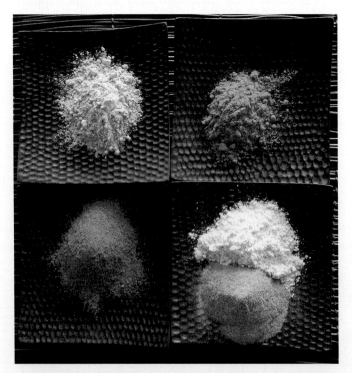

▶ **Figure 6.4** Different clays. Top right: bentonite; top left: yellow Argiletz; bottom left: Moroccan red; bottom right: kaolinite (top) and French green (bottom).

wool clothing where it absorbed lanolin, human body oils, and the dirt attached to them. The clay was shaken out and the piece of clothing was "fluffed up," or "fulled" (Ashworth and Little, 2001a). Fullers were, in fact, the precursors to dry cleaners, and the clay was called "Fuller's earth."

Fuller's earth is mined in many areas of the United States, including Georgia, Florida, Texas, and Illinois. It is also mined in England and Japan. Today, Fuller's earth is used therapeutically for its ability to draw oils in masks for oily skin and to treat acne (*Encyclopedia Britannica,* 2008a).

PEAT

For the past 200 years, peat has been used therapeutically in baths and packs. Peat is an organic soil that contains minerals, organic material, water, and trapped air. It is formed by the decomposition of layers of plants, mainly mosses, and animal matter under bodies of water. The properties of the different peats depend on the local flora and fauna that made up the layers. Most peats used in spa therapies are a combination of moss and sedge, a marshland plant. Peats are mostly cultivated in Ireland, Austria, Germany, the Czech Republic, and other Eastern European countries.

The substances in peat that contribute to its therapeutic effectiveness are organic acids and minerals. These include fulvic acid, humic acids, sulfur compounds, magnesium, manganese, and iron. Low-moor peats are so called because they are in the deeper layers of peat; they are thought to have a greater amount of the acids and minerals. High-moor peats are in the shallower layers of peats; they are thought to have a lesser amount of the organic acids and minerals (Food and Agricultural Organization of the United Nations, 2001; Torv Forsk, Swedish Peat Research Foundation, 2008).

The acids contribute to peat's ability to draw and absorb toxins from the body. Physically, peat contains micropores, which allow it to take in water like a sponge. Like muds, peat can form a covering that acts as an insulator on the body. It keeps heat from radiating away from the body while also keeping water from evaporating from the body. Thus, peats are excellent warming and hydrating treatments. The heat also increases local blood and lymph circulation.

Peats are used to help relieve aching muscles and joints, as well as pain from muscle injuries and noninflammatory stages of arthritis, and to soothe skin disorders (Moor Spa, 2008). ▶Figure 6.5 visually compares mud, peat, and clay.

Moor Mud

Moor mud is a type of peat that is also known as "black mud," because of its appearance. It is the mineral-rich sedimentation that is deposited at the bottom of lakes and rivers fed by both hot and cool springs. The hot springs contribute volcanic ash to the mixture of plant material settling to the bottom of the water. The lakes from which moor mud is taken maintain a temperature around 86°F, but the combination of hot and cool water creates much circulation in the lake. This enhances the decomposition of organic material; layers and layers build up over time. The Neydharting Moor is in a glacial valley that was once a lake, and the moor has been developing for more than 20,000 to 30,000 years. Neydharting Moor mud is an organic mud and is known for being pure and nutrient-rich (SpaElegance.com, 2001).

Moor mud has a very low pH, usually around 3.54. The application of moor mud can assist in the regeneration of the acid mantel of the skin, which protects the body from harmful bacteria. High-grade moor muds come from Austria, Germany, Hungary, and the Czech Republic. In fact, the town of Torf Krasno in the Czech Republic is renowned for its famous organic moor mud. Torf Krasno is the largest supplier of medicinal mud and peat in the Czech Republic and provides mud and peat to clinics and spas worldwide (Lynch, 2000). In North America, Canadian moor is known for its mineral-rich qualities. See ▶Figure 6.6 for an example of moor mud.

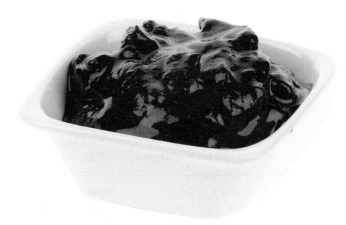

▶ **Figure 6.6** Hungarian moor mud can assist in the regeneration of the acid mantel of the skin, which protects the body from harmful bacteria. *(Photo courtesy of Universal Companies, Inc.)*

TREATMENTS

Body Wraps

Body wraps can be used in conjunction with many different substances. Seaweed, crèmes, muds, clays, and peats are all commonly used materials, as well as sheets soaked in an herbal infusion (discussed more in Chapter 8). It is important to note, though, that new wraps are being continually developed. For example, avocado, aloe, and chocolate wraps are currently popular. Spas and individual therapists can offer site-specific specialties such as, perhaps, a prickly pear gel wrap in the Southwest. As more and more organic substances are discovered to have healing properties, innovations in body wrap materials are inevitable.

It is always important to begin with an exfoliation. Removing the dead skin cells enables the substance being used to work more efficiently. This can be done with any of the treatments outlined in Chapter 5. The quick-prep dry-brushing technique is a standard exfoliation that can be done before any body wrap, or the full-body dry brushing can be performed if clients desire a longer treatment.

There are many opportunities for creativity, depending on what the client chooses or what is included or offered on the spa treatment menu. For example, a desert mineral salt scrub may be offered before a desert herbal wrap; a

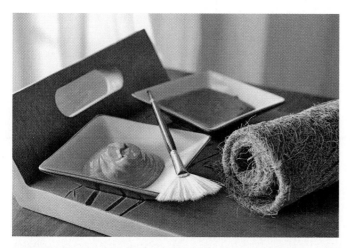

▶ **Figure 6.5** Top, mud; right, peat; left, clay

CLINICAL ALERT !

Practitioners and clients can be allergic to any or all substances used in body wraps. It is important for the practitioner to find out from clients any allergies they may have, and note them on an intake form, so there is written documentation. Practitioners allergic to any or all body wrap substances should never use them on clients even when requested to do so, either by clients or employers.

People can develop allergies throughout their lives; therefore, every time a client arrives for a treatment, the practitioner should do a quick allergy update. Before any treatment is performed, the substance should be applied to a small area on the client's skin and on the practitioner's skin, usually the forearm, to see if there is an allergic reaction.

sea salt glow can be coupled with a seaweed body wrap; a coffee scrub can be offered along with a chocolate wrap.

There are many ways to perform wraps. Practitioners who work in spas should note that each spa has its own body wrap protocols and trains its practitioners accordingly. What is presented in this chapter may or may not be consistent with how individual spas perform their wraps. However, by practicing the procedures in this chapter, practitioners, whether they work in a spa, clinic, or private practice, will acquire foundational skills, become comfortable handling supplies and equipment, and become able to knowledgeably discuss body wrap options with clients.

The body wrap treatment itself typically takes 35 to 40 minutes. The treatment time can be extended to 60 or 90 minutes when supplemented with other bodywork treatments such as a full-body dry brushing, massage therapy, shiatsu, acupressure, reflexology, and so forth. Some body wraps use crèmes and gels, such as aloe vera, cocoa butter, shea butter, and so forth. An ideal way to conclude the wrap is to perform a short gliding massage so the body wrap substance is evenly distributed and absorbed.

It is important that the practitioner inform the client that portions of the treatment have less conservative draping than a regular massage does. If a wet table and Vichy shower or other water source will be used to remove the body wrap substance, the practitioner needs to inform clients that the clients will have minimal covering during the showering process. Although the practitioner is used to this, clients may not be. Clients need to be given the opportunity to decline the treatment if they are not comfortable with this.

The equipment and supplies for body wraps can be purchased at local stores or online; the body wrap substance needs to be purchased through a spa treatment supply store.

Masks

Masks can be performed using many different substances. Seaweed, crèmes, muds, clays, and peats are all commonly used materials. A mask treatment should always begin with an exfoliation, since removing the dead skin cells enables the mask substance being used to work more efficiently. This can be done with any of the treatments outlined in Chapter 5, with the exception of a salt glow that uses coarse salt. The coarse salt would be too abrasive on the delicate skin of the face. However, a polish using a fine grain salt is much less abrasive and could be used if the client tolerates it. A brush used for the facial exfoliation should be softer than one used on the rest of the body.

There are many opportunities for creativity, depending on what the client chooses or what is included or offered on the spa treatment menu. For example, a desert mineral salt scrub may be offered before a Sedona clay mask, or a sea salt glow can be coupled with a marine clay mask.

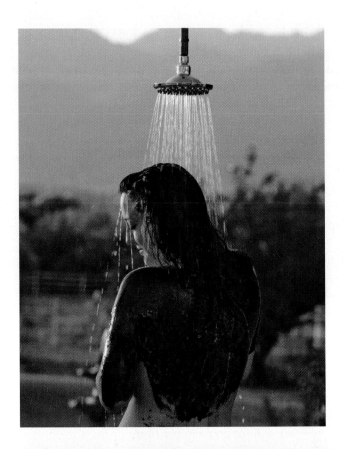

TO GET YOU STARTED

Mud or Clay Mask For Oily Skin
1–2 tsp mud; mud powder mixed with water, mud gel, or crème; clay or clay powder mixed with water
½–1 tsp honey
water
3–4 drops tea tree essential oil

Exfoliate the face. Add enough water to make a thin paste out of the mud or clay. Stir in honey and tea tree essential oil until well mixed. Apply to face and let dry for 10 to 15 minutes. Remove with warm water and washcloth. Gently blot skin dry and apply a moisturizer.

Mud and Clay Back Treatment
Masks can also be applied to the back.
½ cup clay (bentonite, Fuller's earth, or any green or white clay)
1 cup moor mud gel
plastic wrap
towel
small blanket

Exfoliate the back. Mix the clay and mud gel together. Apply the mixture evenly on the back. Cover the application with plastic, then a towel, and then a small blanket. Leave on for 20 to 25 minutes. Remove with a moist, warm towel and gently blot the skin dry. Apply moisturizing lotion to the back.

TREATMENT 6.1

Mud or Peat Body Wrap

Rationale

A mud or peat body wrap can be done for any or all of the following physiological effects:

- Absorptive: a small amount of minerals pass through the skin
- Tonifier: strengthens vitality and the immune system
- Vasodilator: increases local blood flow
- Analgesic: relieves pain
- Detoxifier: elimination of toxins
- Emollient: soothing to the skin
- Sedative: induces a state of deep relaxation
- Thermodynamic: sends deep, penetrating heat into muscles and joints

Indications

- tight joints (from noninflammatory conditions)
- muscle spasms, tightness, or strain
- skin disorders such as eczema and psoriasis
- need to balance skin's pH
- need for relaxation
- need for detoxification
- need for skin cleansing

Contraindications

- heart conditions
- untreated hypertension
- inflammation
- vascular disease, including varicose veins
- numbness/loss of sensation in area
- skin conditions made worse by heat
- intolerance to heat
- broken or irritated skin
- high body temperature (fever)
- claustrophobia
- pregnancy

Equipment and Supplies (see ▶Figures 6.7 a and b)

- exfoliation tools or ingredients for a scrub
- mud, mud powder mixed with water, mud gel or crème, or peat (¼ to ½ cup)
- small, nonmetal bowl—nonmetal because mud and peat react chemically with metal and their properties will change; likewise, mud and peat should not be stored in metal containers
- three cloth sheets (one fitted and two flat)
- insulating sheet (rubber, plastic, Mylar, etc.)
- wool blanket
- one beach towel, approximately 35″ × 65″
- two large towels, approximately 30″ × 60″
- If there is access to a shower, textured washcloth or bath scrubby the client can use to remove the mud or peat
- If there is no access to a shower, a basin of warm water and three to four towels, approximately 18″ × 30″, for substance removal are needed (a towel cabi or crock pot filled with moist towels can also be used; more than three to four towels may be necessary for clients who have a large body size or a lot of body hair, since it may be more difficult to remove mud or peat from the hair)
- washcloth
- small bowl
- cool water

TREATMENT 6.1 CONTINUED

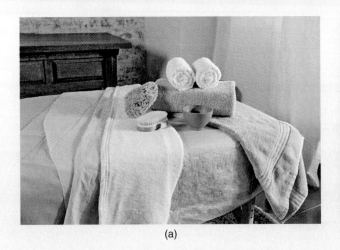
(a)

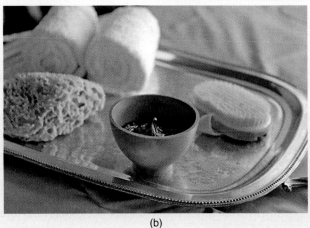
(b)

▶ **Figure 6.7**

Preparation

1. Layer the table in the following order (see ▶Figure 6.8):
   - Fitted sheet to protect table
   - One large towel placed horizontally across the head of the table
   - Wool blanket placed horizontally across the table, on top of the towel, leaving enough room for the head to rest on the towel
   - One large towel placed horizontally across the end of the table, on top of the wool blanket
   - Flat sheet placed horizontally on top of the wool blanket
   - Insulating sheet placed horizontally on top of the cloth sheet
   - One flat sheet placed lengthwise on top of the insulating sheet
   - Beach towel placed lengthwise on top of the flat sheet

2. Place the mud or peat in the small bowl; position the bowl within easy reach.
3. If working in a dry room and using a crock pot or cabi, turn it on to warm the towels for substance removal at the end of the treatment. Moisten the three to four (or more) 18″ × 30″ towels and put them in

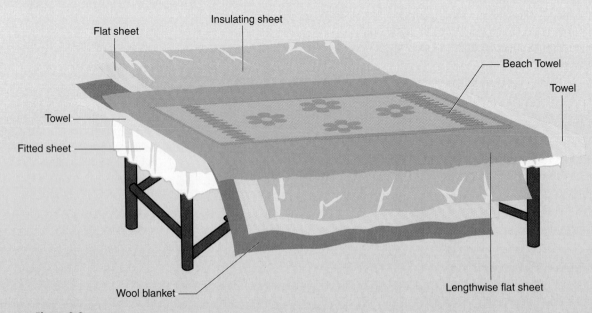

▶ **Figure 6.8**

the crock pot or cabi. If using the basin of warm water and towels, place the basin in a convenient place to fill it with warm water during the treatment.

4. Fill the small bowl with cool water and place the washcloth in it. Position it within easy reach.
5. Leave the room while the client gets on the table under the beach towel, lying prone.

Procedure

Perform a pre–body wrap exfoliation. The quick-prep dry-brushing procedure from Chapter 5 is described here, but any of the exfoliation treatments in Chapter 5 can be performed. If the large towel is used for draping, then there will be no need to undrape the extremities to perform the exfoliation.

Standing at the foot of the table, undrape the client's left leg and gluteal region. Working toward the client's heart, start brushing at the feet, move up the leg, and include the gluteals. Redrape the client's left leg. Move to the client's right leg. Undrape and brush the foot, leg, and gluteal region the same as for the left leg. Redrape the client's right leg.

CLINICAL ALERT !

Check with the client about pressure and adjust as necessary.

2. Move to the client's left arm and undrape it. Brush the palm of the client's hand and fingers. Beginning at the client's wrist, brush up the arm, stroking from the wrist toward the client's heart. Redrape the client's left arm. Move to the client's right arm. Undrape and brush the hand and arm the same as for the left arm. Redrape the client's right arm.

3. Move to the head of the table and undrape the back. Starting at the neck and shoulders, brush down to the client's mid-back. Move to the right side of the table. Reaching across the client's back, brush the client's left lumbar to mid-back area, using angling, upward strokes toward the client's heart. Move to the left side of the table. Brush the client's right lumbar to mid-back area the same as for the left side. Redrape the back.

4. Help the client turn over.

5. Standing at the foot of the table, undrape the client's right leg. Working toward the client's heart, start brushing at the feet and move up the leg. Redrape the client's right leg. Move to the client's left leg. Undrape and brush the foot and leg the same as for the right leg. Redrape the client's left leg.

6. Move to the client's abdomen and drape the large towel across the client's chest area. Have the client hold it firmly as you pull the sheet inferiorly until the client's abdomen is undraped. Using smaller strokes, brush the client's abdomen in a clockwise direction. Finish the abdomen by brushing up each side and coming to the center of the abdomen.

7. Redrape the client's abdomen by pulling the sheet up over the client's abdomen and the draping towel on the client's chest area. Move to one side of the client and, while the client holds the sheet firmly, gently pull the draping towel out from under the sheet.

8. Move to the client's right arm and undrape it. Brush the back of the client's hand and fingers. Beginning at the client's wrist, brush up the arm, stroking from the wrist toward the client's heart. Redrape the client's right arm. Move to the client's left arm. Undrape and brush the hand and arm the same as for the right arm. Redrape the client's left arm.

9. Move to the head of the table. To brush the client's upper chest area, start at the right clavicle and brush downward three times; then brush downward three times from the left clavicle.

Application of mud or peat

Remove the sheet immediately under the client. Ask the client to lift the head slightly. Reach across the client and grasp the sheet on both sides; gently pull down. Have the client lay the head back down, and lift the shoulders, then shoulders down and lift the hips, then hips down as you continue to pull the sheet down toward the foot of the table (▶ Figures 6.9 a, b, and c). Set the sheet aside. Make sure that the client's shoulders are slightly below the top of the insulating sheet.

TREATMENT 6.1 CONTINUED

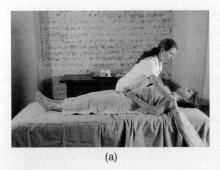
(a)

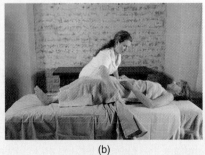
(b)

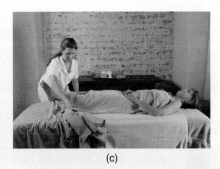
(c)

▶ **Figure 6.9**

2. Help the client sit up and quickly apply the mud or peat to the back with long, smooth strokes, covering the area thoroughly (▶Figures 6.10 a, b, c, and d). Help the client lie back down.

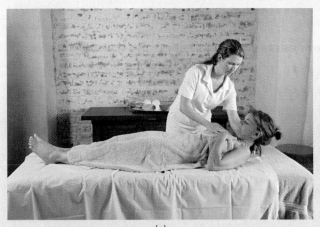
(a)

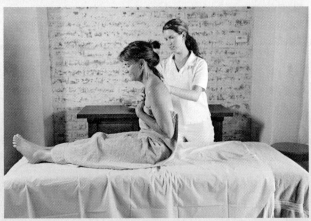
(b)

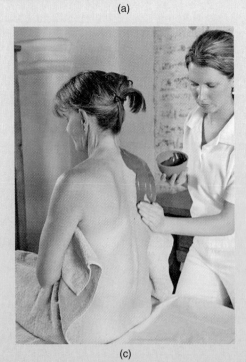
(c)

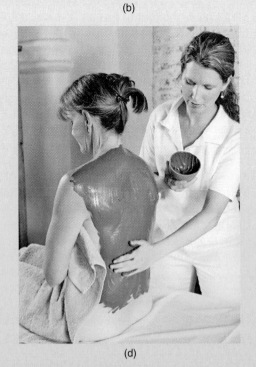
(d)

▶ **Figure 6.10**

TREATMENT 6.1 CONTINUED

3. Move to the client's left leg and ask the client to flex the knee while draping carefully and securely (▶Figures 6.11 a, b, and c). To stabilize the client's leg, gently sit on the foot.

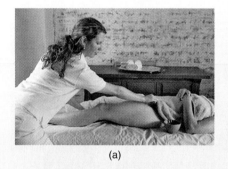 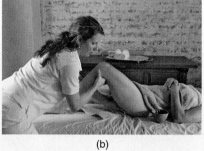 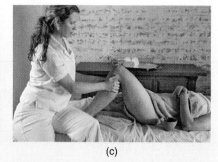

(a)　　　　　　　　　　(b)　　　　　　　　　　(c)

▶ **Figure 6.11**

Apply the mud or peat to the client's posterior leg with one smooth stroke. Grasp the client's ankle and lay the leg flat (▶Figures 6.12 a and b).

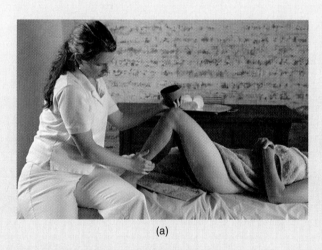 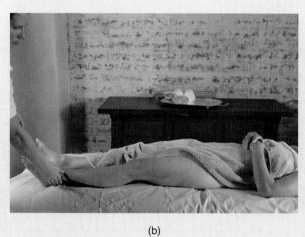

(a)　　　　　　　　　　(b)

▶ **Figure 6.12**

TREATMENT 6.1 CONTINUED

4. Apply the mud or peat to the client's left anterior leg with long, smooth strokes. Cover the client's left leg with the insulating sheet to prevent chilling (▶Figures 6.13 a, b, c, and d).

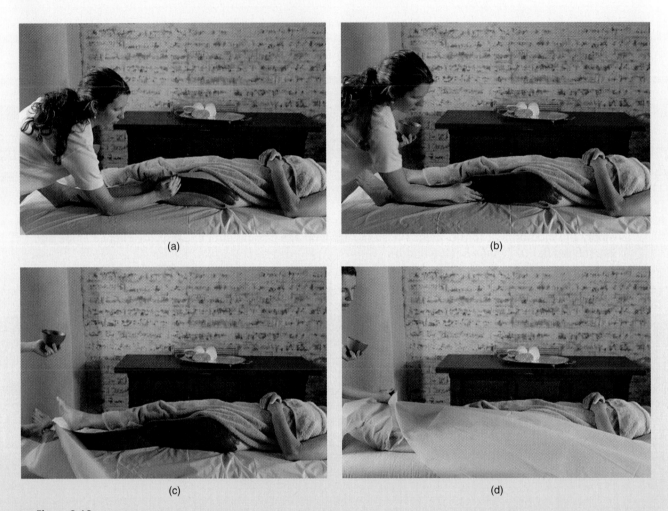

(a)

(b)

(c)

(d)

▶ **Figure 6.13**

5. Move to the client's right leg and apply the mud or peat to the posterior and anterior leg in the same manner as for the left leg. Cover the client's right leg with the insulating sheet to prevent chilling.

TREATMENT 6.1 CONTINUED

6. Move to the client's abdomen and drape one of the large towels across the client's chest area and have the client hold it firmly. Pull the bottom, draping towel inferiorly until the client's abdomen is undraped. Apply the mud or peat to the abdomen in a clockwise motion (▶Figures 6.14 a, b, and c).

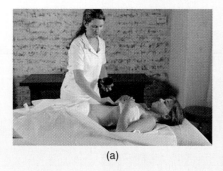
(a)

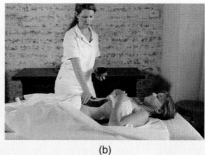
(b)

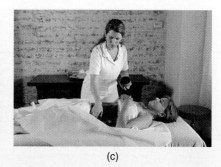
(c)

▶ **Figure 6.14**

7. Move to the client's left arm and apply the mud or peat to the posterior and anterior arm with long, smooth strokes (▶Figures 6.15 a, b, and c). Cover the client's left arm and abdomen with the insulating sheet to prevent chilling. Move to the client's right arm and apply the mud or peat the same as for the left arm. Cover the client's right arm with the insulating sheet to prevent chill.

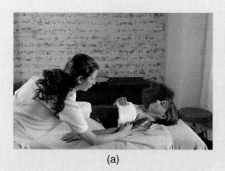
(a)

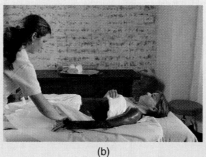
(b)

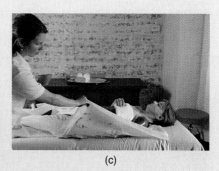
(c)

▶ **Figure 6.15**

8. Move to the head of the table and apply the body wrap substance to the client's upper chest (▶Figure 6.16).

9. Wrap the client securely with each of the layers on the table, one at a time, except the bottom sheet (▶Figures 6.17 a, b, c, d, e, f, and g).

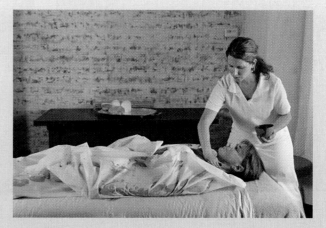

▶ **Figure 6.16**

TREATMENT 6.1 CONTINUED

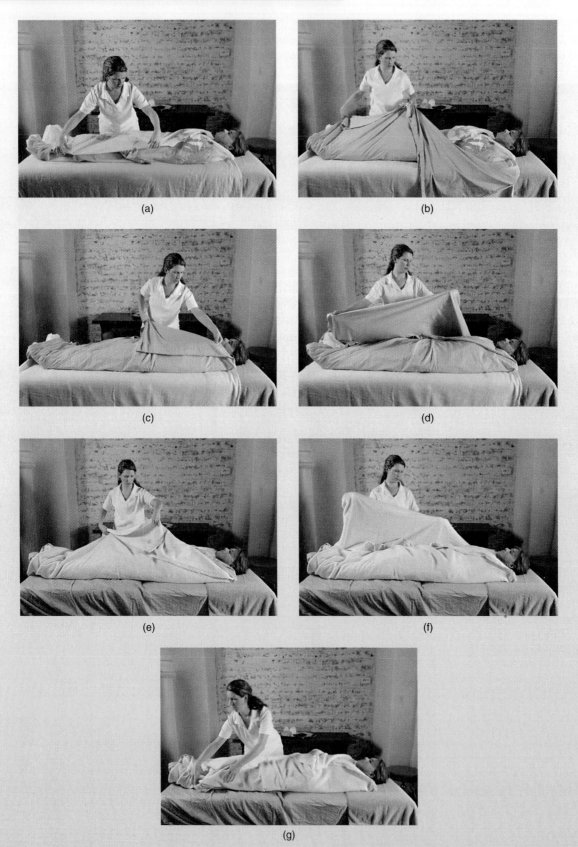

(a)

(b)

(c)

(d)

(e)

(f)

(g)

▶ **Figure 6.17**

TREATMENT 6.1 CONTINUED

10. Use the towel at the head of the table to wrap securely around the client's neck (▶Figures 6.18 a and b).

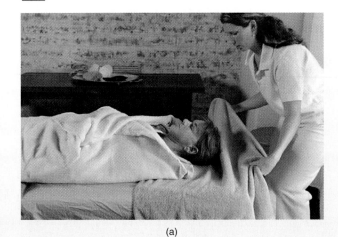
(a)

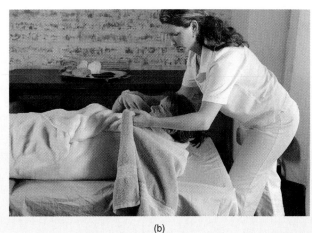
(b)

▶ **Figure 6.18**

11. Make sure the client is comfortable, using bolsters, pillows, or other props as needed. An extra blanket can be added for more warmth. The client should remain wrapped for 25 to 30 minutes. During this time a scalp and facial massage can be given (▶Figure 6.19), or the client's feet can be unwrapped for a foot massage. Another option is to sit quietly at the head or foot of the table. Place a cool, moist washcloth on the client's face or forehead if needed.

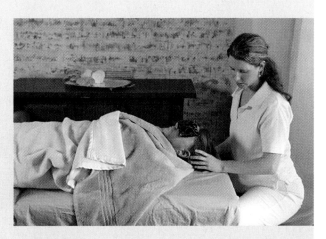

▶ **Figure 6.19**

CLINICAL ALERT !

It is important to stay near the client; some clients may become claustrophobic or overheated and need to have the wrappings removed as soon as they start feeling uncomfortable.

TREATMENT 6.1 CONTINUED

12. When the time is up, unwrap each of the layers until the client is covered by just the plastic sheet (and the towels with which the client was initially draped). Place a large towel lengthwise over the client (▶Figures 6.20 a, b, and c).

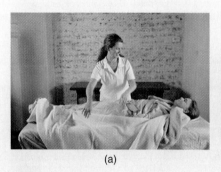
(a)

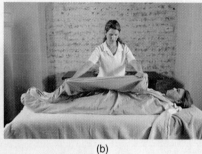
(b)

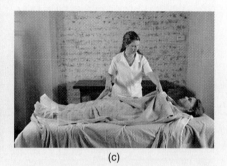
(c)

▶ **Figure 6.20**

Gently pull the plastic sheet out from underneath the towel (▶Figures 6.21 a and b).

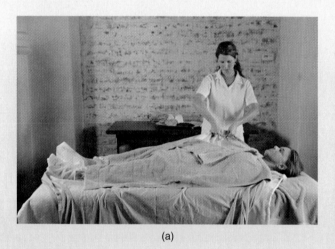
(a)

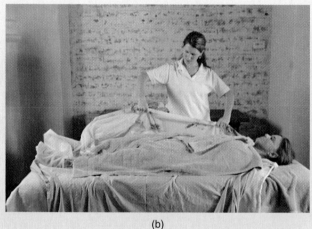
(b)

▶ **Figure 6.21**

13. Help the client sit up and hang the legs off the side of the table (▶Figure 6.22). Use a warm, moist towel to remove the mud or peat residue from the client's back.

14. If using a wet table or Vichy shower, rinse the client thoroughly to remove residue from the mud or peat on the client's skin. If there is a separate shower facility, help the client off the table, offering the bathrobe or draping the large towel around for modesty. Give the client the textured washcloth or bath scrubby (to remove residue on the client's skin), and guide the client to the shower and then back to the massage table after rinsing off. If working in a dry room, with no access to a shower, use the dry room removal technique. Once the residue has been removed from the client's skin, help the client off the table.

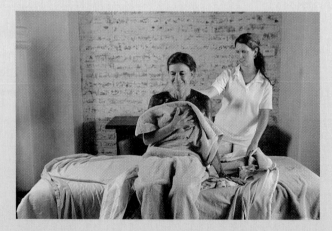

▶ **Figure 6.22**

TREATMENT 6.1 CONTINUED

DRY ROOM REMOVAL TECHNIQUE

The dry room removal technique described here is from Chapter 5. If the mud or peat body wrap is being done in a dry room with no access to a shower, the residue on the client's skin can be removed by placing a warm, moist towel on the area for a few seconds.

▶ Remove a towel from the crock pot, cabi, or basin and wring it out if it is too wet.

▶ Apply the towel to the client's body and pat down firmly; then remove the substance with one firm, smooth stroke. Do not scrub or wipe with the towel.

▶ Use a new towel from the crock pot, cabi, or basin for each area of the body from which residue is removed.

▶ To prevent chilling, cover each part of the client's body immediately after removing the residue.

After the Treatment
Encourage the client to rest and drink plenty of water after treatment. The client's skin may show a slight flush since the mud or peat greatly improves circulation and retains heat. This allows increased blood flow to the surface of the skin.

Hygiene
Any leftover mud or peat should be discarded after each client. The sheets and towels should be laundered with hot water and detergent after each use. Clean the insulating sheet by spraying it with alcohol or other disinfectant. It can also be washed with soap and water, but it should still be sprayed with alcohol after that. If brushes were used for the exfoliation, wash them in warm, soapy water and rinse. After rinsing, place them in rubbing alcohol for at least 20 minutes, then let them air dry. The tools can also be washed in a dishwasher. Store them in an airtight container. If the exfoliation was done using a natural substance, any leftover exfoliation mixture should be immediately discarded. All bowls should be washed in warm, soapy water and rinsed between each use. The washcloth or bath scrubby should be either given to the client to take or discarded; it should never be used by more than one client. The towel cabi should be washed out daily and sprayed with disinfectant. Used towels should never be placed back in it. If a crock pot is used, it should be washed in warm, soapy water, rinsed, and sprayed with disinfectant after each use.

There are many ways to perform masks. What follows is a basic procedure. Once practitioners are skilled at this, they can develop more creative treatments and build their treatment menus. Practitioners who work in spas should note that each spa has its own mask protocols and trains its practitioners accordingly. What is presented in this chapter may or may not be consistent with how individual spas perform masks. However, by practicing the procedures that follow, practitioners will acquire foundational skills, become comfortable handling supplies and equipment, and become able to knowledgeably discuss mask options with clients.

The equipment and supplies for a mask can be purchased at local stores or online; the mud, peat, or clay needs to be purchased through a spa treatment supply store.

CLINICAL ALERT ❗

Practitioners and clients can be allergic to any and all substances used in masks. It is important for the practitioner to find out from clients any allergies they may have, and note them on an intake form, so there is written documentation. Practitioners allergic to any or all mask substances should never use them on clients even when requested to do so, either by clients or employers.

People can develop allergies throughout their lives; therefore, every time a client arrives for a treatment, the practitioner should do a quick allergy update. Before any mask is performed, the substance should be applied to a small area on the client's skin and on the practitioner's skin, usually the forearm, to see if there is an allergic reaction.

TREATMENT 6.2

Mud, Peat, or Clay Mask

For masks, mud, peat, or clay can be used directly on the face when moistened with water.

Rationale
A mud, peat, or clay mask can be performed any or all of the following physiological effects:

- Vasodilator: increases local blood flow
- Thermodynamic: warms the face
- Sedative: induces a state of relaxation and stress relief
- Tonifier: strengthens vitality and the immune system
- Extractor: draws impurities from the skin
- Buffer: balances pH of skin

Equipment and Supplies (see ▶Figures 6.23 a, b, and c)

- exfoliation tools or ingredients for a gentle facial scrub
- small, nonmetal bowl—nonmetal because mud, peat, and clay react chemically with metal and their properties will change; likewise, mud, peat, and clay should not be stored in metal containers
- water
- mud; mud powder mixed with water, mud gel, or crème; peat; clay or clay powder mixed with water (1/3 cup) (see ▶Figure 6.23 d)
- small paint brush (optional)
- cucumber slices (optional)
- one washcloth
- one towel, approximately 18″ × 30″
- small crock pot or electric warmer if warming the mud, peat, or clay; if using a small electric warmer, another bowl will be needed

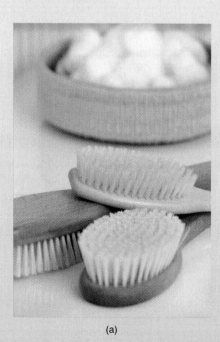

(a)

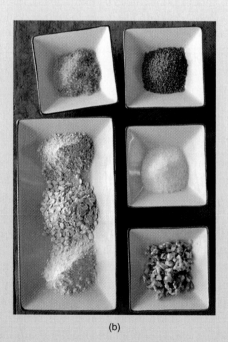

(b)

▶ **Figure 6.23** *(Photo (a) courtesy of John Davis © Dorling Kindersley)*

TREATMENT 6.2 CONTINUED

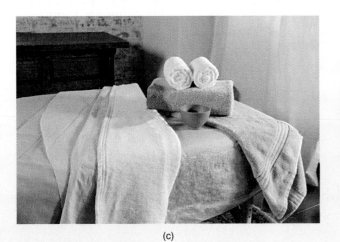

(c)

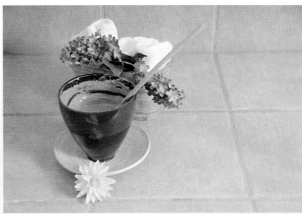

(d) Image © iStockphoto.com/Yanik Chauvin.

▶ **Figure 6.23** (*cont.*)

Indications

- skin disorders such as psoriasis and eczema
- acne
- need for skin cleansing
- need to balance the skin's pH

Contraindications

- numbness or loss of sensation in the face
- high body temperature (fever)
- skin conditions made worse by heat
- local inflammation
- broken or irritated skin
- intolerance to heat

Preparation

1. The mud, peat, or clay can be either warmed or used at room temperature, depending on the client's preference. Mud, peat, and clay should never be warmed by microwaving; this destroys their therapeutic properties. To warm these substances using a crock pot, place the mud, peat, or clay in a small bowl; then put the bowl in a small crock pot with 1 inch of hot water (see ▶Figure 6.24). If using a small electric warmer, place mud, peat, or clay in a small dish, and then put that dish inside another dish that has about 1 inch of water in it; place both bowls on the warmer.
2. Position the mud, peat, or clay and water within easy reach.

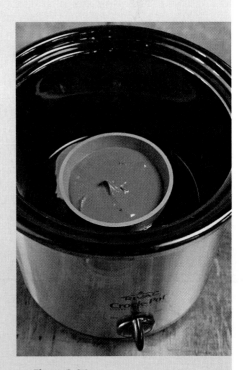

▶ **Figure 6.24**

TREATMENT 6.2 CONTINUED

Treatment

1. Perform a gentle exfoliation of the client's face. ▶Figures 6.25 a, b, and c show an exfoliation using a soft brush. Use small, gentle strokes from the client's chin to the forehead.

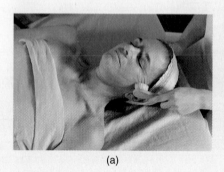
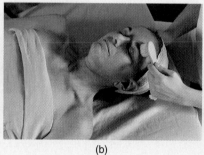
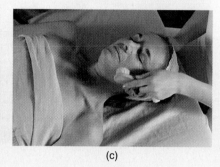

(a)   (b)   (c)

▶ **Figure 6.25**

2. Moisten mud, peat, or clay with enough water to make a thin paste.

3. Apply mixture evenly over the client's face, avoiding the eye area. Application can be done with the hands or using a small paintbrush. Be sure to spread the mixture evenly (▶Figures 6.26 a, b, c, and d).

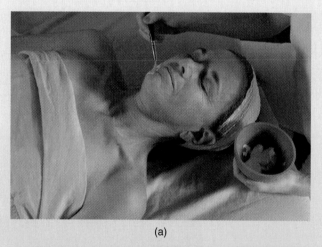
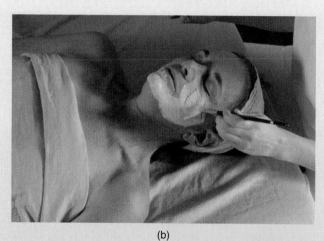

(a)   (b)

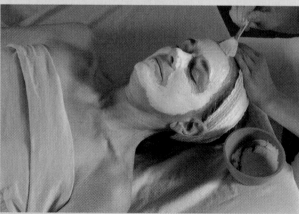
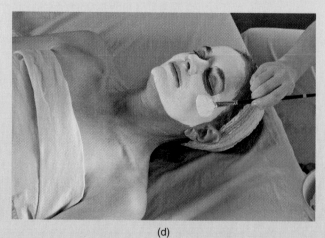

(c)   (d)

▶ **Figure 6.26**

TREATMENT 6.2 CONTINUED

Cucumber slices can be placed over the eyes for added refreshment (▶Figure 6.27).

4. Leave the mask on for 15 minutes. During this time, a scalp massage can be given, or the client's hands, shoulders, or feet can be massaged.

5. Soak the washcloth in warm water, and then wring it out. Remove the mask by wiping the client's face with the warm, moist washcloth. A gentle splash of cold water on the client's face is a good way to finish the treatment.

6. Dry the client's face by gently blotting with the towel.

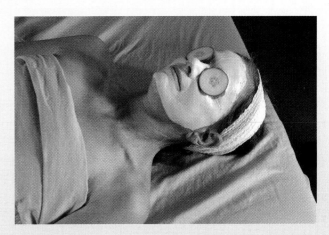

▶ **Figure 6.27**

After the Treatment

Encourage the client to drink plenty of water after the treatment. The skin may show a slight flush since the mud, peat, or clay greatly improves circulation and retains heat, which allows increased blood to flow to the surface of the skin.

Hygiene

Any leftover mud, peat, or clay should be discarded after each client. The face cloth and towel should be laundered with hot water and detergent after each use. The small bowl should be washed in warm, soapy water and rinsed between each use. If a crock pot is used, it should be washed in warm, soapy water, rinsed, and sprayed with disinfectant after each use.

Moor Peat Packs

Moor peat packs consist of organic moor peat sealed between layers of a permeable material and plastic (see ▶Figures 6.28 a and b). The permeable layer allows almost direct contact between the skin and the peat, while preventing the peat from sticking to the skin, and the plastic traps heat or cold and keeps it from leaving the body. These are sometimes called "foment pads."

A moor peat pack can be used locally for either a cold or heat treatment. Cold treatments are usually used for acute (meaning less than 3 days old) conditions such as:

▶ inflammation
▶ muscle pain
▶ muscle spasm

The pack is refrigerated until it is chilled, approximately 1 hour. It should not be frozen because that destroys the therapeutic properties of the mud. The peat pack is placed on the body so that the side with the permeable material is touching the skin. Another cool pack, such as a gel pack, is placed on top of the peat pack to maximize the cooling effect. The packs are left in place for a maximum of 20 minutes; any longer than that and the body's tissues can be damaged by the cold.

A moor peat pack heat treatment is used for people who have:

▶ tight joints (from noninflammatory conditions)
▶ muscle spasms, tightness, or strain
▶ skin disorders such as psoriasis and eczema
▶ need for detoxification
▶ need for skin cleansing

A moor peat pack heat application should not be used on people who have:

▶ heart conditions
▶ untreated hypertension
▶ numbness or loss of sensation in area
▶ inflammation
▶ intolerance to heat
▶ broken or irritated skin

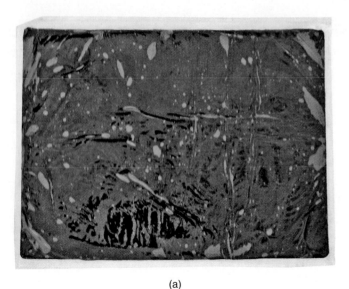

(a)

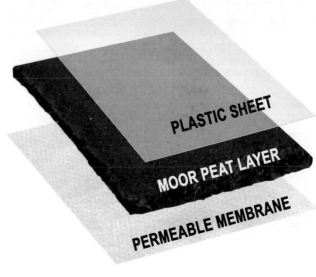

(b)

▶ **Figure 6.28** A moor peat pack can be used locally for a cold or a heat treatment. Each pack consists of organic moor peat sealed between layers of a permeable material and plastic, which allows almost direct contact between the skin and the peat while preventing the peat from sticking to the skin. The plastic traps heat or cold and keeps it from leaving the body. *(Images courtesy of Torf Spa Moor products (www.torfspa.com))*

- ▶ high body temperature (fever)
- ▶ vascular disease, including varicose veins (the heat pack should not be placed over the varicose veins; however, it may be used elsewhere on the body if there are no other conditions prohibiting its use)
- ▶ become pregnant

To warm the peat pack before application, a warm towel can be placed on it for 1 minute, but the pack should not be warmer than body temperature before it is applied; the pack loses some of its heat-penetrating abilities if it is too warm before being applied. After it is placed on the body, a piece of thick cloth such as flannel or a towel is placed over it, then another heat source—a heating pad, hydrocollator pad, warmed gel pack, or hot water bottle—is placed on top of the flannel. The peat pack is usually left in place for 20 to 30 minutes. If the heat becomes intolerable before 20 minutes is up, the pack should be removed immediately to prevent burning.

After the treatment

The skin may show a slight flush since the peat greatly improves circulation and retains heat, which allows increased blood to flow to the surface of the skin. The client should drink plenty of water afterward. If the peat pack was used in a spa or massage and bodywork office, the area can be massaged afterward if warranted and appropriate, for example, if the peat pack was applied to loosen tight back muscles.

Hygiene

The moor peat pack is designed for one-time use and should be discarded after the treatment; it should never be reused on another client. The towel or piece of flannel should be laundered with hot water and detergent after each use. If a hydrocollator pad was used, place it back into the hydrocollator. (At an average temperature of 160°F, the hydrocollator water is hot enough to sterilize the pad.) If a heating pad or gel pack was used, wash the cover after each use. If a hot water bottle was used, wipe it down with a disinfectant between uses.

Mud or Peat Bath

Baths are simple yet incredibly effective for resting, relaxing, and rejuvenating. Some spas have the facilities for clients to bathe in mud baths; those located near hot mineral springs have hot muds in which clients can submerge themselves.

Without traveling to mud bath spas, people can still experience the therapeutic benefits of mud and peat baths. Some day spas have mud-bathing facilities. If municipal regulations allow it, massage and bodywork practitioners may choose to install a bathtub in their clinic or office. A major consideration is the disposal of mud and peat when the tubs are drained. Special plumbing may need to be installed.

Practitioners can also instruct clients on how to have a mud or peat bath in their own homes and give them samples of mud or peat. Unless mud or peat baths are

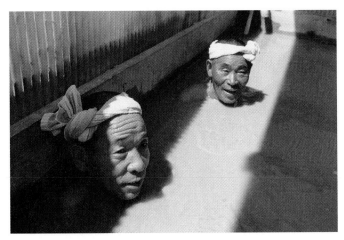

used quite frequently by clients at home, there should not be any plumbing issues. The amount of mud or peat used in a single bath is relatively small.

As with a body wrap, it is always important to begin with an exfoliation since removing the dead skin cells enables the mud or peat to work more efficiently. This can be done manually through dry brushing or using natural substances such as a salt or sugar scrub. More information about these is found in Chapter 5.

Either a full-immersion or foot bath can be taken. In either case, the bath itself typically takes 20 to 25 minutes. If done in a spa or massage and bodywork office, the client can also receive a complementary treatment such as massage therapy, shiatsu, acupressure, reflexology, and so forth.

Among the many benefits of a mud or peat bath are:

- strengthened vitality and immune system
- increased blood and lymphatic flow
- pain relief from tight joints and muscle spasms, tightness, or strain
- detoxification
- cleansed skin
- soothed skin, especially for eczema and psoriasis
- relaxation and stress relief
- deep, penetrating heat sent into muscles and joints
- balanced pH of the skin

There are some conditions, however, that warrant caution in taking a mud or peat bath. They should not be taken by people who have:

- heart conditions
- untreated hypertension
- vascular disease
- inflammation, including inflammatory joint disorders
- high body temperature (fever)

- intolerance to heat
- broken or irritated skin
- numbness or loss of sensation in an area
- become pregnant

The equipment and supplies for a mud or peat bath can be purchased at local stores or online; the mud, peat, or clay needs to be purchased through a spa treatment supply store. The supplies needed are:

- exfoliation tools or ingredients for a scrub
- bath tub for a full-immersion bath; basin large enough to hold water up to mid-calf for a foot bath
- 6 to 8 ounces of mud or peat for a full immersion bath; ⅓ cup mud or peat for a foot bath. The mud or peat should not be stored in metal containers because it may react chemically with metal, changing its properties.
- towels for drying

Before taking the bath, perform an exfoliation. Then fill the tub or basin with comfortably hot water to the desired level. While the tub is filling, add the mud or peat by putting it under the running water. No soaps should be used, but essential oils could be added to the water. Soak in the soothing bath for 20 to 25 minutes, adding hot water as needed. Dry off with the towels.

After the bath, rest and drink plenty of water. The skin may show a slight flush since the mud or peat greatly improves circulation and retains heat. This allows increased blood to flow to the surface of the skin.

Hygiene
The peat and mud bath water should be drained after use. The tub or basin should be scrubbed thoroughly with soap, water, and a disinfectant. If exfoliation tools were used, they should be washed in warm, soapy water and rinsed. After rinsing, place them in rubbing alcohol for at least 20 minutes, then let them air dry. Store them in an airtight container. If an exfoliation mixture was used, any leftover should be immediately discarded. The bowl in which it was mixed should be washed in warm, soapy water and rinsed between each use. Towels should be laundered in hot water and detergent between uses.

Rasul Spa Treatment

Rasul (Rhassoul) clay is found deep under the Atlas Mountains in Morocco, and it takes substantial effort to mine it. Because of this, it has been highly prized throughout the centuries. It was used by nobility in ancient Rome and Egypt for beauty care. Hammams in Turkey, discussed in

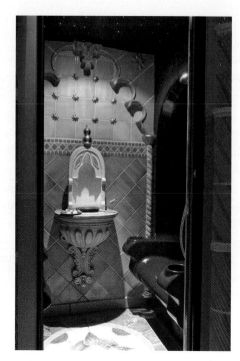

▶ **Figure 6.29** Clients sit on heated seats within a Rasul spa chamber. Clients are covered with multiple muds, which are then moistened by steam and vapor, allowing them to be rubbed into the skin. Then the client can rinse with a gentle rain shower spray.

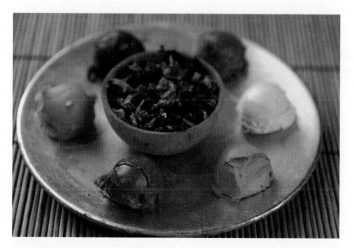

▶ **Figure 6.30** Several different colors of mud are used on clients in a Rasul spa chamber.

Chapter 1, have also used it in specialty treatments. Today, the treatments traditionally done in hammams are being adapted for use in contemporary spas.

A Rasul (Rhassoul) chamber is a small, vaulted steam room, typically inlaid with decorative Turkish tiles with a canopy of tiny twinkling lights (see ▶Figure 6.29). In this chamber, two to four heated seats are positioned across from one another. Several different colored muds are applied to the body (see ▶Figure 6.30). After 10 minutes of being in the chamber, soft clouds of steam and herbal vapors are released into the chamber. As the mud becomes moist, clients are encouraged to massage it into the skin to help exfoliate. A gentle rain shower spray completes the treatment and washes away the mud.

Mud, Peat, and Clay Poultices

Poultices are treatments applied to a specific area of the body. They are soft, moist masses of substance that are applied either directly or encased in a clean cloth such as flannel, cheesecloth, or muslin. The poultice is then covered and left for a period of time. Today's body wraps evolved from the use of poultices. The procedures are the same: a substance is applied to the body then covered by cloth. In fact, a body wrap can be thought of as a poultice applied to the entire body. For more information on mud, peat, and clay poultices, see Appendix 1.

EARTH SALTS

Even before modern science discovered the body's many physiological needs for salt, people have always craved salt and have been instinctively drawn to sources of it. These sources were highly prized and protected. In addition to maintaining health, salt has been used, and is still being used, by many cultures to cure foods before modern food preservation methods were developed. Salt has also played roles in economics, been involved in wars, and been part of religious rituals.

In the West African city of Timbuktu, twelfth-century merchants valued salt as highly as gold. During his travels, Venetian trader and explorer Marco Polo (1254–1324) noted that in Tibet, small tablets of salt bore the images of the Great Khan (emperor) and were used as coins. Outrage over a salt tax instituted in 1259 was in fact, one of the factors that led to the French Revolution in the 18th century. New York State's Erie Canal, dug in 1825, was partially paid for with revenues from salt taxes.

In the Shinto religion, salt is used to purify an area, such as that inside a temple. The Pueblo Native American tribe has a deity named the Salt Mother. In ancient times, Jewish temple offerings included salt, and salt is mentioned throughout the Bible for rituals such as baptisms and the blessing of holy water (Cargill, 2007).

Salts have two main origins. Some are from ancient oceans that once covered the Earth. As the water retreated and evaporated, it left behind rich salt beds and underground deposits. As geological shifts and volcanic eruptions occurred, strata of salts were trapped between layers of rock and volcanic ash, sealing the deposits from pollutants that were later introduced into the environment. Salt deposits are found and mined on every continent (Salt Institute, 2008).

DID YOU KNOW?

The word *salary* comes from the Latin word *salarium,* which is thought to have meant the salt allowance Roman soldiers were given.

The other origin of salt is through water. Seawater is, of course, quite salty, and salt is harvested from it using solar evaporation, either naturally or with the use of technology. Other water sources of salt include landlocked lakes, such as the Dead Sea and the Great Salt Lake in Utah. These are considered "terminal" lakes, meaning that tributaries carry water into them, but there are no outlets carrying water out. The water coming into these lakes contains minerals, among which are salts. Since there are no water outlets, the minerals (and salts) accumulate in the lake, and as the lake water evaporates, the concentration of minerals increases (Williams, 1999).

Salt is an essential element for the body because it plays important roles in maintaining homeostasis, including:

▶ helping balance pH
▶ being vital for nerve impulses
▶ being necessary for nutrient absorption from the digestive tract into the bloodstream
▶ assisting in clearing mucus from the bronchial tubes and the sinuses
▶ facilitating muscle contractions and preventing muscle cramps (Tortora and Derrickson, 2006)

Hippocrates (circa 460–370 BC), the "Father of Modern Medicine" (see Chapter 1) used salt in many of his healing regimens. One example is inhalation treatments of steam from salt water to soothe inflamed sinuses and respiratory passageways. Greek medicine also incorporated the topical use of salt for skin lesions and infections and drinking salty or mineralized waters to alleviate digestive disorders.

Additionally, salt is an excellent substance to use in spa and hydrotherapy treatments because it:

▶ is a natural antibacterial agent
▶ can draw impurities out of the skin
▶ can ease certain skin disorders such as eczema and psoriasis
▶ makes an excellent exfoliant (Nikkola, 1997; Williams, 2007)

Types of Earth Salts

The major types of earth salts use in spa and hydrotherapy treatments are Dead Sea salts; desert mineral salts, which are harvested from desert soils and include borax and Redmond salt; and Epsom salts, which are derived from Epsom, England. It is important to note that another major type of salt is sea salt. Since seawater and sea products have their own special properties and effects on the body, they are covered in Chapter 7.

Dead Sea Salts

The Dead Sea is actually a saline (salt) lake filled with the one of the highest concentrations of salts on Earth. It is located between the West Bank of Israel and Jordan, in a deep hollow in the Jordan Valley, and is fed by the Jordan River. At its deepest point, it is 1,371 feet below sea level, and it gets saltier with increasing depth.

The Dead Sea has a salt concentration of 33 percent. In comparison, the Great Salt Lake in Utah contains a 22 percent concentration of salt, while the ocean's concentration is 3 percent. It is called the Dead Sea because the high concentration makes it impossible for anything, except certain bacteria and microbial fungi, to live in it. For thousands of years, people have sought the healing powers of the Dead Sea. King David used it as a haven for health; Herod the Great established one of the first health resorts at the Dead Sea; Egyptians made balms for the mummification process from the mineral muds (Williamson, 2003). The magnesium and potassium in Dead Sea salts (see ▶Figure 6.31) have cleansing, detoxification, and restorative properties, especially for the skin and muscles (Proksch, Nissen, Bremgartner, and Urquhart, 2005; Williams, 2007; Williamson, 2003).

The Dead Sea Research Center (DSRC) is a nonprofit organization that has been recognized as an official research agency by the Israeli Ministry of Science. Prominent Israeli, American, and European scientists collaborate to research the therapeutic effects of Dead Sea bathing and pelotherapy in relation to, for example, disorders of the skin, joints, lungs, heart, digestive tract, and eyes. Other

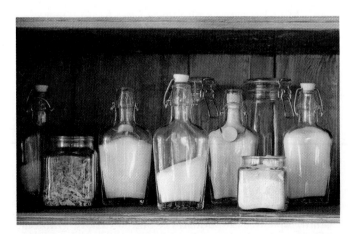

▶ **Figure 6.31** Types of salt. Left to right: jar of herbs, Epsom salt, fine sea salt, Redmond salt, borax, and Dead Sea salt.

areas of research include meteorology, air pollution, and allergens. More information about the Dead Sea and the DSRC, including an extensive list of its research publications, can be found on its website: deadsea-health.org.

Desert Mineral Salts

Desert mineral salts are gathered from deserts that are the remnants of prehistoric oceans. The most common desert mineral salt is borax. Borax, or sodium borate, is a complex mineral, mined near Death Valley, CA, as well as in Tibet and Italy. It is a mineral salt that is naturally fine grained and is frequently used in lotions and face cremès; added to soaps, ointments, and eye solutions; and can be added to a bath or used for a body polish to soften and soothe the skin. Borax is also an **emulsifier,** which is a chemical that breaks large drops of fat into smaller drops so they mix better in a solution; it is often added to other products (*Encyclopedia Britannica,* 2008a; Santa Clarita Valley History, 2008).

Redmond salt is another type of desert mineral salt. It gets its name from the part of the world in which it was initially discovered, Redmond, UT. Redmond is about 200 miles south of Salt Lake City. Redmond salt contains more than fifty trace minerals, which give it a slight pink color. It is certified kosher and comes in many grain sizes that can be used internally or externally. It is perfect for salt baths and exfoliations. More information can be found on the Redmond RealSalt website: http://www.realsalt.com/about.cfm.

Epsom Salt

Epsom salt is named for the mineral-rich waters of Epsom, England, where it was first discovered in 1618. People traveled long distances to bathe in and drink from the wells in Epsom. They did not know what the water contained; they just knew it made them feel better. By the seventeenth century, Epsom was England's first spa town. Modern science pinpointed the healing factor in Epsom's water as magnesium sulfate, a mineral salt. Originally Epsom salt was obtained by boiling down the water in the town, but today the salt is manufactured. Epsom salt can be used for exfoliation, soothing stress-reducing soaks, and reducing inflammation and muscle aches and pains. Some magnesium can be absorbed through the skin to remineralize the body. It is a natural emollient and can be used internally as well as externally. The magnesium helps alleviate irritability, anxiety, and muscle cramps. The terms *Epsom salt* and *Epsom salts* are both commonly used and mean the same thing (*Enclyopedia Britannica,* 2008b; Epsom Salt Industry Council, 2008; Nikkola, 1997; Sinclair, 2008).

TREATMENTS

Unrefined salt is always the best choice to use in spa treatments because it has no additives nor has it undergone chemical processing. Dead Sea salt, sea salt, and natural mineral salts come in different size grains. A fine- or medium-grain salt is best for a salt glow exfoliation or body polish. Larger-grained salts are fine for taking salt baths.

Salt Bath

If there is a bathtub available within the spa or massage and bodywork office, another option is a salt bath. Practitioners can also instruct clients on how to have a salt bath in their own homes and can send them home with salt samples. The best salts to use are ones that are unrefined because their properties have not been altered. Dead Sea salts, desert mineral salts, and Epsom salt are all good choices for a detoxifying bath. For a skin softening and smoothing bath, borax can be added to the bath water.

In contrast to a mud or peat bath, an exfoliation should not be performed before having a salt bath. The salt would be painful on the freshly exfoliated skin.

Either a full-immersion or foot bath can be taken. In either case, the bath itself typically takes 20 to 30 minutes. If done in a spa or massage and bodywork office, the client can also receive a complementary treatment such as massage therapy, shiatsu, acupressure, reflexology, and so forth.

CLINICAL ALERT !

Practitioners and clients can be allergic to any or all salts. It is important for the practitioner to find out from clients any allergies they may have, and note them on an intake form, so there is written documentation. Practitioners allergic to any or all salts should never use them on clients even when requested to do so, either by clients or employers.

People can develop allergies throughout their lives; therefore, every time a client arrives for a treatment, the practitioner should do a quick allergy update. Before any treatment is performed, the salt should be applied to a small area on the client's skin and on the practitioner's skin, usually the forearm, to see if there is an allergic reaction.

TREATMENT 6.3

Salt Glow

Rationale
A salt glow can be applied for any or all of the following physiological effects:

- Exfoliant: removes dead skin cells
- Vasodilator: increases local blood flow
- Stimulant: invigorates the whole body and promotes movement of the digestive tract
- Tonifier: strengthens vitality and the immune system

Equipment and Supplies (see ▶Figure 6.32)

- small, nonmetal bowl for salt—nonmetal because the salt may react chemically with metal, changing the properties of the salt
- ¼–½ cup of salt; use 50 percent fine salt and 50 percent medium-grain salt (sea salt, Epsom salt, Dead Sea salt, desert mineral salt)
- essential oil(s) of choice; if using an essential oil, a couple drops of a carrier oil will also be needed
- warm water or oil (to mix with the salt)
- one cloth sheet and two large towels, approximately 30″ × 60″
- If there is no access to a shower, a basin of warm water and three to four towels, approximately 18″ × 30″, for salt removal are needed. A towel cabi or crock pot filled with moist towels can also be used. More than three to four towels may be necessary for clients who have a large body size or a lot of body hair (since it may be more difficult to remove the salt from the hair).

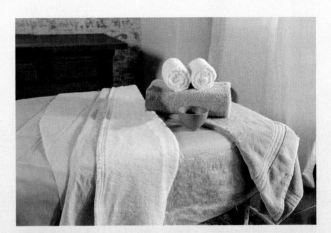

▶ **Figure 6.32**

Indications

- need for exfoliation
- need for detoxification
- fatigue
- low endurance
- beginning or ending of a cold or flu

Contraindications

- broken or irritated skin
- contagious skin condition
- rashes
- sunburn
- allergy to salt
- athlete's foot—only the feet would be contraindicated; the rest of the body could be exfoliated
- recent tattoo
- area shaved within 24 hours prior to treatment

Preparation

1. Place the cloth sheet and two large towels, lengthwise on top of the table.
2. Position the salt, water or oil, and small bowl within easy reach.
3. If working in a dry room and using a crock pot or cabi, turn it on to warm the towels for substance removal at the end of the treatment. Moisten the three to four (or more) 18″ × 30″ towels and put them in the crock pot or cabi. If using the basin of warm water and towels, position the basin in a convenient place to fill it with warm water during the treatment.

TREATMENT 6.3 CONTINUED

Procedure

1. Have the client get on the table in supine position underneath the top large towel.

2. Measure equal parts fine- and medium-grain salt into the small bowl. Make a little depression in the center of the salt. Use just enough warm water or oil to make the salt the consistency of snow; blend the mixture with your fingers (▶Figure 6.33).

If desired, add essential oil to the salt mixture. First, add a couple drops of a carrier oil, then add a drop or two of essential oil; mix well.

3. Take the bowl of mixture to the foot of the table.

4. Undrape the client's right leg.

5. Pour some water in your hands then, starting at the client's right foot, apply it up the client's leg (▶Figures 6.34 a and b).

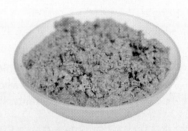

▶ **Figure 6.33** (*Ruth Jenkinson © Dorling Kindersley*)

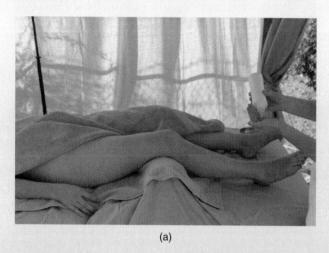
(a)

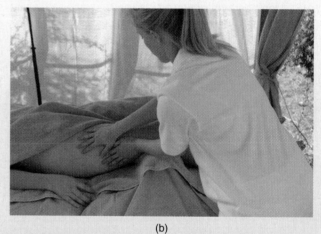
(b)

▶ **Figure 6.34**

6. Take a small amount of the salt mixture and rub it between your hands. Take more as needed during the treatment (▶Figures 6.35 a and b).

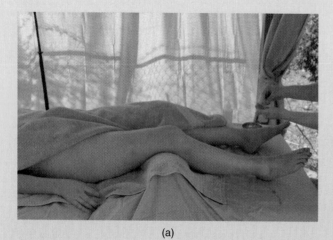
(a)

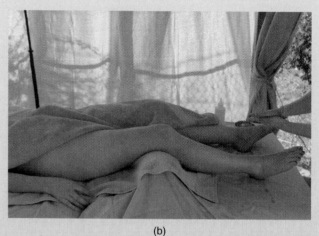
(b)

▶ **Figure 6.35**

TREATMENT 6.3 CONTINUED

7. Apply the salt mixture to the dorsal surface of the client's foot using small circular strokes to thoroughly exfoliate it (▶Figure 6.36).

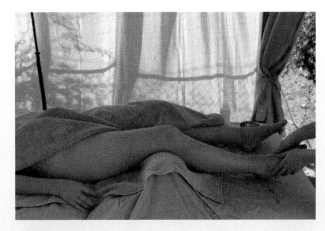

▶ **Figure 6.36**

CLINICAL ALERT !

Check with client about pressure, and adjust it as necessary.

---

8. Continue using small circular strokes up the ankle and anterior right leg (▶Figures 6.37 a and b). Redrape the client's right leg.

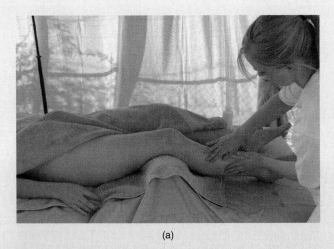

(a)

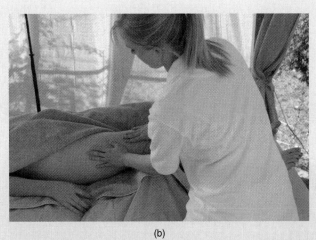

(b)

▶Figure 6.37

9. Move to the client's left leg. Undrape and exfoliate the foot and leg the same as for the right leg. Redrape the client's left leg.

TREATMENT 6.3 CONTINUED

10. Move to the client's right arm and undrape it. Use small circular strokes to thoroughly exfoliate the client's right hand and arm, up to the shoulder (▶Figures 6.38 a and b). Redrape the client's right arm.

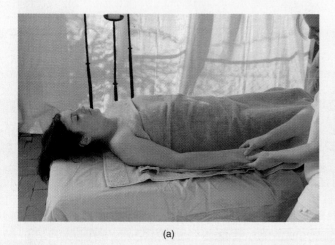

(a)

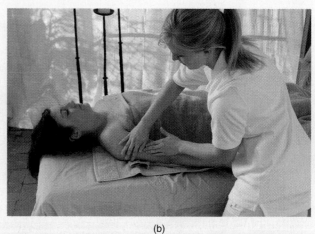

(b)

▶ **Figure 6.38**

11. Move to the client's left arm. Undrape and exfoliate the hand and arm the same as for the right arm. Redrape the client's left arm.

12. Move to the client's abdomen. Fold the large towel like an accordion cross-wise over the client's chest area and grasp the top of the large, length-wise towel on top of the client. As you unfold the cross-wise towel, fold down the length-wise towel until the client's chest is draped by the cross-wise towel, and the abdomen is undraped (▶Figures 6.39 a, b, c, and d).

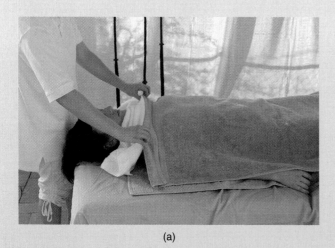

(a)

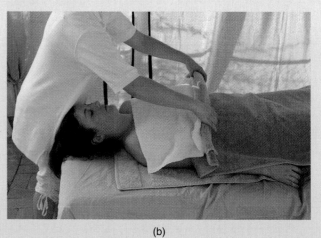

(b)

▶ **Figure 6.39**

TREATMENT 6.3 CONTINUED

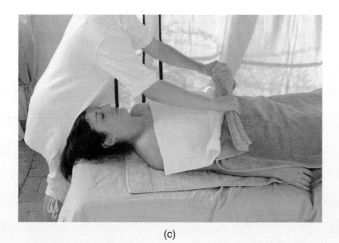

(c)

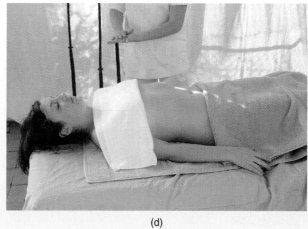

(d)

▶ **Figure 6.39 (*cont.*)**

13. Stand at the side of the table. Using smaller movements and a lighter touch, stroke in a clockwise direction (▶Figures 6.40 a and b).

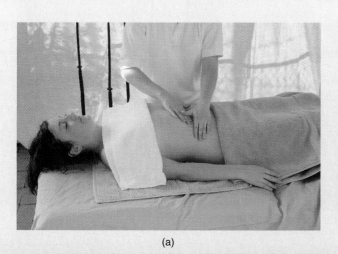

(a)

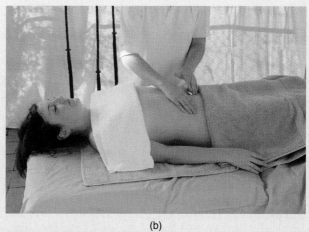

(b)

▶ **Figure 6.40**

Finish by exfoliating each of the client's sides and coming to the center of the abdomen (▶Figure 6.41).

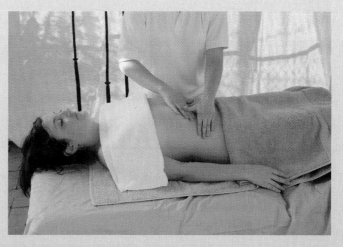

▶ **Figure 6.41**

TREATMENT 6.3 CONTINUED

14. Pull the towel up over the client's abdomen and draping towel on the client's chest area. Gently pull the draping towel out from under the sheet (▶Figure 6.42).

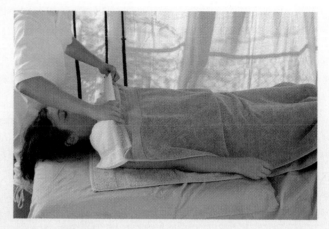

▶ **Figure 6.42**

15. Move to the head of the table. To exfoliate the client's upper chest area, use smaller movements and a lighter touch, working downward from the clavicles (▶Figures 6.43 a and b).

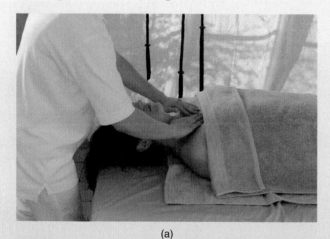
(a)

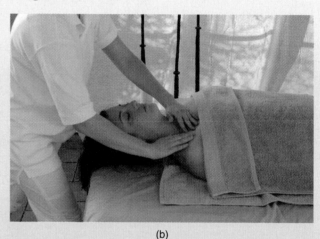
(b)

▶ **Figure 6.43**

16. If the client's face is to be included, use a light touch. With small gentle strokes, exfoliate from the client's chin to forehead.

17. Before the client turns over, the salt should be removed. If using a wet table or Vichy shower, rinse the client thoroughly. If working in a dry room, use the dry room removal technique.

DRY ROOM REMOVAL TECHNIQUE

The dry room removal technique described here is from Chapter 5. If the salt glow is being done in a dry room with no access to a shower, the residue on the client's skin can be removed by placing a warm, moist towel on the area for a few seconds.

- ▶ Remove a towel from the crock pot, cabi, or basin and wring it out if it is too wet.
- ▶ Apply the towel to the client's body and pat down firmly, and then remove the substance with one firm, smooth stroke. Do not scrub or wipe with the towel.
- ▶ Use a new towel from the crock pot, cabi, or basin for each area of the body from which residue is removed.
- ▶ To prevent chilling, cover each part of the client's body immediately after removing the residue.

TREATMENT 6.3 CONTINUED

18. Help the client turn over.

Move to the foot of the table. Standing at the foot of the table, undrape the client's left foot and leg. Exfoliate the sole of the client's foot using small circular strokes (▶Figure 6.44).

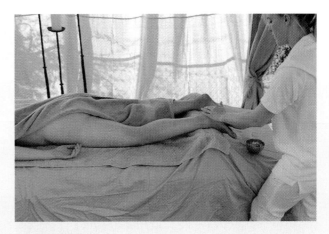

▶ **Figure 6.44**

20. Continue using small circular strokes up the posterior left leg, including the gluteal area (▶Figures 6.45 a and b). Use less pressure on the back of the client's knee. Redrape the client's left leg.

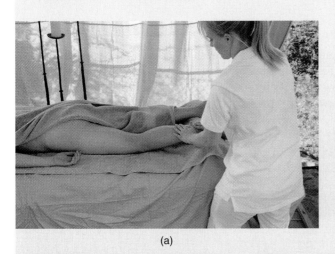

(a)

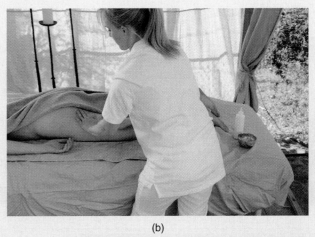

(b)

▶ **Figure 6.45**

21. Move to the client's right leg. Undrape and exfoliate the foot and leg the same as for the left leg. Redrape the client's right leg.

TREATMENT 6.3 CONTINUED

22. Move to the head of the table and undrape the client's back. Using small, circular strokes, exfoliate the client's neck and back (▶Figure 6.46 a) and move around to the side of the table to include the lateral sides of the back. (Figure 6.46 b).

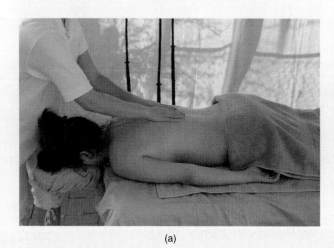
(a)

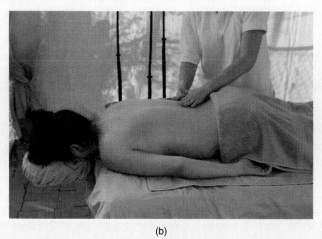
(b)

▶ **Figure 6.46**

23. Once the exfoliation is complete, the salt needs to be removed. If using a wet table or Vichy shower, rinse the client thoroughly. If there is a separate shower facility, help the client off the table, draping the top sheet around for modesty. Guide the client to the shower and then back to the massage table after rinsing off. If the exfoliation is being done in a dry room, with no access to a shower, use the dry room removal technique and skip to Step 26.

24. While the client is in the shower, remove the top of the two remaining sheets on the massage table, uncovering the fresh sheet underneath.

25. When the client returns, apply a moisturizing oil or lotion to the body.

26. If the exfoliation is being done in a dry room, remove the top of the two remaining sheets from underneath the client using the dry room sheet removal Technique.

DRY ROOM SHEET REMOVAL TECHNIQUE

The dry room removal technique described here is from Chapter 5. If the mud or peat body wrap is being done in a dry room with no access to a shower, the residue on the client's skin can be removed by placing a warm, moist towel on the area for a few seconds.

▶ Remove a towel from the crock pot, cabi, or basin and wring it out if it is too wet.
▶ Apply the towel to the client's body and pat down firmly, and then remove the substance with one firm, smooth stroke. Do not scrub or wipe with the towel.
▶ Use a new towel from the crock pot, cabi, or basin for each area of the body from which residue is removed.
▶ To prevent chilling, cover each part of the client's body immediately after removing the residue.

---

27. When the sheet is removed, apply a moisturizing oil or lotion to the body.

TREATMENT 6.3 CONTINUED

After the Treatment
Once the exfoliation is completed, another treatment can be performed, such as a massage or body wrap. Otherwise, assist the client off the table, provide plenty of water to drink, and encourage rest.

Hygiene
Any leftover salt mixture should be immediately discarded. The sheets and towels should be laundered with hot water and detergent after each use. The bowl should be washed in warm, soapy water and rinsed after each use. Since a towel cabi holds multiple towels, it should be washed out daily and sprayed with disinfectant. Used towels should *never* be placed back in a towel cabi. If a crock pot is used, it should be used only for only one treatment. It should be washed in warm, soapy water, rinsed, and sprayed with disinfectant after use.

Among the many benefits of taking a salt bath are:

- increased blood and lymphatic flow
- pain relief
- detoxification
- soothed skin
- relaxation and stress relief
- muscle spasm relief
- relief from congestion

Among the many reasons to consider taking this bath is to:

- relieve joint tightness and achiness from noninflammatory conditions
- relieve muscle spasms, tightness, or strain
- soothe skin disorders such as eczema and psoriasis
- detoxify
- reduce stress and help with insomnia

- relieve chest and sinus congestion from colds, flu, and bronchitis
- relieve headache

There are some conditions, however, that warrant caution in taking a salt bath. They should not be taken by people who have:

- an allergy to salt
- inflammation
- intolerance to heat
- broken or irritated skin
- rashes
- a recent tattoo
- sunburn

The equipment and supplies for a salt bath can be purchased at local stores or online; certain salts, such as Dead Sea salt and desert mineral salts, need to be

TO GET YOU STARTED

To customize salt scrubs for clients, here are some essential oil blends to try.

Relaxing
2 drops lavender
1 drop Roman chamomile

Stimulating
2 drops rosemary
1 drop peppermint
2 drops citrus—lemon, orange, grapefruit or tangerine
1 drop peppermint

Rejuvenating
2 drops eucalyptus

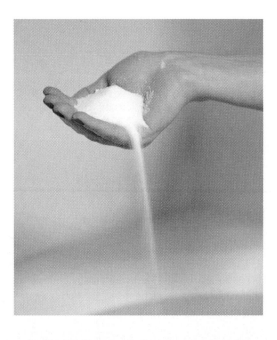

purchased through a spa treatment supply store. The supplies needed are:

- ▶ bathtub for a full immersion bath; basin large enough to hold water up to mid-calf for a foot bath
- ▶ 2 cups of salt for a full immersion bath; ½ cup salt for a foot bath
- ▶ towels for drying

Fill the tub or basin with comfortably hot water to the desired level. While the tub is filling, add the salt by putting it under the running water. No soaps should be used, but essential oils could be added to the water at this time, if desired. Soak in the soothing bath for 20 to 30 minutes, adding hot water as needed. Dry off with the towels.

After the bath, rest and drink plenty of water. The skin may show a slight flush since the salt increases circulation and retains heat. This allows increased blood to flow to the surface of the skin.

Hygiene

The salt bath water should be drained after use. The tub or basin should be scrubbed thoroughly with soap, water, and a disinfectant. Towels should be laundered in hot water and detergent between uses.

PARAFFIN

Paraffin (see ▶Figure 6.47) is a wax that is used for heat treatments. Waxes are excellent insulators because they have a high heat capacity (recall from Chapter 4 that a high heat capacity means that in comparison to most other substances, wax can absorb or release a large amount of heat without

much change in its own temperature). The paraffin is applied in a hot liquid form to the body, and, as it cools, it hardens and forms a shell. The heat from the cooling paraffin is driven into the body because the waxy shell forms a seal over the applied area (*Diracdelta Science and Engineering Encyclopedia*, 2006; *Encyclopedia Britannica,* 2008d). The heat increases blood flow into the area, which enhances healing of damaged tissues. Parafango, the combination of volcanic mud and paraffin, combines the properties of both to increase heat penetration into the body (see ▶Figure 6.48).

Paraffin and parafango applications are used to:

- ▶ soften the skin
- ▶ relieve muscle pain and joint tightness
- ▶ loosen old scarring
- ▶ relieve pain from old sprains and strains

Paraffin and parafango treatments can be done in the spa and massage therapy setting as long as practitioners follow the manufacturer's instructions for operating the paraffin heating unit. Since high temperatures are involved in applying paraffin, practitioners must be careful to apply the paraffin properly and follow all safety precautions listed under Treatment 6.4.

Clients can purchase paraffin heating units for home use. It is important, however, for clients to be knowledgeable about the high temperatures used in paraffin and parafango and to know that they could easily be burned if they are not cautious. Practitioners should instruct their clients on the proper way to use the unit and apply the paraffin.

The equipment and supplies for paraffin application can be purchased at local stores or online, although the unit itself may need to be purchased in a pharmacy. Soy waxes are also available for use, but these generally do not

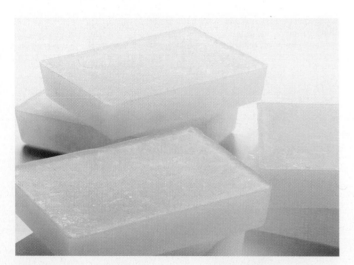

▶ **Figure 6.47** Paraffin wax is used for hydrotherapy treatments because its high heat capacity forces heat into the body. *(Photo courtesy of Universal Companies, Inc.)*

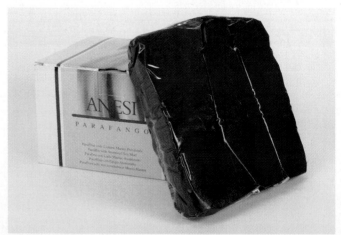

▶ **Figure 6.48** Parafango combines the properties of volcanic mud and paraffin to increase heat penetration into the body. *(Photo courtesy of Universal Companies, Inc.)*

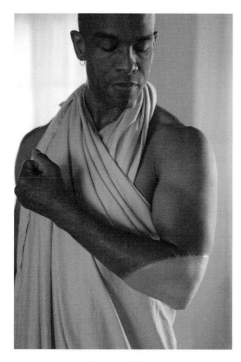

work as well as genuine paraffin. They are not as oily and tend to be sticky and difficult to remove from the skin.

Paraffin Treatment

The paraffin treatment is a useful treatment for joint stiffness from noninflammatory arthritis, as well as tight muscles, ligaments, and tendons. Because it is effective at loosening soft tissues, it can be used before performing massage on tight muscles and fascia. The paraffin is melted and applied to the body in a temperature range of 125 to 130°F. The methods of application are painting and dipping, and both methods are outlined under Treatment 6.4. The treatment time for the painting method requires 10 minutes to paint, and the paraffin is then left on for 20 to 30 minutes. The dipping method requires approximately 10 minutes of dipping time to build up the paraffin shell; it too is then left on for 20 to 30 minutes.

Parafango

Fango mud is from the thermal ponds of Battaglia near Padua in Northern Italy (*fango* is Italian for "mud"). Therapeutic uses of the thermal mud of Battaglia can be traced back to the 1300s. The use of the Fango di Battaglia for treatments on a larger scale began in the early 1900s. It is a treatment combining the rich thermal mud and paraffin wax. The application of hot parafango to parts of the body or to the entire body allows for a deep, slow release of heat, which means the parafango can be left on the body longer than paraffin, for up to 60 minutes. There is no absorption of either the mud or the paraffin by the body.

Prepared parafango bars are available from spa supply stores and can be melted and heated to a temperature of 120 to 125°F. The temperature is lower than that for paraffin alone because the mud adds an additional heating quality. The mixture can then be painted anywhere on the body—the hands, feet, shoulders, knees, backs, hips, or the entire body to provide a slow release of healing warmth. Packs are also available for treating local areas. Commercial parafango kits that include everything needed to do a full body treatment are available.

The physiological effects of a parafango treatment are the same as those for a paraffin treatment, except that there may be additional fluid loss from the body, giving the client a slimmer appearance. The indications, contraindications, equipment, and treatment procedure are the same as for a paraffin treatment. (More information can be found on the Health-Enhancement-Accessories-Training Spa Kur Development, Inc. website: http://www.h-e-a-t.com/library.html; in the left menu scroll down to choose Parafango Therapy.)

GEOTHERMAL THERAPY

Geothermal therapy is the use of stones for therapeutic purposes. Stones have unique properties that make them suitable for use in hydrotherapy. Basically, a stone is a collection of minerals with a dense structure. The main type of stone used in hot stone therapy is basalt (see ▶Figure 6.49) because its chemical structure makes it ideal for retaining heat. Marble, jade, or sardonyx (see ▶Figures 6.65 a and b on p. 221) is used quite often for cold stone therapy because its chemical structure retain coolness quite well.

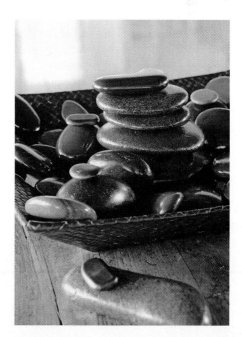

▶ **Figure 6.49** Basalt is used most frequently in hot stone therapy because of its heat-retention capabilities. Round, smooth basalt stones are heated and then tucked around the client. The practitioner also uses basalt stones to massage the client.

TREATMENT 6.4

Paraffin Applications

> **CLINICAL ALERT** !
>
> It is important that clients understand that paraffin is a treatment that uses heat at a relatively high temperature. Only clients who can tolerate heat or do not have contraindications to heat should receive paraffin treatments.

Rationale

A paraffin treatment can be performed for any or all of the following physiological effects:

- Vasodilator: increases systemic blood and lymphatic flow in area
- Analgesic: relieves pain
- Emollient: soothes the skin
- Sedative: induces a state of relaxation and stress relief
- Thermodynamic: sends deep, penetrating heat into muscles and joints

Equipment and Supplies (see ▶Figure 6.50)

- paraffin heating unit with high, medium, and low temperature control
- prepared paraffin for the heating unit
- candy thermometer
- 2 to 3 plastic or cloth sheets (to protect the massage table, floor, and area around the client from dripping wax)
- cloth sheets, if the client needs to be draped while the area of the body has paraffin applied to it, such as the back
- plastic wrap; plastic bags, which are good to use on the hands and feet, come with some heating units (and can be purchased separately); however, plastic wrap is necessary to wrap around the arms and legs and to lay flat on the back
- towel, approximately 18″ × 30″
- chair for the client to sit on, if using the dipping method (optional)

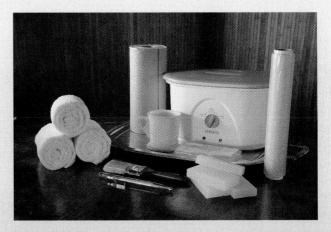

▶ **Figure 6.50**

Additional equipment is needed for the painting method of paraffin application (shown in Figure 6.50):

- ceramic cup, ceramic bowl, or small glass bowl
- any small paint brush, 1″ to 2″

Indications

- tight joints (from noninflammatory conditions)
- muscle spasms, tightness, or strain
- pain from old sprains and strains
- need to loosen scar tissue
- need for stress relief

Contraindications

- heart conditions
- untreated hypertension
- vascular disease, including varicose veins
- numbness or loss of sensation in an area
- skin conditions made worse by heat
- intolerance to heat
- broken or irritated skin
- high body temperature (fever)
- pregnancy

TREATMENT 6.4 CONTINUED

Painting Method

Preparation

1. Place the prepared paraffin in the paraffin heating unit and turn it on approximately 2 hours (or more, depending on the size of the unit and the amount of paraffin) before the treatment in order to have enough time for the paraffin to melt.
2. Lay the cloth or plastic sheets on the massage table and underneath the table to protect the areas from dripping wax. Lay two cloth draping sheets on top of the protective cloth or plastic sheet if the client will need draping during the treatment.
3. Position the ceramic cup, ceramic bowl, or small glass bowl and the paintbrush within easy reach.

Procedure

1. Have the client lie comfortably on the massage table, with the area of the body to be treated easily accessible. If the client needs to be draped, such as to apply paraffin to the back, have the client lie underneath the top sheet.
2. Using the candy thermometer, make sure the melted paraffin is between 125 and 130°F.
3. Dip the cup or bowl in the paraffin and set it aside to cool down to between 120 and 125°F. Be careful not to touch the hot paraffin while doing this. While the paraffin is cooling, perform some complementary therapy on the client, such as massaging the feet or massaging through the sheet the area to be paraffined.

> **CLINICAL ALERT !**
>
> It is absolutely crucial that the paraffin *not* burn the client's skin. The temperature of the first layer of paraffin painted on should be tolerable to the client. Since the paraffin acts as an insulator, subsequent layers can be painted on at a temperature warmer than the initial layer.

4. Paint a small patch of paraffin on the inside of your wrist to see if the temperature is tolerable.
5. When the temperature of the paraffin is tolerable to you, undrape the area of the client's body to be painted.
6. Paint a small patch of paraffin on the client and immediately ask the client about the temperature (▶ Figure 6.51).

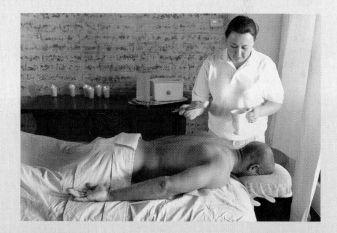

▶ **Figure 6.51**

> **CLINICAL ALERT !**
>
> To avoid startling the client, let the client know when and where the first stroke of paraffin will be applied. It may feel very hot for a second or two to the client, who may then immediately acclimate to it. If, however, the temperature feels too hot to the client after 2 seconds, do not proceed with the treatment. Take a towel and immediately wipe off the patch. Set the paraffin aside until it cools some more. When the temperature of the paraffin is tolerable to the client, proceed with the treatment.

TREATMENT 6.4 CONTINUED

7. Quickly brush on the first layer, extending the painted area approximately one-half inch beyond the targeted treatment area. The first layer of paraffin should be thin enough that you can see the client's skin through it (▶Figures 6.52 a and b).

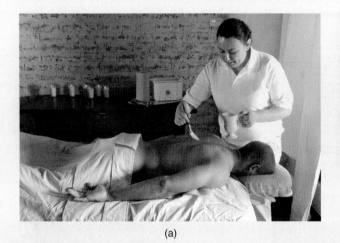
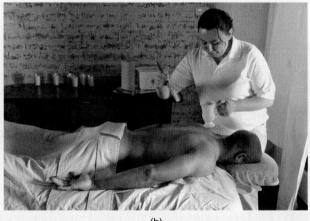

     (a)   (b)

▶ **Figure 6.52**

CLINICAL ALERT ❗

Immediately wipe off any hot wax that drips outside the painted area as it can burn the client.

8. Continue to brush on layers of paraffin until the area is white and the client's skin can't be seen through it (▶Figures 6.53 a and b). (Subsequent painting can be thicker and warmer than the initial layer since, as the paraffin cools and hardens, it becomes an effective insulator.)

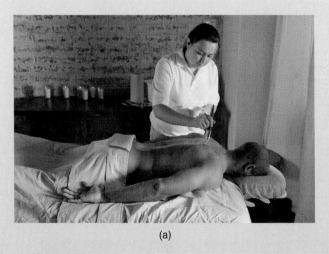
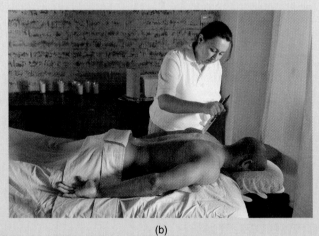

     (a)   (b)

▶ **Figure 6.53**

TREATMENT 6.4 CONTINUED

9. If the paraffin in the cup or bowl begins to cool during the brushing process, add more hot paraffin from the heating unit.

10. Cover the area completely with a single layer of plastic wrap (▶Figures 6.54 a and b). Be careful not to crack the shell of the hardened paraffin. The wrap ensures heat retention.

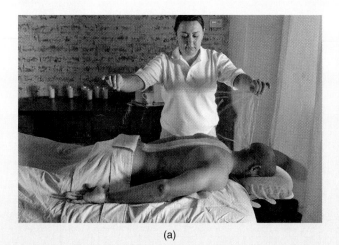

(a)

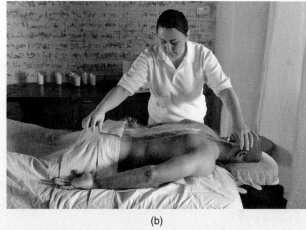

(b)

▶ **Figure 6.54**

11. Place the towel over the plastic wrap to further insulate the area (▶Figure 6.55). The paraffin shell should be left on the client for 20 to 30 minutes.

12. While the heat is being absorbed into the client's body, perform some massage or other complementary therapy on another area of the client's body.

13. After 20 to 30 minutes, remove the towel and plastic wrap from the paraffined area.

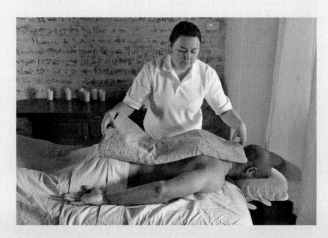

▶ **Figure 6.55**

14. Next, gently slide your fingertips under one edge of the paraffin shell, and then loosen all the way around (▶Figure 6.56).

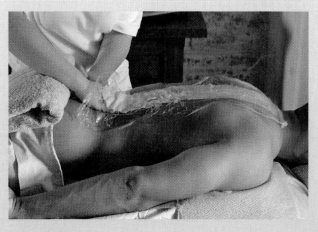

▶ **Figure 6.56**

TREATMENT 6.4 CONTINUED

Slowly peel the paraffin shell off and wrap it in the plastic wrap or bag (▶Figures 6.57 a and b). Discard the plastic wrap or bag and paraffin shell.

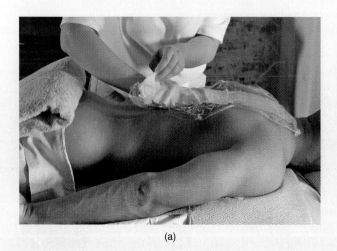

(a)

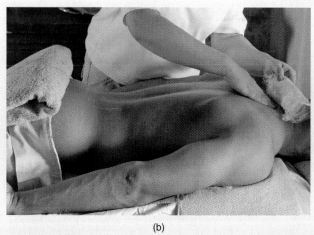

(b)

▶ **Figure 6.57**

15. Clean any remaining paraffin from the client's skin by applying friction with the towel (▶Figure 6.58).

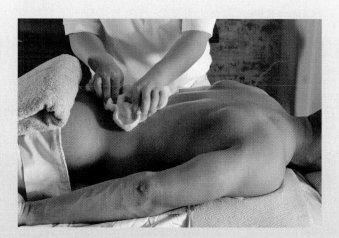

▶ **Figure 6.58**

After the Treatment
Massage the area if it is warranted and appropriate (e.g., if the paraffin was applied to the client's back to loosen tight muscles). Encourage the client to rest and drink plenty of water.

Hygiene
Paraffin that has come off the body should never be remelted and used on another client. Discard any unused paraffin in the cup or bowl; the paraffin in the unit can be reused since it did not come in contact with skin. NOTE: Do *not* pour paraffin down the drain; when it cools, it re-forms into a solid and blocks the drain. Discard the unused paraffin in the wastebasket. Wipe the cooled paraffin off the candy thermometer and paintbrush, and clean them with a disinfectant. Carefully shake out any particles of paraffin from the sheets into a waste can. Clean reusable plastic sheets with a disinfectant after each use. If disposable plastic sheets are used, discard them along with any paraffin particles. The cloth sheets should be laundered with hot water and detergent after each use. Shake out any paraffin particles from the towel into a waste can, then launder with hot water and detergent after each use.

TREATMENT 6.4 CONTINUED

Dipping Method

Preparation

1. Place the prepared paraffin in the paraffin heating unit and turn it on approximately 2 hours (or more, depending on the size of the unit and the amount of paraffin) before the treatment in order to have enough time for the paraffin to melt.
2. Lay the cloth or plastic sheets around the treatment area to protect from dripping wax.

Procedure for Dipping Hands

1. Have the client sit comfortably on the chair or stand.

2. Use the candy thermometer to make sure the melted paraffin is between 125 and 130°F.

3. Ask the client to test the temperature by dipping the fingertips into the paraffin. If the temperature is not to the client's tolerance, have the client remove the fingertips immediately. Wipe the paraffin off with a towel. Turn the heat down on the paraffin unit, and wait 5 to 10 minutes for the paraffin to cool down to between 120 and 125°F.

4. When the temperature is to the client's tolerance, have the client dip the entire hand into the paraffin, and withdraw it after 1 to 2 seconds (▶Figures 6.59 a and b).

> **CLINICAL ALERT** ❗
>
> Tell the client to be careful not to touch the bottom of the paraffin unit since it will be very hot. Make sure the client keeps the fingers relaxed when dipping the hand into the paraffin. This will prevent cracking of the shell that will form when the paraffin cools and will ensure heat retention.

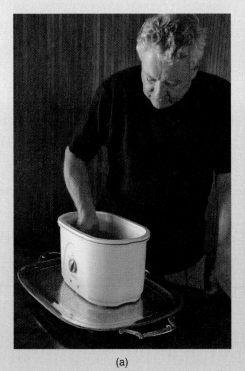
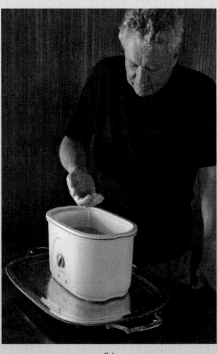

(a)   (b)

▶ **Figure 6.59**

TREATMENT 6.4 CONTINUED

5. Allow the paraffin to cool on the client's hand for 1 to 2 seconds before dipping the hand again. This allows for layers of paraffin to build up. Have the client do successive dips until the paraffin is white, and none of the skin shows through the shell (▶Figure 6.60).

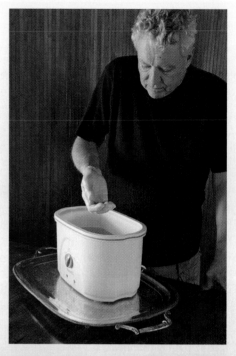

▶ **Figure 6.60**

6. Place the client's entire hand in a bag or wrap with plastic (▶Figures 6.61 a and b). Be careful not to crack the shell of paraffin when moving the client's hand to ensure heat retention.

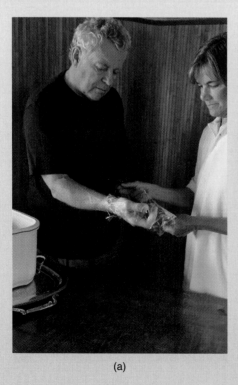
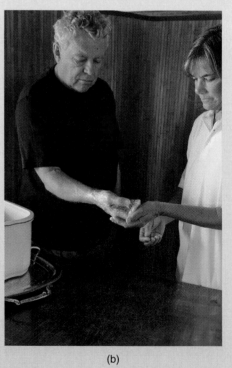

(a)   (b)

▶ **Figure 6.61**

TREATMENT 6.4 CONTINUED

7. Wrap a towel over the plastic to further insulate (▶Figures 6.62 a and b). The paraffin shell should be left on the client for 20 to 30 minutes.

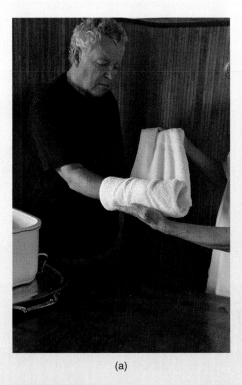
(a)

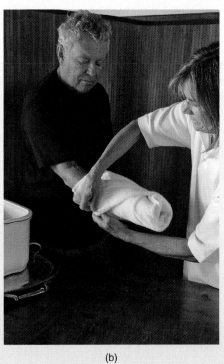
(b)

▶ **Figure 6.62**

8. While the heat is being absorbed into the client's body, perform some massage or other complementary therapy on another area of the client's body.

9. After 20 to 30 minutes, remove the towel and plastic wrap over the paraffined area.

10. Next, gently slide your fingertips under one edge of the paraffin shell, and then loosen all the way around. Slowly peel the paraffin shell off and wrap it in the plastic wrap or bag (▶Figure 6.63). Discard the plastic wrap or bag and paraffin shell.

11. Clean any remaining paraffin off the client by applying friction with the towel.

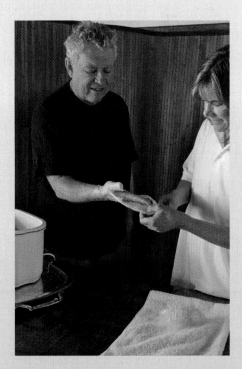

▶ **Figure 6.63**

TREATMENT 6.4 CONTINUED

After the Treatment
Massage the area if it is warranted and appropriate (e.g., if the hand was dipped in paraffin to loosen tight muscles) (▶Figure 6.64). Encourage the client to rest and drink plenty of water.

Hygiene
Discard any unused paraffin from the paraffin unit into the wastebasket after the paraffin has cooled. NOTE: Do *not* pour paraffin down the drain; when it cools, it re-forms into a solid and blocks the drain. Wipe the cooled paraffin off the candy thermometer and clean it with a disinfectant. Carefully shake out any particles of paraffin from the sheets into a waste can. Clean reusable plastic sheets with a disinfectant between uses. If disposable plastic sheets are used, discard them along with any paraffin particles. The cloth sheets should be laundered with hot water and detergent after each use. Shake out any paraffin particles from the towel into a waste can, and then launder with hot water and detergent after each use.

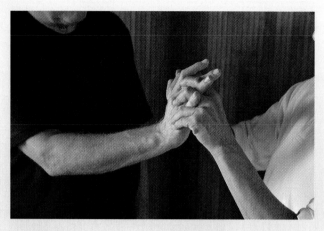

▶ **Figure 6.64**

Procedure for Dipping Feet
Because dirt and oils form a barrier between paraffin and the skin, the client's feet should be cleaned before dipping. They can be freshened with a quick soak or a peppermint spray. Make sure the feet are completely dry before being dipped into the paraffin. The procedure is done much the same way as dipping the hands. The practitioner may need to support the client's leg during dipping of the foot to make sure the toes do not touch the hot bottom of the paraffin unit. Make sure the client keeps the toes relaxed while dipping the foot into the paraffin to prevent cracking the shell that will form when the paraffin cools to ensure heat retention.

After the Treatment
Massage the area if it is warranted and appropriate (e.g., if the foot was dipped in paraffin to loosen tight muscles). Encourage the client to rest and drink plenty of water.

Hygiene
Discard any unused paraffin from the paraffin unit into the wastebasket after the paraffin has cooled. NOTE: Do *not* pour paraffin down the drain; when it cools, it re-forms into a solid and blocks the drain. Wipe the cooled paraffin off the candy thermometer and clean it with a disinfectant. Carefully shake out any particles of paraffin from the sheets into a waste can. Clean reusable plastic sheets with a disinfectant between uses. If disposable plastic sheets are used, discard them along with any paraffin particles. The cloth sheets should be laundered with hot water and detergent after each use. Shake out any paraffin particles from the towel into a waste can, and then launder with hot water and detergent after each use.

Round, smooth basalt stones are heated and then tucked around the client and used in the palms of the practitioner's hands to massage the body. Chilled marble, jade, or sardonyx stones are applied after deep focus work or during deep tissue and trigger-point work.

Mary D. Nelson

Geothermal therapy has been used for thousands of years by various cultures. Native Americans heated stones and applied them to their bodies, and Hawaiian kahunas (reli-

gious leaders and healers) used lava stones in their treatments. In China, using heated stones to relieve sore muscles dates back to before 2000 BC; and in Russia, heated black stones are used to line the bottom of bathtubs.

So, how has it come to have prominence in modern healing modalities? Mary D. Nelson, LMT, MLST, can be credited with bringing Native American hot and cold stone therapy to general use in the hydrotherapy realm. She graduated from the Desert Institute of the Healing Arts, Tucson, AZ, in 1991 with training in massage ther-

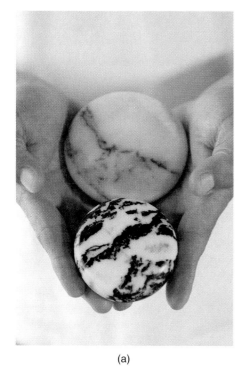
(a)

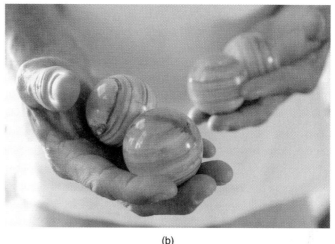
(b)

▶ **Figure 6.65** Marble, jade, and sardonyx are used for cold stone therapy because of their cold-retention capabilities. Chilled marble, jade, or sardonyx is applied after deep focus work or during deep tissue and trigger point work.

apy. Her lifelong interest in the natural healing aspects of Native Americans led her to investigate the geothermal properties of stones. Hot stones, of course, have been used in sweat lodges for thousands of years because the unique dense structure of certain kinds of stones makes them ideal to retain heat. To augment her massage therapy treatments, Nelson started immersing river stones, which are basalt, in hot water, and then applying the stones directly to the body. The weight of the stones helped the heat penetrate deeply into muscles and also affected blood circulation. In 1994, Nelson founded LaStone Therapy™, the original therapeutic stone treatment. Over time, Patricia Warne, an associate of Nelson's, began using cold stones, and the two of them developed treatments that use both hot and cold stones. LaStone™ is also an organization that teaches hot and cold stone therapy in a structured and methodical manner. Nelson continues to research and develop new ways of using stones and alternating temperatures to heal the body (Nelson and Scrivner, 2004).

Benefits of Hot and Cold Stones

The effects of heat from stones include:

▶ increasing blood flow into tightened muscles
▶ lengthening of shortened muscle fibers
▶ loosening of tendons and joints

▶ warming the joints so that they move more easily
▶ creating an overall sense of relaxation

Cold is effective at decreasing inflammation and swelling because it is a vasoconstrictor. The use of cold stones can enhance tissue repair after deep tissue work.

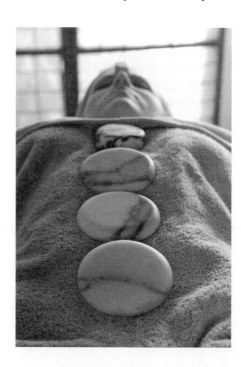

TREATMENT 6.5

Hot and Cold Stone Therapy

The basalt stones need to be heated in water that is 130 to 140°F* for 45 to 60 minutes. Once they are heated, they retain their heat for a relatively long time, compared to other substances. Because the body draws heat from the stones, however, newly heated stones need to be continually reapplied during a treatment.

Cold stones are able to draw a great deal of heat away from the body. Chilling time for stones is about 15 minutes using ice or an hour using a freezer.

Their temperature should be at or just above freezing in order to be effective.

Both hot and cold stones can be used in the same treatment. The weight of the stones also makes them ideal for use because it allows heat to penetrate the body more readily or cold to draw heat from the body more readily.

Rationale

Hot and cold stone therapy can be received for any or all of the following physiological effects:

- Analgesic: relieves pain
- Vasodilator: increases local blood flow
- Vasoconstrictor: decreases local blood flow
- Tonifier: strengthens vitality and the immune system
- Sedative: induces a state of deep relaxation

Equipment and Supplies (see ▶Figure 6.66)

- set of hot stones (basalt)
- set of cold stones (marble, sardonyx, or jade)
- roaster (18 to 20 quart capacity)
- receptacle for cold stones—bowl of ice water or small cooler
- oil for lubricant (jojoba is preferred by many stone therapists; lotion and crème should not be used because they do not have enough glide for the stones to be used properly.)
- 4 to 6 hand towels, approximately 18 ″× 30 ″
- medium-size bowl (to be filled halfway with cool water and used to cool stones that are too hot)
- flat cloth sheet
- one large towel, approximately 50″× 60″
- pillow and bolster
- dial thermometer
- small wrench (to calibrate the thermometer for each treatment)
- spray bottle containing alcohol (cherry almond– or wintergreen-scented alcohols are available)
- insulated gloves
- slotted wooden spoon (optional)
- four mesh drawstring bags (such as lingerie bags) or three mesh bags and one small wire basket
- essential oil (optional)
- sanitizer—Listerine® or Fresh 'N Clear (a sanitizer for whirlpools and hot tubs)
- stone cleaner, such as liquid castille soap, vinegar, or soap and water
- work space large enough to hold the roaster, cooling receptacle, and stones as they are organized

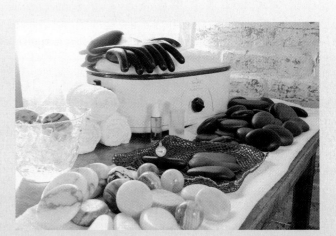

▶ **Figure 6.66**

*If the stones are used at or below 120°, they tend to lose heat rapidly and are not as beneficial. However, 110 to 120° is a good temperature to use on people who are frail or have a low tolerance to heat. When the treatment is being learned, it is best to begin at the lower temperatures (Nelson and Scrivner, 2004).

TREATMENT 6.5 CONTINUED

Indications

- need for deep relaxation
- need for stress relief
- chronic tight muscles
- general aches and pains
- low back pain
- chest or sinus congestion
- noninflammatory stage of arthritis
- noninflammatory joint conditions and pain
- symptoms from premenstrual syndrome
- headache
- insomnia

Contraindications

- heart conditions
- hypertension
- high body temperature (fever)
- vascular disease in area stones would be applied
- numbness or loss of sensation in area stones would be applied
- broken or irritated skin
- inflammation (contraindication for heat)
- pregnancy
- physical frailty
- intolerance to heat
- intolerance to cold

Preparation

Preparation will take approximately 30 to 45 minutes. This includes enough time for the stones to heat to the proper temperature.

1. In the work area, assemble the roaster, cooling receptacle, stones, mesh bags, sanitizer, slotted spoon, and all the other supplies. Leave enough room to organize the stones properly.
2. Calibrate the thermometer; this must be done before each treatment. To do this, use ice water (which is 32°F). Place the thermometer in ice water for a few moments, and then use the small wrench to set the thermometer to 32°. Doing this assures accurate temperature readings.
3. Spread out some hand towels around the work area. These will be used to drain stones after they are lifted out of the heating unit. Keep a few towels within reach for bundling stones and carrying them to the massage table or to set on a stool or chair before placing or using them on the client's body.
4. Place the marble or jade stones in one of the mesh bags and put them in the freezer or refrigerator to cool. Do not put sardonyx stones in the freezer; they will crack. Place the sardonyx stones in the refrigerator or use a bowl of ice water to cool them.
5. Spray the inside of the roaster with alcohol. After it is dry, fold a hand towel in half and place in the bottom of the roaster.
6. Sort the basalt stones according to size and shape. Place them in mesh bags according to size: twelve small stones are in bag one; twelve medium stones are in bag two. The smallest stones, used for the toes and to massage the face, can be placed in either another mesh bag or a small wire basket. The rest of the stones (the ones that are placed under and on the body and in the hands) will be placed in the roaster individually.

TREATMENT 6.5 CONTINUED

7. Place the loose stones in the bottom of the roaster according to the stone placement diagram in ▶Figure 6.67. Place the largest stones in first to anchor the towel. Add 2 to 3 inches of water and turn up the temperature to start the heating process. Place the rest of the loose stones in the roaster. Then place the mesh bags, or mesh bags and wire basket, in the roaster on top of the individual stones as indicated in Figure 6.67.

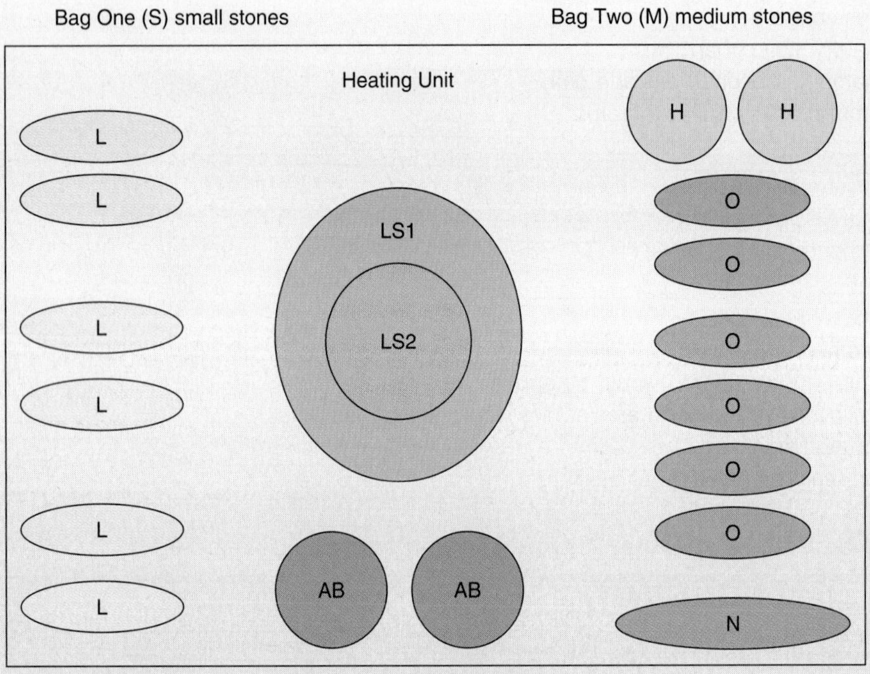

Bag One (S) small stones   Bag Two (M) medium stones

Heating Unit

H H

L

L

L O

LS1 O

L O

LS2 O

O

L O

L AB AB N

KEY:
Hand Stones - H   Abdominal Stones - AB
Large Stones - L   Medium Stones - M
Small Stones - S   Neck Stone - N
Large Stone #1 - LS1   Oval Stones - O
Large Stone #2 - LS2

PLACEMENT -
Bottom of Heating Unit - Large Stones #1 & 2, Pillow stone, Oval stones, 2 AB stones, 6 Large stones & 2 Hand stones

On Top of the Stones in the Bottom of the Heating Unit:
Bag 1 - Small spinal stones - upper left-hand corner of roaster
Bag 2 - Medium stones - center of roaster
Bag 3 - Toe stones, Forehead & Face stones **(wherever they fit)**

▶ **Figure 6.67** Proper placement of stones within the roaster will ensure they heat adequately.

TREATMENT 6.5 CONTINUED

The final result should look like ▶Figure 6.68.

8. Fill the roaster to 1 inch below the top, then add one to two tsp of sanitizer, and mix it into the water. Turn the roaster up to 150°F, and put the cover on. It will take approximately 35 to 40 minutes to reach 130 to 140°F. If essential oil is desired, add ten to twelve drops per ounce of massage oil. The bottle of oil can be warmed by floating in the water in the roaster.

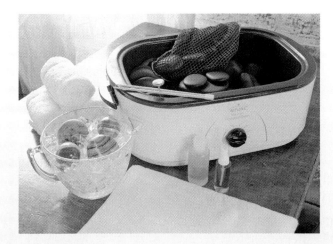

▶ **Figure 6.68**

CLINICAL ALERT !

If the client is frail, has a low tolerance to heat, or is a child, the stones should be used at 110 to 120°F. It is extremely important to check often with the client about the temperature and adjust the treatment as needed.

9. Place the flat sheet on the massage table. Place the large towel lengthwise on the massage table on top of the sheet.

10. Just before the start of the treatment, transfer the cold stones from the refrigerator or freezer to the cooler or bowl of ice water. A freezer pack can be added to the cooler to further cool the stones. An alternative is to have a bowl of ice water to chill the stones.

Procedure

1. Have the client lie prone under the large towel.

2. Apply oil to client's body.

3. Take the large stones out of the roaster (the slotted spoon can be used for this), dry them off, and place one abdominal stone under the client's abdomen, and the other on the towel over the sacrum. Place stones over the towel up the client's back. A stone can be placed in the palms of the client's hands (▶Figure 6.69).

4. Choose a pair of stones to apply to the body, dry them off, and then, to keep from startling the client, touch the client's body with the back of your hand before applying the stone with firm pressure and long gliding strokes. Be careful that the stones stay on the muscle tissue and avoid the bony areas. When the stones start to lose their heat, return them to the heating unit and use another pair. If the stones do not glide easily, apply more oil. The strokes on the client's extremities should always be performed toward the client's heart.

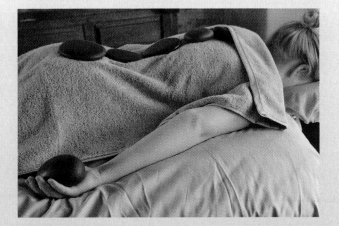

▶ **Figure 6.69**

TREATMENT 6.5 CONTINUED

CLINICAL ALERT !

Immediately check with the client about temperature and make necessary adjustments, such as allowing more cooling time before the stones are applied. When using the stones, make sure to keep gliding them. If they stay too long in one area, the heat may burn the client.

5. Hot stones can be used on the client's back (▶Figures 6.70 a, b, c, and d), posterior arms, posterior legs and gluteals (▶Figure 6.71), feet, and posterior neck (▶Figures 6.72 a and b).

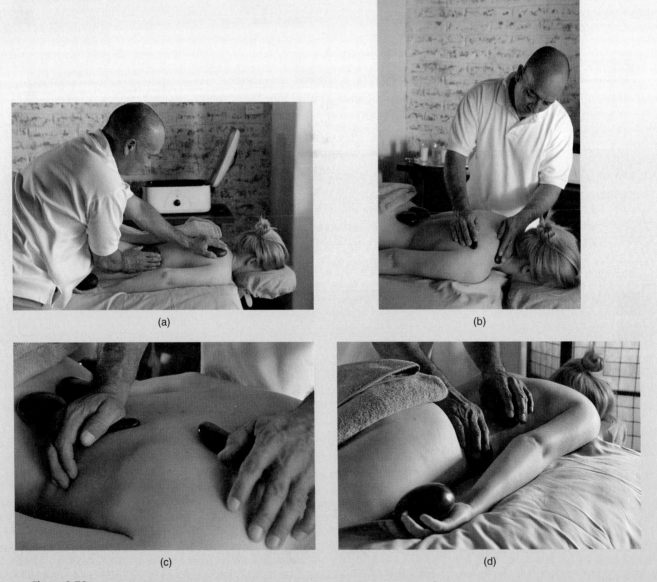

(a)

(b)

(c)

(d)

▶ **Figure 6.70**

TREATMENT 6.5 CONTINUED

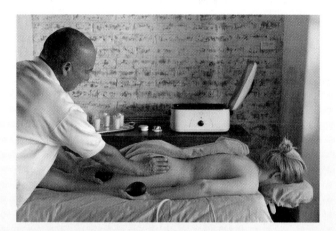

▶ **Figure 6.71**

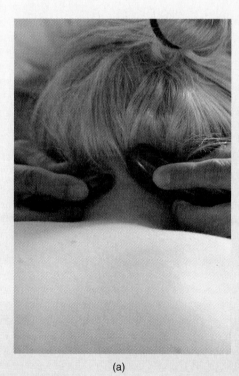

(a)

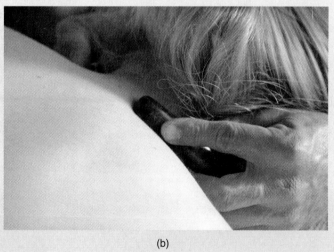

(b)

▶ **Figure 6.72**

TREATMENT 6.5 CONTINUED

Specific work can also be performed with stones (▶Figure 6.73).

6. When finished with the client's posterior side, help the client turning over, making sure the client stays draped.

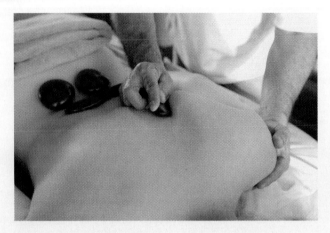

▶ **Figure 6.73**

7. With the client supine, place the hand stones in the client's palms and the toe stones between the client's toes. Cold stones can also be placed along the client's torso and on the client's forehead. (▶Figure 6.74). A hot stone can be placed under the client's neck (▶Figure 6.75).

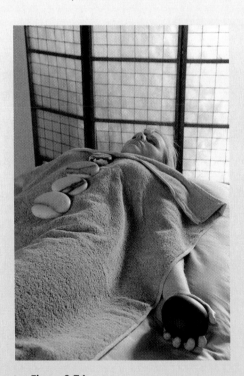

▶ **Figure 6.74**

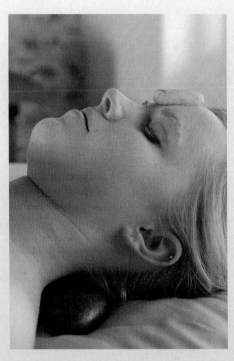

▶ **Figure 6.75**

TREATMENT 6.5 CONTINUED

1. Hot stones can be used to massage the client's anterior arms, hands (▶Figure 6.76), anterior legs (▶Figure 6.77), upper chest (▶Figure 6.78), neck (▶Figures 6.79 a and b), and face (▶Figures 6.80 a and b).

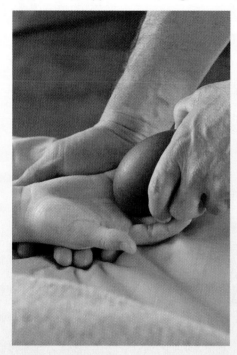

▶ **Figure 6.76**

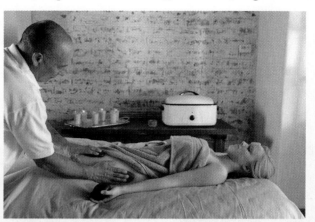

▶ **Figure 6.77**

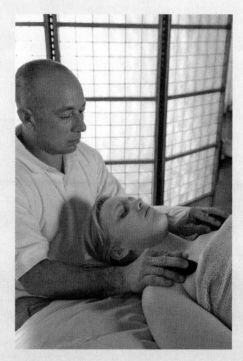

▶ **Figure 6.78**

TREATMENT 6.5 CONTINUED

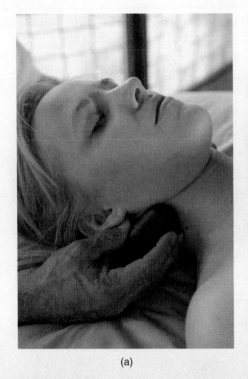
(a)

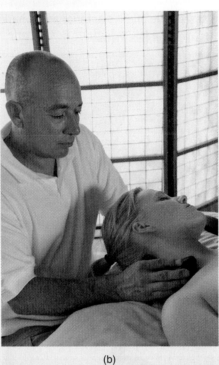
(b)

▶ **Figure 6.79**

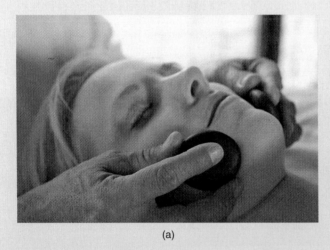
(a)

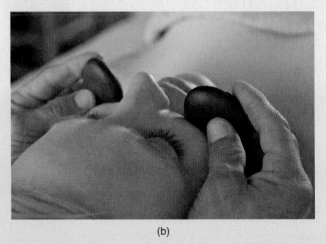
(b)

▶ **Figure 6.80**

9. Finish the treatment by removing the stones placed on the client's body and then performing some long, gliding strokes by hand to close the treatment.

When to Use Cold Stones

Chilled stones can be used in place of heated stones anywhere in the routine. They can be tucked under the abdomen, used in combination with heated stones, or placed along either side of the spine when the client is supine. But they are primarily used following hot stones on a focus area. They are extremely effective when used to chill an area either before or after specific work. The cold stones draw heat from the body and are effective where there is inflammation or to ease the discomfort of sunburn.

As a consideration to the client, it is important to verbally announce cold stones before you apply to them to the client's body. Ask the client to take a deep breath as the stone is applied and to let the breath out immediately after the stone is applied. Having the client focus on the breath is a way to draw attention away from the chill of the stone, and breathing deeply helps the client release muscle tension caused by the application of the cold stone. The application of chilled stones is done slowly and gradually, giving the client time to adjust to the change in temperature. Cold stones are applied with firm pressure, held in place momentarily, and then moved slowly until the area is thoroughly chilled.

After the Treatment
After the treatment, offer the client water and encourage rest before resuming activities. This treatment has a huge impact on the body because of the combination of massage and heat. It frequently leaves clients in an extremely relaxed, slightly euphoric state.

Hygiene
At the end of a treatment, turn the roaster off and add a tablespoon of liquid castile soap. Remove stones after 10 minutes of soaking in the soap solution, and then spray each one with alcohol. Lay the stones out on a clean towel and pat them dry. Spray the cold stones individually with alcohol and pat them dry. Pour the water out of the roaster and spray the inside of the unit with alcohol. All the towels, mesh bags, and the sheet should be laundered in hot water and detergent after each use. Wash out the cooling receptacle and bowls with soapy water and rinse. Spray or wipe all the other equipment with alcohol or other disinfectant, that is, the workspace surface, oil bottle, wooden spoon, thermometer, and insulated gloves.

Cold also slows nerve impulses, including pain impulses, which makes it an ideal analgesic. Overall, geothermal therapy is beneficial for:

▶ acute and chronic injuries
▶ muscle spasms
▶ osteoarthritis, tendonitis, and bursitis (cold is good for acute stages of these; heat is good for noninflammatory stages of these)
▶ sprains, strains (cold is good for acute stages of these; heat is good for noninflammatory stages of these)
▶ headache
▶ stress

Many different types of hot and cold stone therapy options exist. Since innovation is the hallmark of the spa and bodywork field, it is easy to understand how the geothermal properties of stones have been adapted in many ways.

Geothermal therapies can range from simple treatments using a few stones to elaborate setups using multiple sets of stones. The stones are adaptable to a variety of modalities. There are custom sets especially for estheticians, reflexologists, practitioners of Asian bodywork, physical therapists, chiropractors, sports massage therapists, and spa therapists (Nelson and Scrivner, 2004).

Summary

Each of the many different types of soils and earth products has its own therapeutic properties. Muds help with deep skin cleansing and aid in the removal of waste products, stimulate local blood and lymphatic flow, and are excellent warming and hydrating treatments. There are many different types of muds. Each has a unique combination of regional sediments and organic materials.

Clays draw impurities from the body, which facilitates deep skin cleansing, aids in the removal of waste products, and tightens the skin. As with muds, this drawing action stimulates local blood circulation and lymphatic flow. Clays are excellent for heat applications as well. There are many ways to classify clays, such as by their structure, their color, and the location in which they were initially discovered.

Peat is an organic soil that contains minerals, organic material, water, and air. It was formed by the decomposition of layers of plants, mainly mosses, and animal matter under bodies of water. Moor mud or "black mud" is a commonly used peat in spa treatments. Peats are used in spa therapies to draw and absorb toxins from the body, as warming and hydrating treatments, and to increase local blood and lymph circulation. Treatments that can be performed using muds, clays, and peat include body wraps, baths, poultices, masks, and applications of moor peat packs.

The major types of earth salts are Dead Sea salts; desert mineral salts harvested from desert soils, including borax and Redmond salt; and Epsom salt, which derives its name from Epsom, England. Salts are minerals and can draw out toxins. They perform a small amount of remineralization for the body and because they are abrasive, they can be used for exfoliation. The spa and hydrotherapy treatments in which they are used are baths and salt scrubs.

Paraffin is a common waxy petroleum by-product. Waxes are excellent insulators; hence, heat from a paraffin treatment goes deep into the body. The heat increases blood flow into the area, which enhances healing of damaged tissues. Parafango is the combination of volcanic mud and paraffin. Paraffin and parafango can be applied to the body with a paint brush or by dipping the hands or feet into it.

Basalt, marble, jade, and sardonyx stones have unique properties that make them suitable for use in hydrotherapy. Heat from basalt stones applied to the body increases blood flow into tightened muscles, causes shortened muscle fibers to elongate, and helps loosen tendons and joints. Cold from marble, jade, or sardonyx stones is very effective at decreasing inflammation and swelling. Cold also slows nerve impulses, including pain impulses, which makes it an ideal analgesic. Hot and cold stones can be used together in a treatment.

Activities

1. List the correct way to layer the massage table when performing a body wrap.

   _____
   _____
   _____
   _____
   _____
   _____
   _____

2. Explain why it is important to perform an exfoliation before performing a body wrap.

   _____
   _____
   _____

3. List three benefits of a mud, peat, or clay body wrap.

   _____
   _____
   _____

4. List three contraindications for a mud, peat, or clay body wrap.

   _____
   _____
   _____

4. List two indications for a mud, peat, or clay mask.

   _____
   _____

5. List three contraindications for a mud, peat, or clay mask.

   _____
   _____
   _____

6. List five benefits of a paraffin treatment.

   _____
   _____
   _____
   _____
   _____

7. List five contraindications for a paraffin treatment.

_____

_____

_____

_____

_____

8. Explain five benefits of hot and cold stone therapy.

_____

_____

_____

_____

9. List five contraindications for hot and cold stone therapy.

_____

_____

_____

_____

_____

10. Receive a mud, peat, or clay body wrap treatment. Describe which type of wrap you received. What did you like about it? What did you not like about it? What would you have done differently? How did you feel 24 hours after the treatment? 48 hours after the treatment?

_____

_____

_____

_____

_____

_____

_____

11. Receive a mud, peat, or clay mask treatment. Describe which type of mask you received. What did you like about it? What did you not like about it? What would you have done differently? How did you feel 24 hours after the treatment? 48 hours after the treatment?

_____

_____

_____

_____

_____

_____

_____

12. Take a salt bath. What did you like about it? What did you not like about it? How did you feel 24 hours after the treatment? 48 hours after the treatment?

_____

_____

_____

_____

_____

_____

_____

13. Receive a paraffin treatment. What did you like about it? What did you not like about it? What would you have done differently? How did you feel 24 hours after the treatment? 48 hours after the treatment?

_____

_____

_____

_____

_____

_____

_____

14. Receive a hot and cold stone treatment. What did you like about it? What did you not like about it? What would you have done differently? How did you feel 24 hours after the treatment? 48 hours after the treatment?

_____

_____

_____

_____

_____

15. Using some of the smaller stones for hot and cold stone treatment, design your own facial and foot protocols.

16. Do some exploring in nature and see if you can find some interesting basalt stones to use for hot stone treatments.

Study Questions

1. Which of the following is a nonswelling clay?
   a. Smectite
   b. Illite
   c. Kaolinate
   d. Bentonite

2. The mineral-rich sedimentation that is found at the bottom of lakes and rivers fed by hot and cool springs is called
   a. Fuller's earth
   b. French green clay
   c. China white
   d. moor mud

3. Which of the following treatments should be performed before a mud wrap?
   a. salt scrub
   b. cold stone therapy
   c. paraffin application
   d. hot foot bath

4. Because clays and muds form emulsions, they are useful for which type of treatment?
   a. exfoliation
   b. cooling
   c. heating
   d. dehydrating

5. Parafango is a combination of paraffin and
   a. peat
   b. stones
   c. red clay
   d. volcanic mud

6. Which of the following has the highest saline content?
   a. Moor mud
   b. Dead Sea mud
   c. Bentonite clay
   d. Fuller's earth

7. Which of the following is contraindication for hot stone therapy?
   a. pregnancy
   b. low back pain
   c. chest congestion
   d. headache

8. Paraffin is effective because its effect on the body includes that it is a(n)
   a. emollient
   b. vasodilator
   c. analgesic
   d. all of the above

9. Which of the following is a contraindication for a salt glow?
   a. need for exfoliation
   b. recent tattoo
   c. fatigue
   d. skin irritation

10. Which of the following should not be used to warm mud, peat, or clay?
    a. crockpot
    b. electric warmer
    c. microwave
    d. double boiler

11. The shallower layers of the moor contain which type of moor peat?
    a. high
    b. low
    c. top
    d. middle

12. Which of the following clays is best for sun-damaged skin?
    a. green
    b. red
    c. yellow
    d. white

13. In a body wrap treatment, the typical length of time a client remains wrapped is how many minutes?
    a. 10–15
    b. 25–30
    c. 30–45
    d. 45–60

14. In which type of bowl should mud, peat, clay, and salt never be placed?
    a. glass
    b. ceramic
    c. metal
    d. wooden

Case Samples

A. Lawrence Melbourne is a 78-year-old retired school teacher. He and his wife, Esther, have been receiving massage from Maggie Garcia for about 5 years. Lawrence was recently diagnosed with degenerative osteoarthritis in his spine, and it's been hurting him quite a bit lately. Maggie would like to recommend that he try one of the pelotherapy treatments she offers.

1. Which pelotherapy treatments would be best for Lawrence to receive?
2. What are the rationale, equipment and supplies, indications, contraindications, preparation, after-treatment care, and hygiene for these treatments?
3. Which questions should Maggie ask Lawrence to determine which treatment would be most beneficial?

B. Larry Levine suffers from osteoarthritis in his knees from long years of playing professional soccer. While on a business trip, he is staying at a hotel with a spa and is curious about the spa treatments.

1. Which treatments could a spa practitioner recommend to help relieve the pain in his knees?
2. What are the rationale, equipment and supplies, indications, contraindications, preparation, after-treatment care, and hygiene for these treatments?
3. Which questions should the spa practitioner ask Larry to determine which treatment would be most beneficial?

C. Alima Bhodran has been "burning the candle at both ends." She is working on her master's degree while struggling to keep up with a thriving private practice in healing touch therapy. She hasn't been eating as well as she normally does and feels depleted.

1. Which spa treatments would help her feel rejuvenated?
2. What are the rationale, equipment and supplies, indications, contraindications, preparation, after-treatment care, and hygiene for these treatments?
3. Which questions should a spa practitioner ask Alima to determine which treatment would be most beneficial?

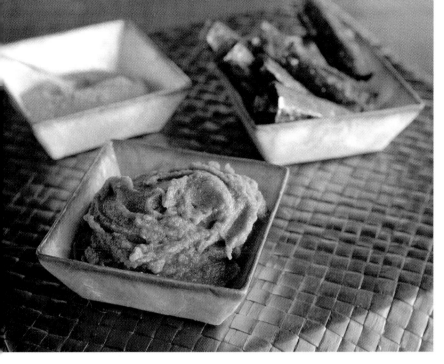

Thalassotherapy

What Is Thalassotherapy?
Elements of Thalassotherapy
Seawater
Sea Products
Treatments
Brine Inhalation Treatment

LEARNING OBJECTIVES

After studying this chapter, the reader will have the information to

1. Trace the history of the use of thalassotherapy.

2. Explain how plasma and ocean water are similar.

3. Discuss the various elements of thalassotherapy—seawater, seaweed, sea mud, and sea salt.

4. Delineate the supplies needed, rationale, indications, contraindications, treatment procedure, hygiene, and after-treatment care for a seaweed or other algae body wrap.

5. Delineate the supplies needed, rationale, indications, contraindications, treatment procedure, hygiene, and after-treatment care for a sea mud body wrap.

6. Delineate the supplies needed, rationale, indications, contraindications, treatment procedure, hygiene, and after-treatment care for a seaweed, other algae, or sea mud mask.

7. Delineate the supplies needed, rationale, indications, contraindications, treatment procedure, hygiene, and after-treatment care for a sea salt glow.

The cure for anything is salt water—sweat, tears, or the sea.
— Isak Dinesen, Danish writer and author of *Out of Africa* and *Babette's Feast*

KEY TERMS

Algae	Green seaweeds	Sea mud	Seawater
Brown seaweeds	Red seaweeds	Sea salt	Thalassotherapy

WHAT IS THALASSOTHERAPY?

Thalassotherapy is the use of the sea and sea products to maintain health and wellness. Thalassa was the Greek personification of the Mediterranean Sea. She was thought to be the creator of all sea life and was known for the life-giving aspect of her sea nature. Thalassotherapy uses all the benefits of the marine environment—the air, the water, seaweed, marine extracts, and sea salt—to treat and prevent illness. Spa and hydrotherapy treatments use **seawater** and seaweed in many different types of relaxing, detoxifying, and revitalizing therapies, such as hydro baths, jet spray, and seaweed wraps.

Early Use of Thalassotherapy

In the fifth century BC, the ancient Romans, Egyptians, and Greeks built temples of healing along the coasts, near both warm and cold springs. The Romans also thought of using marine mud in mud baths for healing. These could be thought of as the earliest seawater spas. Hippocrates, Galen, Plato, and Aristotle recommended the use of seawater for treating various ailments. They encouraged their fellow healers to have patients with aching muscles and arthritis immerse themselves in seawater. The belief in the curative uses of seawater was affirmed in 480 BC when Euripedes said, "The sea washes all men's illnesses" (Jouan, 2008).

In 1750, British physician Richard Russell published his treatise, *A Dissertation on the Use of Seawater in the Affections of the Glands,* the culmination of much research on the benefits and healing properties of seawater. He stated, "It is necessary to drink some seawater, to have baths in seawater, and to eat any sea product where its virtue is concentrated" (Ball, 2008). This work helped usher in the modern era of sea bathing and interest in sea products. More and more doctors and scientists began studying seawater to determine its healing components (Ball, 2008; Lauste, 1974).

Soon after Dr. Russell's work was published, the first hydrotherapy center devoted to using seawater and sea products opened in England. People traveled from all over to be treated for arthritis, lack of vitality, and many other disorders. The sea environment was seen as therapeutic, and many seaside towns in England, such as Brighton, came to be known as destinations for a "sea cure." People with asthma, tuberculosis, and nervous disorders are just some of those who sought relief at the ocean (Minton, 2008a). Word of sea bathing traveled across the English Channel to the French coast, where immersion in the open sea became popular as well. Small wooden structures were provided to individual bathers out in the water so they could enjoy the benefits of seawater with privacy (Turcke Bilgi, 2008).

With the expansion of the railway system in both England and France, travel to seaside resorts from inland cities became more and more fashionable. Around 1820, the individualized bathing cabins in the open sea gave way to buildings (hydrotherapy centers) with the baths inside. Men and women bathed separately, and the different social classes were also separated (Walton, 2005).

Modern Thalassotherapy

In 1865, French physician Joseph de la Bonnardiere, who had a practice in the sea bathing resort in the town of Arcachon, coined the word *thalassotherapy* to encompass the treatments based on the healing benefits of the sea. In 1899, the first medical thalassotherapy center was opened in Roscoff, France.

In 1906, Rene Quinton, a French marine biologist, wrote a book called *L'Eau de Mer, Milleu Organique (Seawater, Organic Medium).* Through his years of research and experiments, he came to several revolutionary conclusions, one of which is that the internal environment of each living creature is a reflection of the external environment of primordial life. Based on his studies of human blood plasma and lymph, Quinton discovered that seawater is chemically identical to both. Plasma, lymph, and seawater contain almost identical amounts of mineral salts, proteins, and trace elements, and in almost the same concentrations (Crebbin-Baily, Harcup, and Harrington, 2005; Minton, 2008a).

The study of the curative effects of thalassotherapy continued in France, and in 1960, the French Medical Academy officially defined thalassotherapy as a therapy that "uses seawater, seaweed, sea mud, or other sea resources and/or the marine climate for the purpose of medical treatment or treatment with a medicinal effect" (Williams, 2007, p. 195). Using seawater as a curative medium was brought into popular focus by Frenchman Louison Bobet, a Tour-de-France cyclist who was injured in a car accident. He achieved great recovery results through the use of the seawater in Roscoff, France. He was so impressed that he decided to pursue developing the use of thalassotherapy. In 1964, he opened the first contemporary establishment for seawater therapy (Crebbin-Baily, Harcup, and Harrington, 2005).

Since then, there has been a steady increase in interest in this ancient healing method, which has led to the flourishing sea therapy industry of today. In France, thalassotherapy has continued to be viewed as medicinal, with medical insurance covering treatments for many conditions, including hydrotherapy using seawater, seaweed, and sea mud poultices and wraps and eating seaweed and seafood. Many of these treatments are in use in European spas and have been adapted, in varying degrees, in Amer-

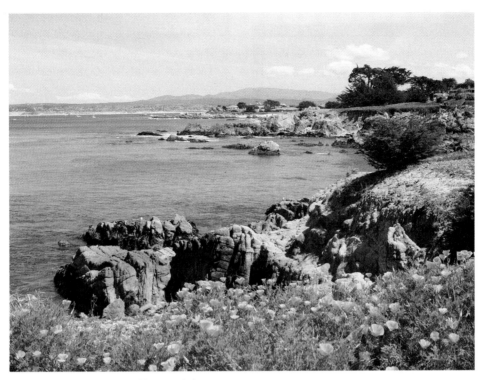

(Geri Engberg/Geri Engberg Photography)

ican spas as well. The focus in the United States, however, has been more toward the toning, moisturizing, and detoxifying effects of thalassotherapy on the skin.

ELEMENTS OF THALASSOTHERAPY

Seaweed and other sea products are organic materials that have more than sixty salts, vitamins, and other trace elements essential to the body. These trace elements include sulfate ion (SO_4^{++}), Mg^{++}, iodine, K^+, and other salts and vitamin A, B vitamins, and vitamins C, D, E, and K. The salts account for seawater's buoyancy. The salts are minerals, and, as discussed in Chapter 4, the more minerals water has, the denser the water is, and the easier it is to float in it. This is why relaxing in seawater is so refreshing, and why exercises performed in seawater can be so effective. Sea air is rich in ozone, and just breathing it has a revitalizing and tonifying effect. It is easy to understand why so many people are drawn to oceans and beaches for rejuvenation.

In addition to seawater, other sea substances are used in spa and hydrotherapy treatments, including seaweed, **sea mud,** and **sea salt.** For simplicity's sake, seaweed, sea mud, and sea salt will be referred to by the collective term *sea products* throughout the rest of the chapter.

In general, sea products have a number of qualities that are beneficial to the body, including:

- being antibacterial agents; the minerals and salts in sea products kill certain bacteria
- firming the skin; water is drawn from the skin to the salts in the sea products (which also gives the body a slimmer appearance)
- helping to eliminate toxins; the water drawn from the skin to the salts in the sea products carries wastes with it
- stimulating blood circulation; some of the small mineral salts in the sea products are able to enter the skin and go into the blood (water is drawn to the higher ion content in the blood so blood volume increases, and this stimulates blood circulation)
- being nourishing; certain small mineral salts and trace elements pass from the skin into the bloodstream (Barron, 2003; Minton, 2008a; Williams, 2007).

SEAWATER

Bathing in seawater can help remineralize the body to a limited extent, which may, in turn, help balance aspects of the body's metabolism, leaving the person feeling invigorated. As a result of the drawing properties of its minerals, seawater baths can be detoxifying as well as stimulating to blood and lymphatic flow. Some spas have seawater baths available, and seawater can also be used in hydrotherapy tubs while practitioners perform therapeutic techniques on clients.

CLINICAL ALERT !

Practitioners and clients can be allergic to any or all sea products, including seawater. Clients who are allergic to shellfish or iodine should *never* receive thalassotherapy treatments; practitioners who are allergic to shellfish or iodine should *never* perform thalassotherapy treatments. Clients may not realize that an allergy to shellfish or iodine also means allergies to sea products, so it is important for the practitioner to find out from clients any allergies they may have, and note them on an intake form, so there is written documentation. Practitioners allergic to any or all sea products should never use them on clients even when requested to do so, either by clients or employers.

People can develop allergies throughout their lives; therefore, every time a client arrives for a treatment, the practitioner should do a quick allergy update. Before any treatment is performed, the substance should be applied to a small area on the client's skin and on the practitioner's skin, usually the forearm, to see if there is an allergic reaction.

SEA PRODUCTS

Seaweed

The word *seaweed* has become an umbrella term for any marine plant or algae. However, seaweed is not technically a true plant. Although it does have chlorophyll, which allows it to produce oxygen as plants do, it does not have true roots, stems, or leaves. It is actually **algae.** Algae are groups of aquatic organisms that perform photosynthesis. They are found in almost every habitat in the world. Species of algae range in size from single celled and microscopic, such as plankton, to multicellular and huge, such as a brown seaweed that has fronds (leaves) 200 feet long. Sometimes the terms *algae* and *seaweed* are used interchangeably. There are many different types of seaweed, and they are used for many different things:

▸ Seaweed is harvested for food, especially in Asian countries. For example, Japan does not have a lot of land mass to grow food, so it looks to the sea to help feed its people. It is also farmed for food in China, the British Isles, and Iceland.

▸ Certain seaweeds are processed to make a gelatin used in foods, cosmetics, and hair care products, as well as in the textile industry.

▸ Some seaweeds are sources for vitamin and mineral supplements for humans and livestock and are used in medicines and even fertilizer.

Some seaweeds are harvested from beaches where they have washed up, some are harvested from the water close to shore, and some are harvested from the deep oceans (Ellis, 2000).

Types of Seaweed

The three major categories of seaweed are based on their colors: green, brown, and red. **Green seaweeds** (see ▸Figure 7.1) are found near shores in shallow waters. They usually grow in threadlike filaments, sheets, or branching fronds. One of the most common green seaweeds used in spa treatments is sea lettuce (*Ulva lactuca*), which is used in spa and hydrotherapy treatments to relieve inflammation and muscle soreness.

Brown seaweeds (see ▸Figure 7.2) have a brown pigment that masks the green of the chlorophyll. They are the most numerous of the seaweeds in moderate and polar climate regions and grow at depths of 50 to 75 feet. There are two major groups of brown seaweeds used in spa treatments:

▸ *Laminaria* species: commonly known as kelp, generally large and leathery, found worldwide
▸ *Fucus* species: commonly known as wracks, the most common seaweed along the Atlantic coasts of Europe and North America, and along the California coast

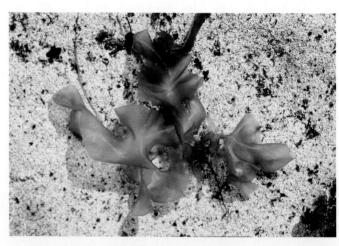

▸ **Figure 7.1** Green seaweeds are often used in spa and hydrotherapy treatments to relieve inflammation and muscle soreness. *(Laurie Campbell/Photoshot/NHPA Limited)*

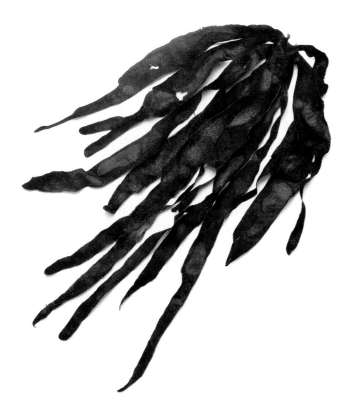

▶ **Figure 7.2** Brown seaweeds are used in spa and hydrotherapy treatments for detoxification, revitalization, slimming, and skin tightening. *(Karl Shone © Dorling Kindersley)*

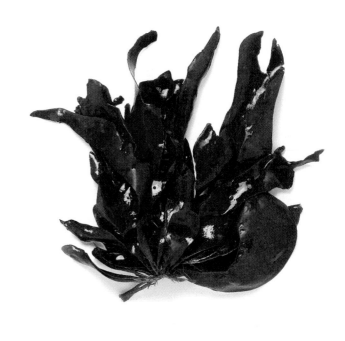

▶ **Figure 7.3** Red seaweeds are used in spa and hydrotherapy treatments for detoxification, revitalization, slimming, skin tightening, moisturizing, and exfoliation. *(Tim Ridley © Dorling Kindersley)*

Brown seaweeds are used in spa and hydrotherapy treatments for detoxification, revitalization (through increased local blood and lymph circulation), slimming, and skin tightening.

The **red seaweeds** (see ▶Figure 7.3) are mostly delicate and fernlike. Many grow at great depths, down to 879 feet; their red pigment allows them to absorb the small amount of blue and violet light that penetrates to this level and use this light to produce oxygen. Red seaweed grows abundantly along the Atlantic coasts of Europe and North America, in the Northern Pacific Ocean, and in parts of the Mediterranean. One red seaweed, *Chondrus crispus,* actually grows in more shallow waters, especially around the British Isles. Because it is harvested extensively in Ireland, it is called Irish moss. Another name for it is carragen (or carragen moss). One of the products made from processing carragen is carrageenan, which is a thickener used in many foods. Irish moss is used in spa and hydrotherapy treatments for detoxification, revitalization (through increased local blood and lymph circulation), slimming, skin tightening, and moisturizing.

Lithothamnium is another type of red algae that can be used in spa treatments. It is a delicate, small seaweed that grows off the southwestern coast of Ireland. It leaves behind a calcified skeleton when it dies. The skeletons of

this algae are harvested when they wash closer into shore. When ground, they make an excellent natural exfoliation substance (Ellis, 2000; Williams, 2007).

DID YOU KNOW?

During the great potato famine in the mid-1800s, many families who lived along the coasts of Ireland were able to avoid starvation by eating Irish moss. After it was dried and bleached by the sun, it yielded a highly nutritious jelly (carrageenan) that was used in soups, stews, and puddings. This same drying and sun-bleaching process for carrageenan is used today.

Other Algae

Other algae that are not seaweed are also used in spa therapy treatments. These include spirulina, a type of blue-green algae (see ▶Figure 7.4), and white algae, which is really lichen. Lichens are actually a combination of a fungus and an organism, usually a type of green algae, that produces food for the lichen from sunlight. Spirulina and white algae treatments are used in spas for detoxification, revitalization (through increased local blood and lymph

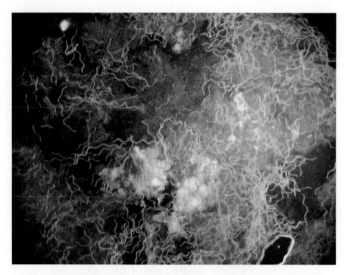

▶ **Figure 7.4** Spirulina treatments are used in spa treatments for detoxification, revitalization, slimming, skin tightening, and moisturizing. *(Photo by Jesse Brouse)*

circulation), slimming, skin tightening, and moisturizing (Abel, 2005).

Sea Mud

Sea mud is collected from beaches at low tide and mixed with seawater. Like all sea products, it is used for its analgesic, warming, and sedative properties, as well as for detoxification. Sea mud can be used by itself or mixed with clays or paraffin. Body wraps, masks, and baths are just some of the ways it can be used in spa and hydrotherapy treatments.

Sea Salt

Sea salt is formed by the natural evaporation of ocean water. It is harvested when seawater is left to dry in the sun. Sea salt can be used for salt scrubs, baths, and inhalation treatments.

TREATMENTS

Body Wraps

There are many ways to perform wraps. Practitioners who work in spas should note that each spa has its own body wrap protocols and trains its practitioners accordingly. What is presented in this chapter may or may not be consistent with how individual spas perform their wraps. However, by practicing the procedures in this chapter, practitioners, whether they work in a spa, clinic, or private practice, will acquire foundational skills, become comfortable handling supplies and equipment, and become able to knowledgeably discuss body wrap options with clients.

The body wrap treatment itself typically takes 35 to 40 minutes. The treatment time can be extended to 60 to 90 minutes when supplemented with other bodywork treatments, such as full-body dry brushing, massage therapy, shiatsu, acupressure, reflexology, and so forth. For example, a seaweed or sea mud wrap could be paired with a sea salt glow.

It is important that the practitioner inform the client that portions of the treatment have less conservative draping than a regular massage. If a wet table and Vichy shower or other water source will be used to remove the body wrap substance, the practitioner needs to inform clients that they will have minimal covering during the showering process. Although the practitioner is used to this, clients may not be. Clients need to be given the opportunity to decline the treatment if they are not comfortable with this.

The equipment and supplies for the following body wraps can be purchased at local stores or online; the sea products (see ▶Figure 7.5) need to be purchased through a spa treatment supply store.

Poultices

Poultices are treatments applied to a specific area of the body. They are soft, moist masses of substance that are applied either directly or encased in a clean cloth such as flannel, cheesecloth, muslin. The poultice is then covered and left for a period of time. Today's body wraps evolved from the use of poultices. The procedures are the same: a substance is applied to the body and then covered by cloth. In fact, a body wrap can be thought of as a poultice applied to the entire body. For more information on seaweed and sea mud poultices, see Appendix 1, "Poultices."

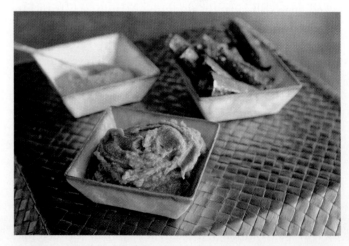

▶ **Figure 7.5** Clockwise from top right: seaweed, sea mud, and sea salt.

TREATMENT 7.1

Seaweed or Other Algae Body Wrap

Rationale

A seaweed or other algae body wrap can be done for any or all of the following physiological effects:

- Absorptive: a small amount of minerals pass through the skin
- Tonifier: strengthens vitality and the immune system
- Vasodilator: increases local blood flow
- Detoxifier: eliminates toxins
- Emollient: soothes the skin
- Sedative: induces a state of deep relaxation
- Buffer: balances pH of skin

Equipment and Supplies (see ▶Figures 7.6 a and b)

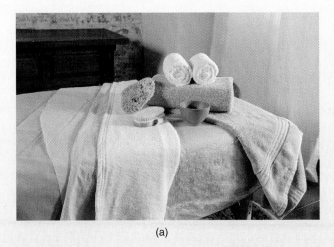
(a)

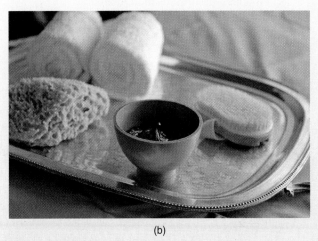
(b)

▶ **Figure 7.6**

- exfoliation tools or ingredients for a scrub
- seaweed, kelp, or other algae powder mixed with water, seaweed, or other algae gel, or crème (¼ to ½ cup)
- small, nonmetal bowl—nonmetal because seaweed reacts chemically with metal, causing properties of the seaweed to change; likewise, seaweed should not be stored in metal containers
- three cloth sheets (one fitted and two flat)
- insulating sheet (rubber, plastic, Mylar, etc.)
- wool blanket
- one beach towel, approximately 35″ × 65″
- two large towels, approximately 30″ × 60″
- If there is access to a shower, textured washcloth or bath scrubby for client use to remove the seaweed or other algae
- If there is no access to a shower, a basin of warm water and three to four towels, approximately 18″ × 30″, for substance removal are needed. A towel cabi or crock pot filled with moist towels can also be used. More than three to four towels may be necessary for clients who have a large body size or a lot of body hair (since it may be more difficult to remove seaweed from the hair).
- washcloth
- small bowl
- cool water

TREATMENT 7.1 CONTINUED

Indications

- need for detoxification
- muscle tightness
- skin disorders such as eczema and psoriasis
- need to balance skin's pH
- need for stress relief and relaxation
- need to increase metabolism

Contraindications

- heart conditions
- untreated hypertension
- allergy to iodine or shellfish
- inflammation
- vascular disease, including varicose veins
- numbness/loss of sensation in area
- skin conditions made worse by heat
- intolerance to heat
- broken or irritated skin
- high body temperature (fever)
- claustrophobia
- pregnancy

Preparation

1. Layer the table in the following order (see ▶ Figure 7.7):

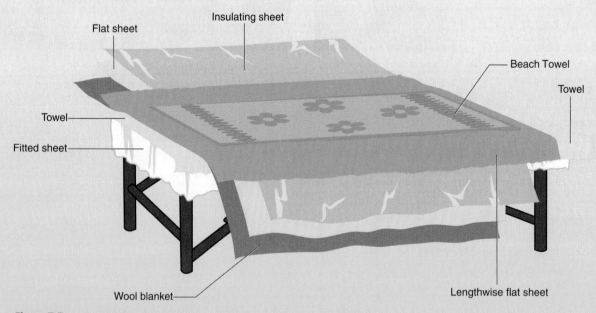

▶ **Figure 7.7**

- Fitted sheet to protect table
- One large towel placed horizontally across the head of the table
- Wool blanket placed horizontally across the table, on top of the towel, leaving enough room for the head to rest on the towel
- One large towel placed horizontally across the end of the table, on top of the wool blanket

- Flat sheet placed horizontally on top of the wool blanket
- Insulating sheet placed horizontally on top of the cloth sheet
- 1 flat sheet placed lengthwise on top of the insulating sheet
- Beach towel placed lengthwise on top of the flat sheet

2. Place the seaweed in the small bowl; position the bowl within easy reach.
3. If working in a dry room and using a crock pot or cabi, turn it on to warm the towels for substance removal at the end of the treatment. Moisten the three to four (or more) 18″ × 30″ towels and put them in the crock pot or cabi. If using the basin of warm water and towels, place the basin in a convenient place to fill it with warm water during the treatment.
4. Fill the small bowl with cool water and place the washcloth in it. Position it within easy reach.
5. Leave the room while the client gets on the table under the beach towel, lying prone.

Procedure

Perform a pre–body wrap exfoliation. The quick-prep dry-brushing procedure from Chapter 5 is described here, but any of the exfoliation treatments in Chapter 5 can be performed. If the large towel is used for draping, then there will be no need to undrape the extremities to perform the exfoliation.

Standing at the foot of the table, undrape the client's left leg and gluteal region. Working toward the client's heart, start brushing at the feet, move up the leg, and include the gluteals. Redrape the client's left leg. Move to the client's right leg. Undrape and brush the foot, leg, and gluteal region the same as for the left leg. Redrape the client's right leg.

CLINICAL ALERT !

Check with the client about pressure and adjust as necessary.

2. Move to the client's left arm and undrape it. Brush the palm of the client's hand and fingers. Beginning at the client's wrist, brush up the arm, stroking from the wrist toward the client's heart. Redrape the client's left arm. Move to the client's right arm. Undrape and brush the hand and arm the same as for the left arm. Redrape the client's right arm.

3. Move to the head of the table and undrape the back. Starting at the neck and shoulders, brush down to the client's mid-back. Move to the right side of the table. Reaching across the client's back, brush the client's left lumbar to mid-back area, using angling, upward strokes toward the client's heart. Move to the left side of the table. Brush the client's right lumbar to mid-back area the same as for the left side. Redrape the back.

4. Help the client turn over.

5. Standing at the foot of the table, undrape the client's right leg. Working toward the client's heart, start brushing at the foot and move up the leg. Redrape the client's right leg. Move to the client's left leg. Undrape and brush the foot and leg the same as for the right leg. Redrape the client's left leg.

6. Move to the client's abdomen and drape the large towel across the client's chest area. Have the client hold it firmly as you pull the sheet inferiorly until the client's abdomen is undraped. Using smaller strokes, brush the client's abdomen in a clockwise direction. Finish the abdomen by brushing up each side and coming to the center of the abdomen.

Redrape the client's abdomen by pulling the sheet up over the client's abdomen and the draping towel on the client's chest area. Move to one side of the client, and while the client holds the sheet firmly, gently pull the draping towel out from under the sheet.

8. Move to the client's right arm and undrape it. Brush the back of the client's hand and fingers. Beginning at the client's wrist, brush up the arm, stroking from the wrist toward the client's heart. Redrape the client's right arm. Move to the client's left arm. Undrape and brush the hand and arm the same as for the right arm. Redrape the client's left arm.

9. Move to the head of the table. To brush the client's upper chest area, start at the right clavicle and brush downward three times, then brush downward three times from the left clavicle.

TREATMENT 7.1 CONTINUED

Application of seaweed

1. Place a large towel over the top sheet lengthwise along the client. Have the client hold the towel firmly in place while you reach across the client and grasp the top sheet on both sides. Gently pull the top sheet out from underneath the towel and set the sheet aside. Having the client draped with the towel will make it easier to apply the seaweed.

2. To remove the sheet on which the client is lying, ask the client to lift the head slightly. Reach across the client and grasp the sheet on both sides; gently pull down. Have the client lay the head back down, and lift the shoulders, then shoulders down and lift the hips, then hips down as you continue to pull the sheet down toward the foot of the table. (▶Figures 7.8 a, b, and c) Set the sheet aside. Make sure that the client's shoulders are slightly below the top of the insulating sheet.

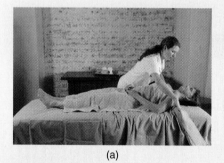
(a)

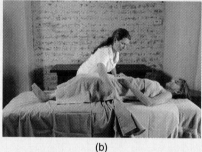
(b)

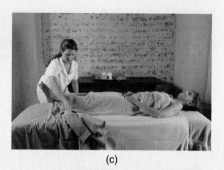
(c)

▶ **Figure 7.8**

3. Help the client sit up and quickly apply the seaweed to the back with long, smooth strokes, covering the area thoroughly (▶Figures 7.9 a, b, c, and d). Help the client lie back down.

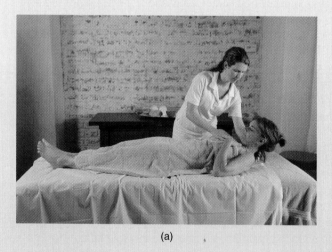
(a)

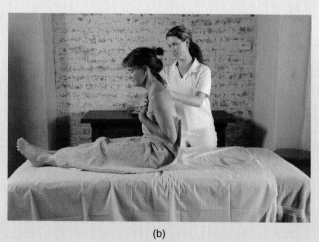
(b)

▶ **Figure 7.9**

TREATMENT 7.1 CONTINUED

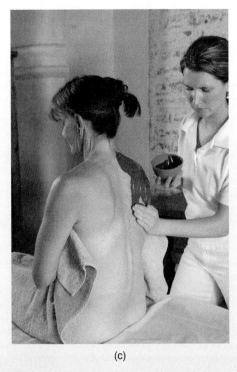

(c)

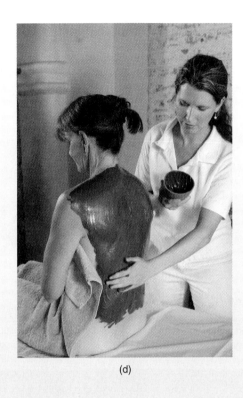

(d)

▶ **Figure 7.9 (*cont.*)**

4. Move to the client's left leg and ask the client to flex the knee while draping carefully and securely (▶Figures 7.10 a, b, and c). To stabilize the client's leg, gently sit on the foot. Apply the seaweed to the client's posterior leg with one smooth stroke.

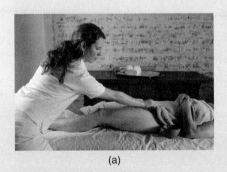

(a)

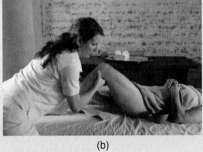

(b)

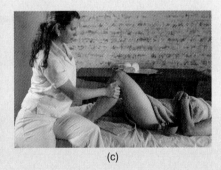

(c)

▶ **Figure 7.10**

TREATMENT 7.1 CONTINUED

Grasp the client's ankle and lay the leg flat (▶Figures 7.11 a and b).

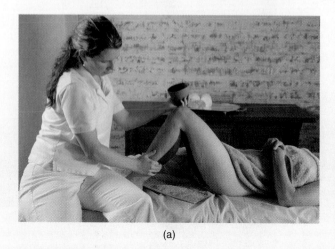

(a)

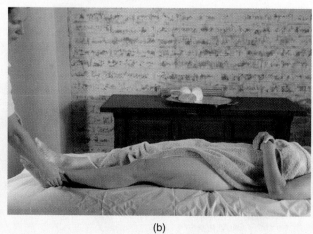

(b)

▶ **Figure 7.11**

5. Apply the seaweed to the client's left anterior leg with long, smooth strokes. Cover the client's left leg with the insulating sheet to prevent chilling (▶Figures 7.12 a, b, c, and d).

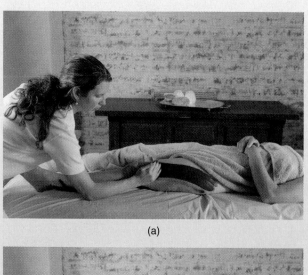

(a)

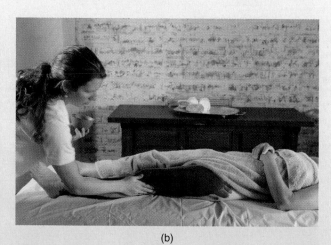

(b)

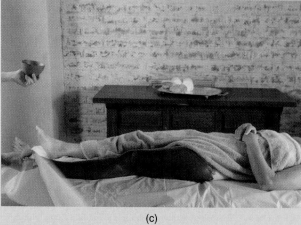

(c)

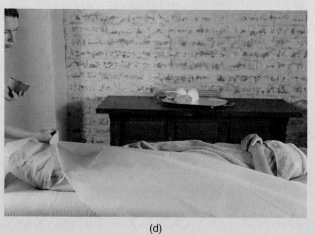

(d)

▶ **Figure 7.12**

TREATMENT 7.1 CONTINUED

6. Move to the client's right leg and apply the seaweed to the posterior and anterior leg in the same manner as for the left leg. Cover the client's right leg with the insulating sheet to prevent chilling.

7. Move to the client's abdomen and drape one of the large towels across the client's chest area and have the client hold it firmly. Pull the bottom, draping towel inferiorly until the client's abdomen is undraped. Apply the seaweed to the abdomen in a clockwise motion (▶Figures 7.13 a, b, and c).

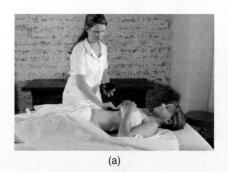
(a)
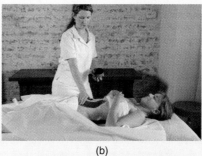
(b)
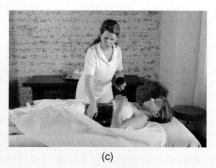
(c)

▶ **Figure 7.13**

8. Move to the client's left arm and apply the seaweed to the posterior and anterior arm with long, smooth strokes (▶Figures 7.14 a, b, and c). Cover the client's left arm and abdomen with the insulating sheet to prevent chilling. Move to the client's right arm and apply the seaweed the same as for the left arm. Cover the client's right arm with the insulating sheet to prevent chill.

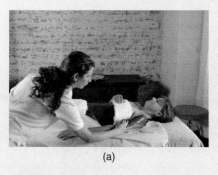
(a)
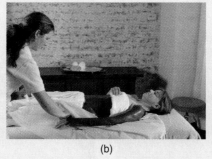
(b)
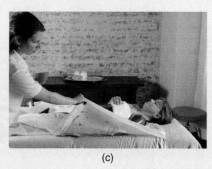
(c)

▶ **Figure 7.14**

9. Move to the head of the table and apply the seaweed to the client's upper chest (▶Figure 7.15).

10. Wrap the client securely with each of the layers on the table, one at a time, except the bottom sheet (▶Figures 7.16 a, b, c, d, e, f, and g).

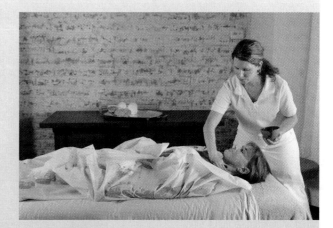

▶ **Figure 7.15**

TREATMENT 7.1 CONTINUED

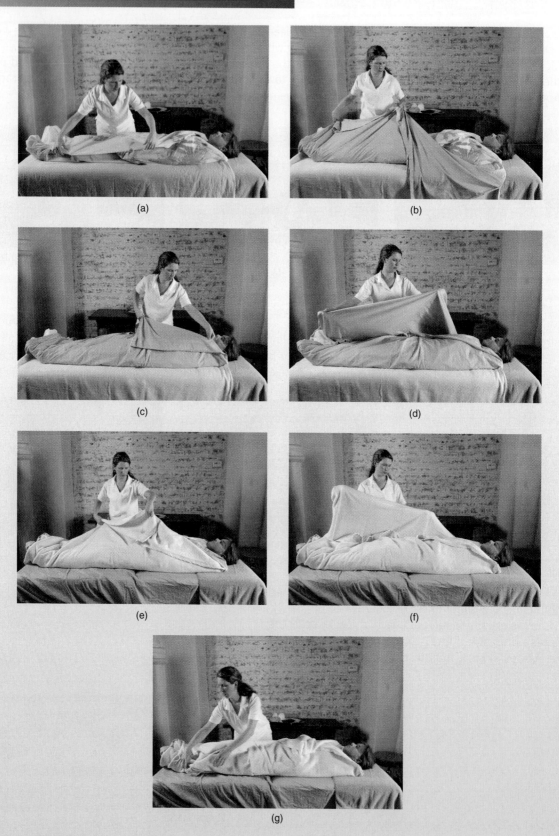

(a)

(b)

(c)

(d)

(e)

(f)

(g)

▶ **Figure 7.16**

TREATMENT 7.1 CONTINUED

11. Use the towel at the head of the table to wrap securely around the client's neck (▶Figures 7.17 a and b).

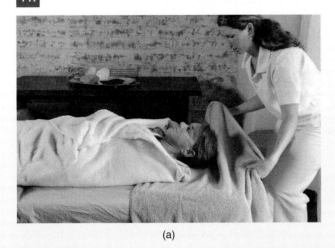
(a)

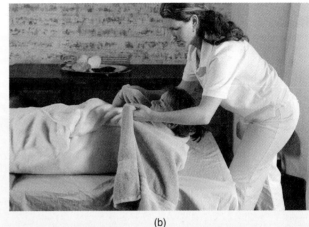
(b)

▶ **Figure 7.17**

12. Make sure the client is comfortable using bolsters, pillows, or other props as needed. An extra blanket can be added for more warmth. The client should remain wrapped for 25 to 30 minutes. During this time, a scalp and facial massage can be given (▶Figure 7.18), or the client's feet can be unwrapped for a foot massage. Another option is to sit quietly at the head or foot of the table. Place a cool, moist washcloth on the client's face or forehead if needed.

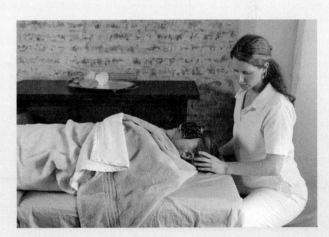

▶ **Figure 7.18**

CLINICAL ALERT !

It is important to stay near the client; some clients may become claustrophobic or overheated and need to have the wrappings removed as soon as they start feeling uncomfortable.

TREATMENT 7.1 CONTINUED

13. When the time is up, unwrap each of the layers until the client is covered by just the plastic sheet (and the towels with which the client was initially draped). Place a large towel lengthwise over the client (▸Figures 7.19 a, b, and c).

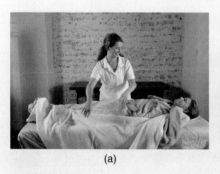

(a)

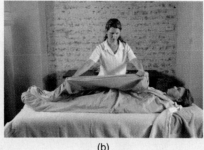

(b)

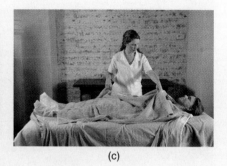

(c)

▸ **Figure 7.19**

Gently pull the plastic sheet out from underneath the towel (▸Figures 7.20 a and b).

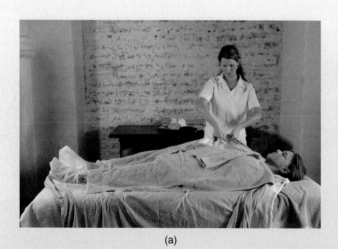

(a)

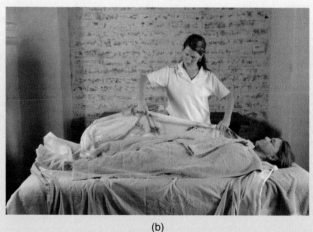

(b)

▸ **Figure 7.20**

14. Help the client sit up and hang the legs off the side of the table (▸Figure 7.21). Use a warm, moist towel to remove the seaweed residue from the client's back.

15. If using a wet table or Vichy shower, rinse the client thoroughly to remove residue from the seaweed or other algae on the client's skin. If there is a separate shower facility, help the client off the table, offering a bathrobe or draping a large towel for modesty. Give the client the textured washcloth or bath scrubby (to remove residue on the skin), and guide the client to the shower and then back to the massage table after rinsing off. If working in a dry room with no access to a shower, use the dry room removal technique. Once the residue has been removed from the client's skin, help the client off the table.

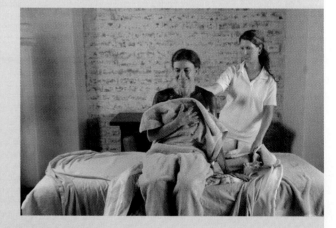

▸ **Figure 7.21**

TREATMENT 7.1 CONTINUED

DRY ROOM REMOVAL TECHNIQUE

The dry room removal technique described here is from Chapter 5.

If the seaweed body wrap is being done in a dry room with no access to a shower, the residue on the client's skin can be removed by placing a warm, moist towel on the area for a few seconds.

▶ Remove a towel from the crock pot, cabi, or basin and wring it out if it is too wet.
▶ Apply the towel to the client's body and pat down firmly, and then remove the substance with one firm, smooth stroke. Do not scrub or wipe with the towel.
▶ Use a new towel from the crock pot, cabi, or basin for each area of the body from which residue is removed.
▶ To prevent chilling, cover each part of the client's body immediately after removing the residue.

After the Treatment
Encourage the client to rest and drink plenty of water after treatment. The client's skin may show a slight flush since the seaweed greatly improves circulation and retains heat. This allows increased blood flow to the surface of the skin.

Hygiene
Any leftover seaweed should be discarded after each client. The sheets and towels should be laundered with hot water and detergent after each use. Clean the insulating sheet by spraying it with alcohol or other disinfectant. It can also be washed with soap and water, but it should still be sprayed with alcohol after that. If brushes were used for the exfoliation, wash them in warm, soapy water and rinse. After rinsing, place them in rubbing alcohol for at least 20 minutes, then let them air dry. The tools can also be washed in a dishwasher. Store them in an airtight container. If the exfoliation was done using a natural substance, any leftover exfoliation mixture should be immediately discarded. All bowls should be washed in warm, soapy water and rinsed between each use. The washcloth or bath scrubby should be either given to the client to take or discarded; it should never be used by more than one client. The towel cabi should be washed out daily and sprayed with disinfectant. Used towels should never be placed back in it. If a crock pot is used, it should be washed in warm, soapy water, rinsed, and sprayed with disinfectant after each use.

Masks

TO GET YOU STARTED

Seaweed Clay Mask
¼ cup seaweed of choice
¼ cup clay of choice

Mix the seaweed and the clay together and apply to the face. Leave on for 15 minutes and then remove with a warm, moist washcloth. Finish with a splash of cold water; then gently blot the skin dry.

Try different combinations of seaweed and clay to see which ones you like the best.

Baths

Sea baths can be rejuvenating, as the popularity of bathing in the ocean shows. Since going to the ocean is not practical for everyone, some spas have the facilities for clients to take seawater baths, either still baths or seawater-filled whirlpools. Other sea products can also be added to bath water. If their municipal regulations allow it, practitioners may choose to install a bathtub in their clinic or office, but they need to be aware that special plumbing may be required to dispose of the seaweed, other algae, and sea mud after the bath water is used.

Practitioners can also instruct clients on how to have a sea product bath in their own homes and they can give their clients samples of seaweed, other algae, sea mud, and sea salt to use. Unless seaweed or sea mud baths are used quite frequently by clients at home, there should not be any plumbing issues from the seaweed and sea mud when tubs are drained. The amount of seaweed and sea mud used in a single bath is relatively small.

As with a body wrap, it is always important to begin with an exfoliation, since removing the dead skin cells enables the sea products to work more efficiently. This can be done manually through dry brushing or using natural substances such as a salt or sugar scrub. More informa-

TREATMENT 7.2

Sea Mud Body Wrap

Rationale

A sea mud body wrap can be done for any or all of the following physiological effects:

- Absorptive: a small amount of minerals pass through the skin
- Tonifier: strengthens vitality and the immune system
- Vasodilator: increases local blood flow
- Analgesic: relieves pain
- Detoxifier: eliminates toxins
- Emollient: soothes the skin
- Buffer: balances pH of skin
- Extractor: draws impurities from the skin
- Sedative: induces a state of deep relaxation
- Thermodynamic: sends deep, penetrating heat into muscles and joints

Equipment and Supplies

The list of equipment and supplies for a sea mud body wrap are the same as for Treatment 7.1. Instead of seaweed, kelp, or other algae, ¼ to ½ cup of sea mud powder mixed with water or ¼ to ½ cup sea mud gel or crème is used.

Indications

- tight joints (from noninflammatory conditions)
- muscle spasms, tightness, or strain
- skin disorders such as eczema and psoriasis
- need to balance skin's pH
- need for detoxification
- need for skin cleansing
- need for stress relief and relaxation
- need to increase metabolism

Contraindications

- heart conditions
- untreated hypertension
- allergy to iodine or shellfish
- inflammation
- vascular disease, including varicose veins
- numbness/loss of sensation in area
- skin conditions made worse by heat
- intolerance to heat
- broken or irritated skin
- high body temperature (fever)
- claustrophobia
- pregnancy

The preparation, procedure, after-treatment care, and hygiene are the same as for Treatment 7.1.

TREATMENT 7.3

Seaweed, Other Algae, or Sea Mud Mask

Rationale

A seaweed, other algae, or sea mud mask can be done for any or all of the following physiological effects:

- Extractor: draws impurities from the skin
- Absorptive: a small amount of minerals passes through the skin
- Tonifier: strengthens vitality and the immune system
- Vasodilator: increases local blood flow
- Detoxifier: eliminates toxins
- Emollient: soothes the skin
- Buffer: balances pH of skin

Equipment and Supplies (see ▶Figures 7.22 a, b, and c)

- exfoliation tools or ingredients for a gentle facial scrub
- small, nonmetal bowl—nonmetal because seaweed and sea mud react chemically with metal, changing the properties of the seaweed or mud; likewise, seaweed and sea mud should not be stored in metal containers
- water
- seaweed, kelp, other algae, or sea mud powder mixed with water, or seaweed, kelp, other algae, or sea mud gel or crème (1/3 cup)
- small paint brush (optional)
- cucumber slices (optional)
- washcloth
- one towel, approximately 18″ × 30″
- small crock pot or electric warmer if warming the seaweed or sea mud; if using a small electric warmer, another bowl will be needed

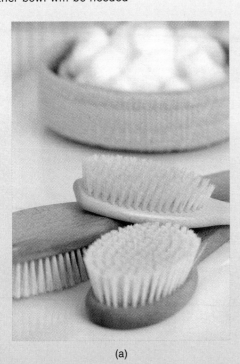

(a)

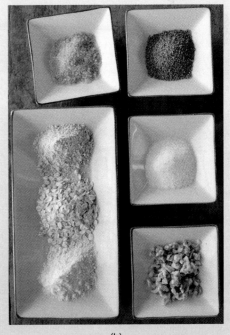

(b)

▶ **Figure 7.22** *(Photo (a) courtesy of John Davis © Dorling Kindersley)*

TREATMENT 7.3 CONTINUED

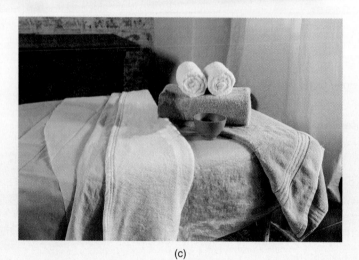

(c)

▶ **Figure 7.22 (*cont.*)**

Indications

- need for detoxification
- muscle tightness
- skin disorders such as eczema and psoriasis
- need to draw impurities from the skin
- mild acne
- need to balance skin's pH
- need for stress relief and relaxation

Contraindications

- allergy to iodine or shellfish
- numbness or loss of sensation in the face
- high body temperature (fever)
- skin conditions made worse by heat
- local inflammation
- broken or irritated skin
- intolerance to heat

Preparation

1. The seaweed or sea mud can be either warmed or used at room temperature, depending on the client's preference. Seaweed and sea mud should never be warmed by microwaving; this destroys their therapeutic properties. To warm these substances using a crock pot, place the seaweed or sea mud in a small bowl, then put that bowl in a small crock pot with one inch of hot water (see ▶Figure 7.23). If using a small electric warmer, place the seaweed or sea mud in a small dish, and then put that dish inside another dish that has about an inch of water in it; place both bowls on the warmer.

2. Position the seaweed or sea mud and water within easy reach.

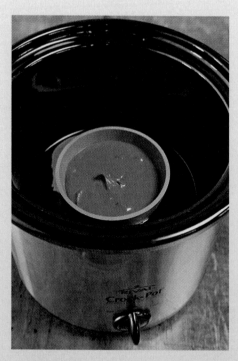

▶ **Figure 7.23**

TREATMENT 7.3 CONTINUED

Treatment

1. Perform a gentle exfoliation of the client's face. ▶Figure 7.24 shows an exfoliation using a soft brush. Use small, gentle strokes from the client's chin to the forehead.

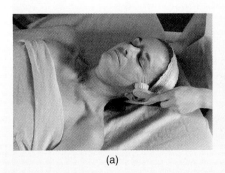

(a)

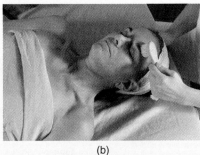

(b)

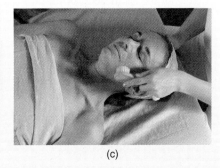

(c)

▶ **Figure 7.24**

2. Moisten the seaweed or sea mud with enough water to make a thin paste.

3. Apply mixture evenly over the client's face, avoiding the eye area. Application can be done with the hands or using a small paintbrush. Be sure to spread the mixture evenly (▶Figures 7.25 a, b, c, and d).

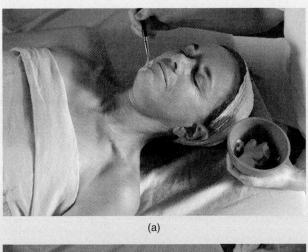

(a)

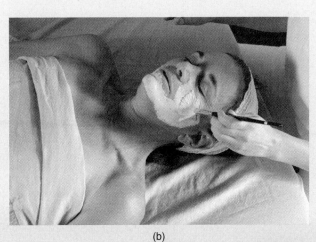

(b)

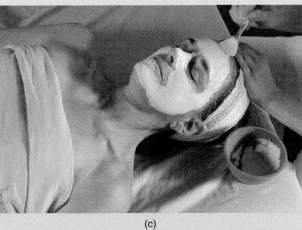

(c)

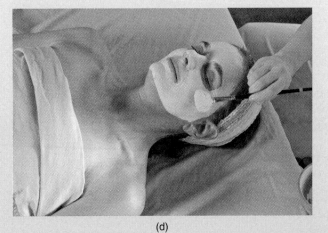

(d)

▶ **Figure 7.25**

TREATMENT 7.3 CONTINUED

Cucumber slices can be placed over the eyes for added refreshment (▶ Figure 7.26).

4. Leave the mask on for 15 minutes. During this time, a scalp massage can be given, or the client's hands, shoulders, or feet can be massaged.

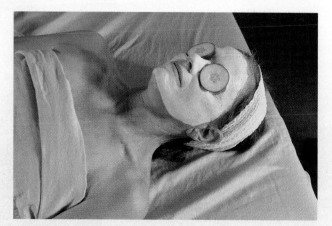

▶ **Figure 7.26**

CLINICAL ALERT: ❗

It is important to stay near the client; if the mask becomes uncomfortable, it needs to be removed immediately.

5. Soak the washcloth in warm water, and then wring it out. Remove the mask by wiping the client's face with the warm, moist washcloth. A gentle splash of cold water on the client's face is a good way to finish the treatment.

6. Dry the client's face by gently blotting with the towel.

After the Treatment

Encourage the client to drink plenty of water after the treatment. The skin may show a slight flush since the seaweed or sea mud greatly improves circulation and retains heat, which allows increased blood to flow to the surface of the skin.

Hygiene

Any leftover seaweed or sea mud should be discarded after each client. The face cloth and towel should be laundered with hot water and detergent after each use. The small bowl should be washed in warm, soapy water and rinsed between each use. If a crock pot is used, it should be washed in warm, soapy water, rinsed, and sprayed with disinfectant after each use.

tion about these is found in Chapter 5. However, an exfoliation should not be done before taking a sea salt bath because of the painful effect the salt will have on the newly exfoliated skin.

Either a full-immersion or foot bath can be taken. In either case, the bath itself typically takes 20 to 25 minutes. If done in a spa or massage and bodywork office, the client can also receive complementary treatments such as massage therapy, shiatsu, acupressure, reflexology, and so forth.

Among the many benefits of taking a seawater or sea product bath are:

▶ strengthened vitality and immune system
▶ increased blood and lymphatic flow
▶ pain relief from tight joints and muscle spasms, tightness, or strain
▶ detoxification
▶ cleansed skin
▶ soothed skin, especially for eczema and psoriasis
▶ relaxation and stress relief
▶ deep, penetrating heat sent into muscles and joints
▶ balanced pH of the skin
▶ decongestion from colds, flu, or bronchitis

TREATMENT 7.4

Sea Salt Glow

Salt glows can be performed using sea salt as well as earth salts, as discussed in Chapters 5 and 6.

Rationale

A sea salt glow can be applied for any or all of the following physiological effects:

- Exfoliant: removes dead skin cells
- Vasodilator: increases local blood flow
- Stimulant: invigorates the whole body and promotes movement of the digestive tract
- Tonifier: strengthens vitality and the immune system

Equipment and Supplies

- small, nonmetal bowl for sea salt—nonmetal because the sea salt may react chemically with metal, which may change the salt's properties
- ¼ to ½ cup of salt; use 50 percent fine salt and 50 percent medium-grain salt (sea salt, Epsom salt, Dead Sea salt, desert mineral salt)
- essential oil(s) of choice; if using an essential oil, a couple drops of a carrier oil will also be needed
- warm water (to mix with the salt)
- one cloth sheet and two large towels, approximately 30″ × 60″
- If there is no access to a shower, a basin of warm water and three to four towels, approximately 18″ × 30″, for salt removal are needed. A towel cabi or crock pot filled with moist towels can also be used. More than three to four towels may be necessary for clients who have a large body size or a lot of body hair (since it may be more difficult to remove the salt from the hair).

Indications

- need for exfoliation
- need for detoxification
- fatigue
- low endurance
- beginning or ending of a cold or flu

Contraindications

- allergy to iodine or shellfish
- allergy to salt
- broken or irritated skin
- contagious skin condition
- rashes
- sunburn
- athlete's foot—only the feet would be contraindicated; the rest of the body could be exfoliated
- recent tattoo
- area shaved within 24 hours prior to treatment

Preparation

1. Place the cloth sheet and two large towels lengthwise on top of the table.
2. Position the salt, water, and small bowl within easy reach.
3. If working in a dry room and using a crock pot or cabi, turn it on to warm the towels for sea salt removal at the end of the treatment. Moisten the three to four (or more) 18″ × 30″ towels and put them in the crock pot or cabi. If using the basin of warm water and towels, position the basin in a convenient place to fill it with warm water during the treatment.

TREATMENT 7.4 CONTINUED

Procedure

Have the client get on the table in supine position underneath the large towel.

1. Measure equal parts fine- and medium-grain salt into the small bowl. Make a little depression in the center of the salt. Use just enough warm water to make the salt the consistency of snow; blend the mixture with your fingers. If desired, add essential oil to the salt mixture. First, add a couple drops of a carrier oil, then add a drop or two of essential oil; mix well.

2. Take the bowl of mixture to the foot of the table.

3. Undrape the client's right leg. Pour some water in your hands. Then, starting at the client's right foot, apply it up the client's leg.

4. Take a small amount of the salt mixture and rub it between your hands. Take more as needed during the treatment. Apply the salt mixture to the dorsal surface of the client's foot using small circular strokes to thoroughly exfoliate it. Continue using small circular strokes up the ankle and anterior right leg. Redrape the client's leg. Move to the client's left leg. Undrape and exfoliate the foot and leg the same as for the right leg. Redrape the client's left leg.

CLINICAL ALERT ❗

Check with client about pressure, and adjust it as necessary.

---

5. Move to the client's right arm and undrape it. Use small circular strokes to thoroughly exfoliate the client's right hand and arm, up to the shoulder. Redrape the client's right arm. Move to the client's left arm. Undrape and exfoliate the hand and arm the same as for the right arm. Redrape the client's left arm.

6. Move to the client's abdomen. Fold the large towel like an accordion crosswise over the client's chest area and grasp the top of the large, lengthwise towel on top of the client. As you unfold the crosswise towel, fold down the lengthwise towel until the client's chest is draped by the crosswise towel, and the abdomen is undraped. Stand at the side of the table. Using smaller movements and a lighter touch, stroke in a clockwise direction. Finish by exfoliating each of the client's sides and coming to the center of the abdomen. Pull the towel up over the client's abdomen and draping towel on the client's chest area. Gently pull the draping towel out from under the sheet.

7. Move to the head of the table. To exfoliate the client's upper chest area, use smaller movements and a lighter touch, working downward from the clavicles.

8. If the client's face is to be included, use a light touch. With small gentle strokes, exfoliate from the client's chin to forehead.

9. Before the client turns over, the salt should be removed. If using a wet table or Vichy shower, rinse the client thoroughly. If working in a dry room, use the dry room removal technique.

DRY ROOM REMOVAL TECHNIQUE

The dry room removal technique described here is from Chapter 5. If the sea salt glow is being done in a dry room with no access to a shower, the residue on the client's skin can be removed by placing a warm, moist towel on the area for a few seconds.

▶ Remove a towel from the crock pot, cabi, or basin and wring it out if it is too wet.

▶ Apply the towel to the client's body and pat down firmly. Then remove the substance with one firm, smooth stroke. Do not scrub or wipe with the towel.

▶ Use a new towel from the crock pot, cabi, or basin for each area of the body from which residue is removed.

▶ To prevent chilling, cover each part of the client's body immediately after removing the residue.

10. Help the client turn over.

11. Move to the foot of the table. Standing at the foot of the table, undrape the client's left foot and leg. Exfoliate the sole of the client's foot using small circular strokes.

12. Continue using small circular strokes up the posterior left leg, including the gluteal area. Use less pressure on the back of the client's knee. Redrape the client's left leg. Move to the client's right leg. Undrape and exfoliate the foot and leg the same as for the left leg. Redrape the client's right leg.

13. Move to the head of the table and undrape the client's back. Using small, circular strokes, exfoliate the client's neck and back and move around to the side of the table to include the lateral sides of the back.

14. Once the exfoliation is complete, the salt needs to be removed. If using a wet table or Vichy shower, rinse the client thoroughly. If there is a separate shower facility, help the client off the table, draping the top sheet around for modesty. Guide the client to the shower and then back to the massage table after rinsing off. If the exfoliation is being done in a dry room with no access to a shower, use the dry room removal technique and skip to the last step.

15. While the client is in the shower, remove the top of the two remaining sheets on the massage table, uncovering the fresh sheet underneath.

16. When the client returns, apply a moisturizing oil or lotion to the body.

17. If the exfoliation is being done in a dry room, remove the top of the two remaining sheets from underneath the client using the dry room sheet removal technique.

DRY ROOM REMOVAL TECHNIQUE

The dry room removal technique described here is from Chapter 5. If the sea salt glow is being done in a dry room with no access to a shower, the residue on the client's skin can be removed by placing a warm, moist towel on the area for a few seconds.

► Remove a towel from the crock pot, cabi or basin and wring it out if it is too wet.
► Apply the towel to the client's body and pat down firmly, and then remove the substance with one firm, smooth stroke. Do not scrub or wipe with the towel.
► Use a new towel from the crock pot, cabi, or basin for each area of the body from which residue is removed.
► To prevent chilling, cover each part of the client's body immediately after removing the residue.

---

18. When the residue is removed, apply a moisturizing oil or lotion to the body.

After the Treatment
Once the exfoliation is complete, another treatment can be performed, such as a massage or body wrap. Otherwise, assist the client off the table, provide plenty of water to drink, and encourage rest.

Hygiene
Any leftover salt mixture should be immediately discarded. The sheets and towels should be laundered with hot water and detergent after each use. The bowl should be washed in warm, soapy water and rinsed after each use. Since a towel cabi holds multiple towels, it should be washed out daily and sprayed with disinfectant. Used towels should *never* be placed back in a towel cabi. If a crock pot is used, it should be used for only one treatment. It should be washed in warm, soapy water, rinsed, and sprayed with disinfectant after use.

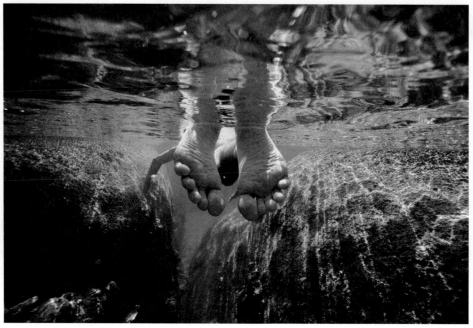

(Heather Perry/National Geographic Image Collection)

Some conditions, however, warrant caution in taking a seawater or sea product bath. They should not be taken by people who have:

- ▶ allergy to iodine or shellfish
- ▶ heart conditions
- ▶ vascular disease
- ▶ numbness or loss of sensation in an area
- ▶ high body temperature (fever)
- ▶ broken or irritated skin
- ▶ inflammation, including inflammatory joint disorders
- ▶ intolerance to heat
- ▶ become pregnant
- ▶ recently exfoliated, shaved, or have a recent tattoo (seawater and sea salt baths in particular are contraindicated)

The equipment and supplies for a sea product bath can be purchased at local stores or online; the sea product needs to be purchased through a spa treatment supply store. The supplies needed are:

- ▶ exfoliation tools or ingredients for a scrub (except for a sea salt bath)
- ▶ bathtub for a full-immersion bath; basin large enough to hold water up to mid-calf for a foot bath
- ▶ for a full immersion bath:
  6 to 8 ounces of seaweed, kelp, or other algae powder
  6 to 8 ounces of sea mud
  OR
  2 cups of sea salt

- ▶ for a foot bath:
  1/3 cup seaweed, kelp, or other algae powder
  1/3 cup sea mud
  OR
  1/3 cup sea salt
  NOTE: The sea products should not be stored in metal containers because they may react chemically with metal, changing the properties of the sea products.
- ▶ towels for drying

Before taking the bath, perform an exfoliation (except for a sea salt bath). Then fill the tub or basin with comfortably hot water to the desired level. While the tub is filling, add the sea product by putting it under the running water. No soaps should be used, but essential oils could be added to the water. Soak in the soothing bath for 20 to 25 minutes, adding hot water as needed. Dry off with the towels.

After the bath, rest and drink plenty of water. The skin may show a slight flush since the sea products greatly improve circulation and retains heat. This allows increased blood to flow to the surface of the skin.

Hygiene

The bath water should be drained after use. The tub or basin should be scrubbed thoroughly with soap, water, and a disinfectant. If exfoliation tools were used, they should be washed in warm, soapy water and rinsed. After rinsing, place them in rubbing alcohol for at least 20 minutes; then let them air dry. Store them in an airtight container. If an exfoliation mixture was used, any leftover should be immediately discarded. The bowl in which the exfoliation

TO GET YOU STARTED

Seaweed Lotion

1 tbsp kelp powder
1 cup distilled, mineral, or floral water
½ cup aloe vera gel
2 tbsp almond oil

Combine kelp powder and water in a nonmetal bowl and mix. Add aloe vera gel and almond oil to the kelp mixture. Add more water to bring to desired consistency. Bottle or jar and refrigerate. Keeps up to 6 months.

Sea Salt Detoxification Bath

2 cups sea salt
2 tbsp oil of choice—sweet almond, apricot kernel, grapeseed, and so on.

Pour ingredients into the tub while the tub is filling and mix well. Soak for 20 to 30 minutes.

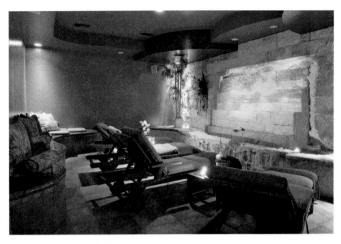

▶ **Figure 7.27** Brine light therapy rooms, such as this one at Touch of Tranquility, Tucson, AZ, have comfortable seating, ambient lighting, beautiful surroundings, relaxing music, and a saltwater flow. This atmosphere can help decrease respiratory inflammation and clear congestion.

substance was mixed should be washed in warm, soapy water and rinsed between each use. Towels should be laundered in hot water and detergent between uses.

BRINE INHALATION TREATMENT

Breathing sea air has many benefits for the respiratory tract, including decreasing inflammation, helping to moisturize, and clearing congestion. Additionally the sea air feels soothing and moisturizing to the skin. Some spas have installed rooms in which clients can experience brine (saltwater) inhalation treatments. As shown in ▶ Figure 7.27, these rooms have comfortable seating, ambient lighting, beautiful surroundings, relaxing music, and a salt water flow. The white along the sides and bottom of the waterfall in the figure is salt buildup, enhancing the briny atmosphere.

Summary

Humans have a long history of using the sea and products from the sea for healing. Although many spas have made use of thalassotherapy throughout the world for several hundred years, it was brought to modern prominence in France, where it remains part of the country's medical system. Contemporary spas and practitioners in private practice are rediscovering the benefits of thalassotherapy. Body wraps, masks, poultices, salt glows, and baths are examples of the ways that sea products are being incorporated into spa and hydrotherapy treatments.

Activities

1. Briefly describe each of the three major types of seaweed used in thalassotherapy. Include the benefits of using each.

_____

_____

_____

2. List five indications for a seaweed or other algae body wrap.

_____

_____

_____

_____

3. List five contraindications for a seaweed or other algae body wrap.

_____

_____

_____

_____

_____

4. Explain three benefits of a sea mud body wrap.

_____

_____

_____

5. List five indications of a sea mud body wrap.

_____

_____

_____

_____

_____

6. List five contraindications of a sea mud body wrap.

_____

_____

_____

_____

_____

7. Explain three benefits of a sea product mask.

_____

_____

_____

8. List three indications for a sea product mask.

_____

_____

_____

9. List three contraindications for a sea product mask.

_____

_____

_____

10. List five benefits of a sea salt glow.

_____

_____

_____

_____

_____

11. List five indications for a sea salt glow.

_____

_____

_____

_____

_____

12. List five contraindications for a sea salt glow.

_____

_____

_____

_____

_____

13. Receive a sea mud or seaweed body wrap treatment. Describe which type of wrap you received. What did you like about it? What did you not like about it? What would you have done differently? How did you feel 24 hours after the treatment? 48 hours after the treatment?

_____

_____

_____

_____

_____

_____

_____

14. Receive a sea salt glow. What did you like about it? What did you not like about it? What would you have done differently? How did you feel 24 hours after the treatment? 48 hours after the treatment?

_____

_____

_____

_____

_____

_____

_____

15. Take a sea salt bath. What did you like about it? What did you not like about it? How did you feel 24 hours after the treatment? 48 hours after the treatment?

_____

_____

_____

_____

_____

_____

_____

Study Questions

1. In which country did the first hydrotherapy center devoted to using seawater and sea products open?
   a. United States
   b. France
   c. England
   d. Ireland

2. Who coined the term *thalassotherapy?*
   a. Dr. Joseph de la Bonnardiere
   b. Rene Quinton
   c. Dr. Richard Russell
   d. Hippocrates

3. Which body fluid most closely resembles seawater?
   a. tears
   b. plasma
   c. mucus
   d. urine

4. Which type of organism is seaweed?
   a. animal
   b. plant
   c. bacteria
   d. algae

5. A contraindication for receiving thalassotherapy is an allergy to which of the following foods?
   a. peanuts
   b. shellfish
   c. milk
   d. tofu

6. Which of the following is most commonly used in spas for seaweed wraps?
   a. *Corallina officinalis*
   b. *Laminaria digitata*
   c. *Chlorella*
   d. *Spirulina maxima*

7. Thalassotherapy treatments include which of the following?
   a. seaweed wraps
   b. sea salt scrubs
   c. marine water filled whirlpool baths
   d. all of the above

8. Which of the following would be a reason for receiving a sea salt glow?
   a. fatigue
   b. skin rash
   c. joint pain
   d. muscle tightness

9. A benefit of sea products on the body is that they
    a. loosen the skin
    b. inhibit blood circulation
    c. help eliminate toxins
    d. all of the above

10. Which of the following makes a good exfoliant?
    a. brown seaweed
    b. red seaweed
    c. blue green algae
    d. white algae

Case Samples

A. Liu Chang is a 23-year-old student and aspiring model. She smoked for six years in order to remain thin. However, she stopped smoking one week ago because of the health risks. She is committed to remaining a nonsmoker and has asked her massage therapist, Jack Martin, for suggestions to help her detoxify from the nicotine. Jack recently completed a program of study in spa and hydrotherapy treatments and said he believes he can help her.

1. Which thalassotherapy treatments would be best for Liu to receive?
2. What are the rationale, equipment and supplies, indications, contraindications, preparation, after-treatment care, and hygiene for these treatments?
3. Which questions should Jack ask Liu to determine which treatment would be most beneficial?

B. Marian Mrotek is a guest at a destination spa. She has been suffering from fatigue and stress after taking a new position at her company; her spa stay is a gift from her husband, Ralph. Which thalassotherapy treatments could the spa practitioner suggest for her and why?

1. What are the rationale, equipment and supplies, indications, contraindications, preparation, after-treatment care, and hygiene for these treatments?
2. Which questions should the spa practitioner ask Marian to determine which treatment would be most beneficial?

C. Tanisha Miller recently moved to the southwest United States. She loves the climate but notices that her skin is always dry and flaky. She applies a moisturizer regularly, but it doesn't seem to help. Her massage therapist, Bertha Valenzuela, has recommended that Tanisha try one of the thalassotherapy treatments Bertha offers.

1. Which thalassotherapy treatments would be best for Tanisha to receive?
2. What are the rationale, equipment and supplies, indications, contraindications, preparation, after-treatment care, and hygiene for these treatments?
3. Which questions should Bertha ask Tanisha to determine which treatment would be most beneficial?

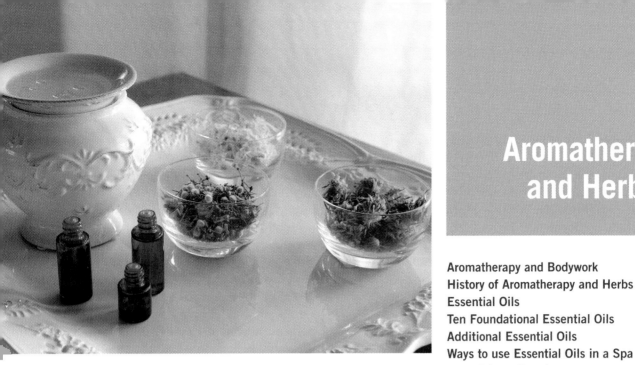

LEARNING OBJECTIVES

After studying this chapter, the reader will have the information to

1. Discuss the history of the use of aromatherapy and herbs.

2. Explain what essential oils are, how they are extracted, and how they affect the body.

3. Delineate precautions for working with essential oils.

4. Explain how to tell if an essential oil is pure, and how to store essential oils.

5. Explain the concept of notes in regard to essential oils.

6. Discuss the characteristics, uses, and cautions of ten foundational essential oils.

7. Outline ways to use essential oils in a spa or private practice.

8. Describe the effects of common herbs on the body.

9. Outline how to make an herbal infusion and what it can be used for in a spa or private practice.

10. Delineate the supplies needed, rationale, indications, contraindications, treatment procedure, hygiene, and after-treatment care for simple inhalation and facial sauna treatments using herbs.

11. Delineate the supplies needed, rationale, indications, contraindications, treatment procedure, hygiene, and after-treatment care for an herbal wrap.

Arranging a bowl of flowers in the morning can give a sense of quiet in a crowded day—like writing a poem, or saying a prayer.

— Anne Morrow Lindbergh

KEY TERMS

Absolute	Distillation	Infusion	Olfactory epithelium
Aromatherapy	Essential oils	Limbic system	Top notes
Base notes	Herbs	Middle notes	Volatile
Carrier oil	Hydrosol	Olfaction	
Centrifugation	Hypothalamus	Olfaction bulbs	

AROMATHERAPY AND BODYWORK

Scents can be used in so many different ways in the spa and bodywork profession, as well as in everyday life, that aromatherapy in popular culture has come to mean anything that is scented in a pleasant way. Air fresheners, candles, and even flower-scented detergents are now called aromatherapy. Scented spray mists to freshen the face or feet, dishes of aromatic beads placed in the treatment room, and lavender lubricants are all examples of what may be considered aromatherapy in the spa and bodywork realm.

With so many products and substances available, practitioners who work in spas and in private practice have much to choose from when deciding to enhance their treatments and treatment spaces with aromas designed to evoke feelings of well-being in their clients. Most products, such as the scented candles, aromatic beads, and fragrance mists, are relatively easy to use and inexpensive to buy commercially. Practitioners can experiment with these to see which scents blend well together and which moods are stimulated.

Two particular types of substances, however, require more research and education than can be found just through experimentation. These are **essential oils** and **herbs** and other plants. Their effects can be so powerful that in order to truly understand how they should be used, it is recommended that practitioners who are interested in becoming aromatherapists attend formal courses in aromatherapy. The National Association for Holistic Aromatherapy (www.naha.org) is a valuable source of information. This is an educational, nonprofit organization dedicated to enhancing public awareness of the benefits of true aromatherapy.

The focus of this chapter is to introduce basic aromatherapy concepts to practitioners who are beginners in the use of essential oils and herbs. Information on common essential oils and herbs is presented. Characteristics, uses, and cautions are included, along with methods of incorporating essential oils and herbs into the spa and bodywork setting and treatments.

It is important to note that practitioners should never go beyond their scope of practice. They need to check their local and/or state regulations regarding the use of essential oils in their practice. Some areas require that anyone who applies essential oils topically to another person be professionally licensed, such as for massage therapy, energy work, cosmetology, and so on. It is recommended that practitioners check with all pertinent regulatory bodies to make sure they are in compliance with the laws that govern them and their practice.

HISTORY OF AROMATHERAPY AND HERBS

Since ancient times, people have lived in close proximity to the earth and plants. It is only natural that they would look to the surrounding flora as a source of healing and well-being. Plant lore developed over generations as ancient tribes learned which plants healed wounds, staved off hunger, and helped with the pain of childbirth. Different parts of plants were used in different ways to heal.

As discussed in Chapter 1, phytotherapy is the therapeutic use of plants. Entire plants, parts of plants, and plant extracts are used for medicinal purposes, and phytotherapy is intertwined with herbal medicine. Phytotherapy and herbal medicine are comprehensive fields of study. However, with some basic knowledge, practitioners can use herbs and other plants as additions to spa and hydrotherapy treatments. Herbs (for simplicity's sake, the term *herb* will be used to mean herbs and other plants throughout the rest of this chapter) and their extracts are used in restorative baths, teas, poultices, and fomentations. They are also used to make massage oils, balms, and salves.

Aromatherapy is the therapeutic use of the preparation of fragrant essential oils extracted from plants. According to the National Association for Holistic Therapy, "Aromatherapy can be defined as the art and science of utilizing naturally extracted aromatic essences from plants to balance, harmonize, and promote the health of the body, mind, and spirit" (NAHA, 2005a). Aromatherapy has many effects on the body and it is because of this that aromatherapy can be used in many different ways.

DID YOU KNOW?

Aroma is Greek for "spice."

Plant Use by Ancient Civilizations

The Aztecs and Native Americans used aromatic oils and made their own herbal remedies for healing and for spiritual practices. They would apply plants or plant parts topically, makes teas out of them, and chew leaves and stems. For healing, the plants would be used for a variety of reasons, such as analgesics, diuretics, and skin emollients. Certain plants were used to induce sacred dreams and, along with oils, in rites of passage. Each Native American tribe had its particular methods of plant use, and many of these traditions are still in use today.

The ancient Egyptians used specific herbs to help with digestion, protect against infection, and build the immune

18, 10, 16

system, and they used fragrant oils for bathing, massage, and embalming their dead (Tisserand, 1985). To extract the oils from aromatic plants, they used the process of **infusion.** One method involves pouring boiling water over the leaves, flowers, or berries of a fragrant plant. The plants are then left to stand for 15 to 30 minutes, or longer for a stronger infusion. An oil infusion involves placing plant parts in oil and leaving them for weeks. The herb or botanical is removed from the oil or water through straining, and the remaining oil or water is then used.

At about the same time the early Egyptians were using aromatics, the ancient Chinese were also using them. Shen Nung's herbal book dating from about 2700 BC includes information on the properties and use of more than 300 plants.

The early Greeks used aromatic oils for medicines and cosmetics. Hippocrates promoted a daily aromatherapy bath and scented massage for good health. His use of aromatic vapors is thought to have played a role in stopping the spread of the plague in Athens. A Greek physician, Pedacius Dioscorides, wrote a book about herbal medicine that became the Western world's medical reference for about 1,200 years. Many of the preparations in the text are still in use today and are part of modern aromatherapy.

The Romans continued the Greek practice of aromatherapy baths followed by massage with scented oils. The need for aromatics, in fact, played a role in the Roman creation of trade routes to India and the Middle East. These gave the Romans the opportunity to import exotic oils and spices. These trade routes continued to be used for hundreds of years and were responsible for the intermingling of cultures.

Throughout the Middle Ages, knowledge of aromatics oils, and the subsequent development of perfumes, continued to spread from India, the Middle East, and Asia. During the Crusades, which lasted from 1096 to 1272, Christian soldiers waged campaigns to try to reclaim

Jerusalem from the Muslims, who had captured it in 1076. Although they were not successful in this endeavor, the Crusaders did introduce aromatic oils and perfumes to Europe. It was also during this time that the Persian physician Ibn Sina (Avicenna) lived (see Chapter 1 for more information on Ibn Sina). In addition to being one of the Islamic world's most well-known scientists and writers, he experimented with the process of distillation and was able to distill the essence of rose. **Distillation** is the process in which a solution consisting of water and a substance such as parts of a plant are boiled (see ▶Figure 8.1). The resulting evaporation is cooled or condensed, forming a liquid, which is then captured. It contains the "essence" of the plant that was distilled. At about the same time that Ibn Sina was distilling using water, Arabs were discovering how to distill alcohol. Perfumes made with alcohol quickly replaced perfumes in the heavy oil base (Keville and Green, 1995).

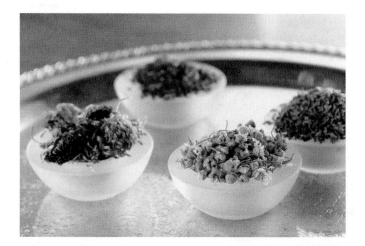

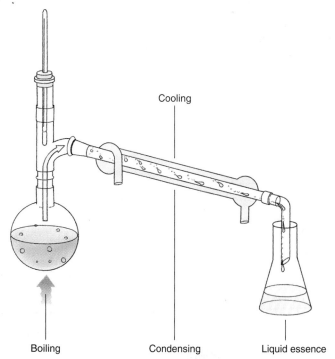

▶ **Figure 8.1** In distillation, a solution of water and plant parts is boiled, cooled, and condensed, capturing the liquid essence of the original plant. (© Dorling Kindersley)

43, 41, 3, 1, 4, 38

Aromatics from the Middles Ages to the Present

During the Middle Ages, bathing had been prohibited by the Catholic Church. As a result, perfumes and herbs were used liberally to freshen the body and the home. For example, people would wear rosemary to keep fleas from feasting on them. Lavender would be put down with rushes on the floor to make homes smell better, and perfumes were used to mask body odor.

The Renaissance brought a surge of interest in new aromas. As explorers traveled to new lands, they brought back new spices, new herbs, new plants and, of course, new aromas. Europeans began to use fragrance everywhere—in their homes; in their clothing, even in their wigs, which were scented with oils. Since modern sanitation and sewer systems would not exist for hundreds of years, small bunches of aromatic plants called *nosegays* were carried to mask the smells of the streets and bodies. In France, lavender and rosemary were burned in hospitals to cleanse the atmosphere of the smell of disease and death (Tisserand, 1985).

Even though the origins of aromatherapy go back as far as the origins of humans, the term itself is relatively new. The term *aromatherapy* was first coined in the early 1900s by French chemist Rene-Maurice Gattefosse, who came from a long line of French perfumers. For some time, he had been gathering information about the antiseptic properties of essential oils. When an explosion in his family's perfume factory severely burned his hand, he plunged it into the nearest cold liquid, a vat of lavender essential oil. He was amazed at the immediate pain relief he felt and, later on, how well his burns healed with no sign of infection and very little scarring. He continued exploring the benefits of essential oils, especially their antimicrobial properties. It became his life's work; he wrote several scientific papers about essential oils, and in 1937, he wrote *Aromatherapie: Les Huiles essentielles, hormons vegetales (Aromatherapy: The Essential Oils, Vegetable Hormones)* (Shutes and Weaver, 2008).

Dr. Jean Valnet, a French physician, further developed Gattefosse's findings. He experimented with essential oils and, during World War II, used them as antiseptics in the treatment of wounded soldiers. At about the same time, Austrian biochemist Marguerite Maury, who was living in France, explored the psychological and physiological benefits from applying essential oils to the skin. She is credited with popularizing the topical application of essential oils and, of special interest to bodyworkers, incorporating the use of essential oils into massage therapy. Her work emphasized that using massage therapy and aromatherapy together created more benefit for the client than if each treatment were applied separately. This helped move aromatherapy into the realm of complementary therapies (Shutes and Weaver, 2008).

Robert Tisserand is a well-known English aromatherapist and massage therapist who wrote the first edition of *The Art of Aromatherapy* in 1977 (the latest edition was published in 1985). This work helped draw attention to aromatherapy in current culture. Tisserand works closely with doctors and herbalists and tracks all published scientific research relevant to essential oils. He lectures around the world and is the author of several more books on aromatherapy such *The Practice of Aromatherapy,* written with Jean Valnet and published in 1996, and *Essential Oil Safety: A Guide for Health Care Professionals* written with Tony Balaz and published in 1995.

Today, the practice of aromatherapy is not viewed the same throughout the world. Often it is seen more as an art form than a bona fide healing science, used complementarily, not as a primary treatment. In France and the United Kingdom, it is incorporated more fully into mainstream medicine. Essential oils are regulated as prescription medications and are used in hospitals, hospices, special care units, and in general practice. Many other European countries include essential oils in their national pharmacopeias. In still other countries, including the United States, aromatherapy is not yet recognized as a science. Nonetheless, interest in aromatherapy and its benefits continues to grow. For example, one area of study is its use in clinics and hospitals for pain relief and to help alleviate anxiety (Price and Price, 2007).

ESSENTIAL OILS

Essential oils are the volatile oils that aromatic plants, trees, and grasses produce. **Volatile** means able to vaporize easily at low temperatures. It is essential oils' volatility that causes their scents to spread so rapidly. These oils can be obtained from any part of the plant. Usually they are distilled from the flowers, roots, rinds of fruits, stalks, sap or resin, nuts, or bark. For example, sandalwood is gathered from the heart of the tree, but only after the tree is at least 40 years old. Eucalyptus is obtained from the leaves of the eucalyptus tree. Neroli, rose, jasmine, and lavender come from the plants' flowers. Various species of frankincense trees grow wild throughout western India, northeastern Africa, and southern Saudi Arabia. The oil is distilled from the gum resin that oozes from incisions made in the bark of the trees. Myrrh comes from a shrub that grows in Ethiopia, Sudan, and Somalia. The shrubs exude a resin that hardens into what is classified as reddish brown "tears"; this is myrrh.

There are three categories of essential oil plant purity. They are based on how and where the plants are grown and harvested:

▶ **Certified Organic:** The plants are grown, harvested, and processed without the use of pesticides, chemical fertilizers, herbicides, Genetically Modified Organisms (GMOs), synthetic chemicals, and growth agents and are free from irradiation and chemical sterilization. All certified organic materials must meet USDA organic certification requirements.

▶ **Wild harvested:** These are plants gathered from their natural environment, such as woodlands, prairies, deserts, and tropical forests. All wild harvested items are taken to specific facilities for further processing, such as drying and package. The best facilities sign a "Wild Take Audit" to ensure that the materials are sustainably gathered with a no more than 10 percent take, and that the plants are reseeded or roots are left to restock native populations.

▶ **Cultivated:** These are conventionally grown plants that may have been cultivated with the use of pesticides, chemical fertilizers, herbicides, and synthetic chemicals, although some are free of pesticide and organophosphate residues. (Shutes and Weaver, 2008)

Essential Oil Extraction

Essential oils are extracted from plants in four main ways:

▶ **Steam distillation:** As described previously in this chapter, hot steam is used to separate the oil from the plant; the oil is then condensed with water. **Hydrosols** are the watery by-products from the distillation of plant products. Common hydrosols are rosewater, lavender water, and orange flower water.

▶ **Infusion:** This process involves steeping plants, much like a tea, in hot water. An example is an infusion of chamomile (and the resulting fluid would be the hydrosol chamomile). Oil infusions are extractions of plants made from placing them in oil for 1 to 2 weeks.

▶ **Pressure and centrifugation:** The pressure method consists of physically pressing a plant to extract the oil. **Centrifugation** is a process in which plants are spun rapidly to separate the oils from the plant matter. It is called centrifugation because centrifugal force is used. Grapefruit oil is extracted from grapefruit rind this way.

▶ **Dissolving in solvent:** In this method, plant parts are placed in a volatile solvent. As the solvent evaporates, it leaves behind a natural wax. The fluid that is then separated from the wax is called an **absolute.** Absolutes are the most concentrated forms of essential oils. An example is rose absolute. (Shutes and Weaver, 2008)

How Essential Oils Work

About 200 different essential oils have been extracted from plants for use in aromatherapy and are employed for many different purposes, including:

▶ antiseptics against viruses, bacteria, and fungi
▶ analgesics
▶ acting on the central nervous system to reduce anxiety and insomnia or to be stimulating and energizing
▶ acting on the endocrine system and metabolism
▶ stimulating the immune system

Essential oil preparations that are taken internally may stimulate the immune system and function as antibiotics. Since these are pharmacological uses of essential oils, recommending internal use of essential oils is beyond the scope of the practice of massage therapists and bodyworkers and will not be discussed in this text.

Other essential oils that are applied to the skin activate thermal (heat) receptors and kill dermal microbes and fungi. They can also be absorbed through the skin from baths, massage treatments, and compresses. Essential oils are readily absorbed through the skin because of their lipid solubility and the small size of the aromatic molecules. The molecules enter the bloodstream quickly and easily cross the blood-brain barrier to have an effect on the brain. The natural oiliness of the skin also enhances the uptake of essential oils (Martin, 2007; Shutes and Weaver, 2008).

Essential oils used for their aromas stimulate a specific part of the brain called the limbic system. The **limbic system** (see ▶Figure 8.2) is located within the higher brain, or cerebrum. It is sometimes referred to as the "emotional brain" because it has a major role in a variety of emotions—pleasure, affection, passivity, fear, sorrow, sexual feelings, and anger. It is also involved in memory and **olfaction,** which is the term for the sense of smell. This is why our sense of smell evokes memories much more strongly than any of our other senses. **Olfaction bulbs,** components of the limbic system, are nervous tissues that play a role in the brain's interpretation and differentiation of all the diverse aromas we are able to detect.

The limbic system is closely associated with the part of the brain called the **hypothalamus,** which controls many physiological functions and plays a major role in the regulation

7, 35, 36, 50.

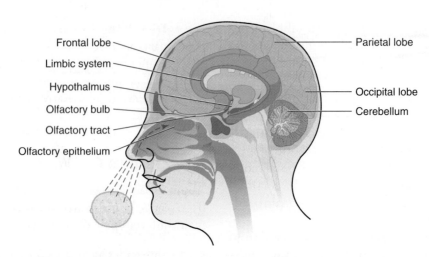

▶ **Figure 8.2** The limbic system, or "emotional brain," plays a major role in a variety of emotions, memory, and the sense of smell.

of homeostasis. It is responsible for, among other things, controlling the autonomic nervous system (discussed in Chapter 2) and regulating emotional and behavioral patterns.

Located in the superior part of the nasal cavity is **olfactory epithelium,** specialized tissue that has thousands of receptors. These receptors are the endings of nerve fibers that carry impulses for the sense of smell into the olfactory bulbs. When aroma particles are inhaled, they travel up to the olfactory epithelium and dissolve in nasal mucus, which makes it easier for them to stimulate the receptors. Stimulating the receptors means that the receptors create nerve impulses that then travel along olfactory nerves into the olfactory bulbs.

From the olfactory bulbs, the impulses travel along the olfactory tract. The olfactory tract extends into parts of the brain that identify odors, so a person can put a name to them, and to parts of the brain that distinguish different odors so a person can sort them out. This tract extends into the part of the brain where conscious awareness of smell begins, as well as into the limbic system and hypothalamus. It is this connection to the limbic system and hypothalamus that accounts for emotional and memory-based responses to aromas (Tortora and Derrickson, 2006).

DID YOU KNOW?

Humans are able to distinguish 10,000 different smells. Dogs, on the other hand, can detect hundreds of thousands; bloodhounds can even detect up to 400,000 different scents. That is because the nasal cavities of dogs have nearly 220 million olfactory receptors in an area that covers about 6″ × 6″. Humans, on the other hand, have smaller nasal cavities with just 5 million receptors in an area that covers ½″ × ½″.

Over time, experimentation with human responses to various essential oils has allowed for them to be categorized as energizing, relaxing, soothing, balancing, and so forth. This categorization is based on the way the majority of people have reacted to the various essential oils. It is important to note, however, that because of individual emotions and memories, not everyone responds the same way to aromas. For example, an aroma that is supposed to be soothing and relaxing may be so for one person because nerve impulses sent along the olfaction pathway stimulate the limbic system to respond with a feeling of pleasure or passivity, and cause the hypothalamus to increase parasympathetic activity. On the other hand, another person may respond to the same odor with anger as nerve impulses generated by the aroma stimulate the limbic system, and a sympathetic response from the hypothalamus.

Precautions for Working with Essential Oils

Essential oils are highly concentrated and volatile, and they need to be handled with care. Only two essential oils can be applied directly to the skin—lavender and tea tree. All other essential oils must be diluted in **carrier oil,** also called *base oil,* before applying to the body. These are typically plant-based oils used to dilute essential oils for use on the skin, as in massage. They can also serve to moisturize the skin and keep essential oils on the skin longer. The carrier oil can be any high-quality vegetable oil such as:

▶ sweet almond
▶ apricot
▶ grapeseed
▶ olive
▶ coconut
▶ sunflower
▶ jojoba

Practitioners and clients can be allergic to any or all essential oils. It is important for the practitioner to find out from clients any allergies they may have, and note them on an intake form so there is written documentation. Practitioners allergic to any or all essential oils should never use them on clients even when requested to do so, either by clients or employers.

People can develop allergies throughout their lives; therefore, every time a client arrives for a treatment, the practitioner should do a quick allergy update. Before any treatment is performed, the oil should be applied to a small area on the client's skin and on the practitioner's skin, usually the forearm, to see if there is an allergic reaction.

- sesame
- canola
- sunflower
- safflower
- peanut

See ▶Table 8.1 for a list of dilutions of common essential oils within a carrier oil.

The following are more precautions to keep in mind as practitioners work with essential oils:

- A skin test should always be done on clients and on practitioners themselves before any essential oil is used, even if the essential oil has been used before. As stated in the Clinical Alert above, people can develop allergies throughout their lives, even to substances to which they have not previously been allergic.
- Essential oils should NEVER be used near the eyes.
- Pregnancy is a consideration, especially the first trimester. A qualified aromatherapist should be

TABLE 8.1	
Dilutions of essential oils in carrier oil	

Dilution	Drops per Ounce of Carrier Oil
1%	5–6
2%	10–12
3%	15–18

consulted for information about essential oils that work well and essential oils that are contraindicated. Some safe oils for use during pregnancy are rose, neroli, lavender, ylang-ylang, chamomile, geranium, sandalwood, spearmint, frankincense, and the citruses. A 1 percent dilution of essential oil to carrier oil should be used on pregnant clients, or one drop added to bath water. When in doubt, however, do not use essential oils.

- Use essential oils cautiously with clients who are fragile, including babies, small children, the aged, and those who have serious health problems such as asthma, epilepsy, or heart disease. No more than a 1 percent dilution of essential oil to carrier oil or one drop added to bath water should be used for these clients. Again, when in doubt, do not use essential oils.
- Caution should be used with essential oils that can result in photosensitivity. For example, bergamot contains a natural chemical called bergaptene that causes the skin to become sensitive to ultraviolet light. If bergamot is applied and the skin is exposed to sunlight or light from sun lamps or tanning beds, the reaction can be anywhere from mild (just reddening of the skin) to severe (acute lesions and brown spots). Mild reactions usually resolve within a day or so. However, severe reactions can take weeks to resolve, with the accompanying brown spots taking months or years to disappear completely. Removing the bergaptene does not hinder the benefits of the essential oil, and it is recommended that bergaptene-free bergamot be used whenever possible.

Practitioners and clients can be allergic to any or all carrier oils. One of the more well-known allergies is to nuts. If the practitioner or client is allergic to nuts, nut-based carrier oils should NOT be used. Oils to avoid because of the most frequent occurrences of allergies are almond, coconut, sunflower, and peanut.

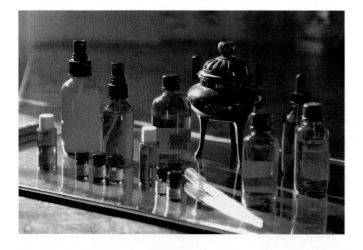

▶ If taking homeopathic remedies, consult a qualified aromatherapist before using essential oils since they may counteract the action of the homeopathic remedy. (Buckle, 2007; Rose, 1999; Shutes and Weaver, 2008)

Purchasing Essential Oils

It is best to buy only pure, organic, good-quality essential oils. *Organic* means that the plant material was grown without the use of pesticides, herbicides, or fungicides made from synthetic chemicals or petrochemicals.

Avoid synthetic fragrance oils. They have no therapeutic value. Labels on bottles may say "organic," "pure," and "natural," but the oil may, in fact, be synthetic. A label that says "fragrant oil," "perfume oil," or "aromatherapy oil" is an indication that the oils are not pure oils and have been mixed with other substances. For example, the oil may have been diluted with vegetable oils. A good way to test for this is to place a couple drops of the essential oil on a piece of paper. If an oily stain is left behind when the essential oil evaporates, it was most likely diluted with vegetable oil.

True essential oils will have the botanical name, not just the common name, on the label. The label will also state that it is a "pure essential oil" or "100% essential oil." If the label is not clear about this information, do not buy it. See ▶ Figure 8.3 for comparison between a typical synthetic essential oil label and a pure essential oil label.

Another way to know whether an oil is natural or synthetic is to research the company that produces it. Find out how long the company has been in business and if it is able to back up claims of purity. The company's catalog should list the country of origin and method of extraction for each of its oils. A good supplier should also be able to produce a "Certificate of Naturalness" about any of its products. This shows the total percentage of the oil involved, a listing of the percentages and types of each additive, and if the oil is truly 100 percent derived from the plant source by a physical process (one of the proper methods of essential oil extraction) (NAHA, 2005b). If the supplier is unable to do this, then practitioners should not buy those oils.

Price can also be an indication. Pure, organic oils cost more than synthetic oils or blends. Some are quite expensive. Whereas orange, lemon, and lime may be reasonably

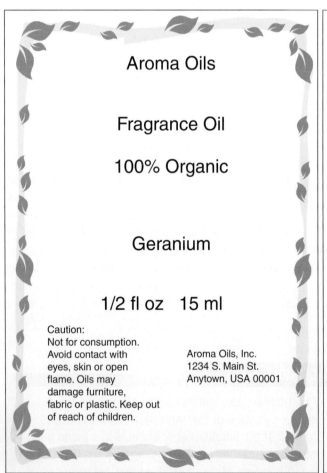

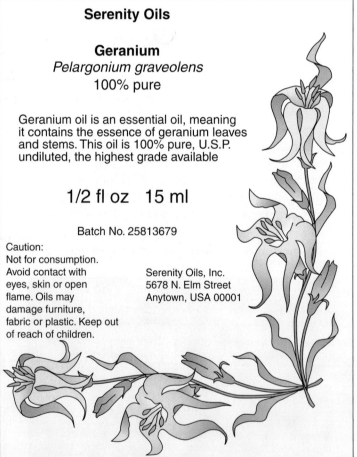

▶ **Figure 8.3** Notice the differences on the labels of synthetic essential oil versus pure essential oil. True essential oils will have the botanical and common names on the label and will state that it is a "pure" or "100%" essential oil.

priced, jasmine, neroli, and rose are costly. The bottle itself can be a guide. The best quality oils will always be in dark glass bottles to protect them from sunlight. A product line of aromatherapy oils in clear glass bottles that are all the same price are most likely synthetic fragrance oils.

Storage and Shelf Life

Essential oils are best stored tightly sealed in amber, blue, or brown glass bottles. Oxygen, sunlight, and heat can damage oils, causing them to lose their therapeutic properties. The average shelf life for most essential oils is 2 years, although the citrus oils have a somewhat shorter life expectancy. Unused oils that have reached the end of their shelf life should be discarded. It is interesting that the heavy, woodsy, resin-type oils such as patchouli and cedarwood can last much longer (up to 6 years) and are said to actually improve with age (Shutes and Weaver, 2008).

Notes

Essential oils have been classified by the French perfume industry according to their "notes," or scent characteristics, and by the rate at which they evaporate. There are top notes (T), middle notes (M), and base (B) notes. Some oils are a combination of top and middle (T/M) or middle and base (M/B) notes.

Top notes have light, fresh, and uplifting qualities. They typically have antiviral properties. Since they evaporate quickly, their scents are usually not long lasting. **Middle notes** comprise the bulk of the essential oils. They have warm, soft fragrances that unfold gradually. They are the balancing and harmonizing scents. **Base notes** are intense, heavy, long-lasting fragrances that evaporate slowly. They are rich and relaxing and usually are the most expensive essential oils. See ▶Table 8.2 for more information on essential oils and notes.

TABLE 8.2

Essential oils and notes

	Top Notes (T)	Middle Notes (M)	Base Notes (B)
Characteristics	Light and airy	Also known as the heart notes	Deep
	Evaporate quickly	Harmonizing	Intense
	Penetrating or sharp scent	Soothing, soft undertones	Powerful
			Long lasting
	Fresh smell	Scent unfolds gradually	Warm
			Sensuous
Examples	peppermint (T/M)	chamomile	rose absolute
	orange	cypress	patchouli
	lemon	marjoram	vetiver
	lime	lavender	jasmine
	tangerine	geranium	myrrh
	grapefruit	dill	frankincense
	melissa	celery	sandalwood
	lemongrass	coriander	benzoin
	mandarin	black pepper	spikenard
	eucalyptus (T/M)	juniper	cedarwood
	basil	thyme	
		rose (M/B)	
		neroli (M/B)	
		rosemary	
		pine	

(Pure Essential, Inc., 2007)

TEN FOUNDATIONAL ESSENTIAL OILS

With almost 200 essential oils (Rose, 1999) from which to choose, practitioners may not know where to start when beginning their work with aromatherapy. Some practitioners may want to learn as much as they can as fast as they can, whereas others may want to find only a few oils they can use regularly and in many different ways.

The ten essential oils profiled have many different uses. Purchasing these oils would give practitioners a good "starter set" of oils without investing a large amount of money. As practitioners become more comfortable working with essential oils, they may discover that they want additional oils in their collection. Or they may discover that having just these is enough for the treatments they perform.

The following information is meant as an introduction to essential oils and does not contain in-depth descriptions. The information is not intended to treat, cure, prevent, or diagnose any disease, disorder, or health condition.

Blending Essential Oils

Essential oils can be used individually, of course, and have powerful effects. Sometimes, though, blending different essential oils can create a more optimal outcome. The main factor to keep in mind when considering which essential oils to blend is the intention behind the blend. For example, if the goal is the creation of pleasant and relaxing ambiance for the treatment area, any essential oils that are soothing can be blended and placed in a diffuser. On the other hand, if a client has muscle pain, other essential oils can be chosen specifically for their muscle tightness—relieving properties, and a muscle relief blend can be created.

The French perfume industry considers a well-rounded blend to contain top, middle, and base notes. Top notes can comprise up to 20 percent of the blend, middle notes approximately 50 to 80 percent of the blend, and the deep base notes up to 5 percent of the blend. Using this guideline, the majority of the blend will contain middle note essential oils because they tend to harmonize best with other oils. Since top note oils are lighter and more quickly detected by the nose, they are used in a lesser amount. Base note oils are intense and longer lasting, so they are usually used in the least amount (Keville and Green, 1995; Pure Essential, Inc., 2007).

For example, if a 2 percent well-rounded blend is desired, 10 to 12 drops of essential oil will be added to one ounce of carrier oil, according to Table 8.1. Of those 10 to 12 drops, 2 can be of a top note oil, 5 to 8 drops can be a middle note oil, and 1 to 3 drops can be a base note oil.

However, all three notes do not always have to be used in a blend; it all depends on the individual properties of the essential oils, what they will be used for, the blender's preference of oils, and what the final product smells like.

PROFILES OF FOUNDATIONAL ESSENTIAL OILS

Bergamot

Citrus bergamia

Characteristics: relaxing, refreshing, uplifting, cooling. This is the flavor of Earl Grey tea. It can be a good substitute for rose oil.

Uses: to reduce allergies, acne, psoriasis and gas; to relieve anxiety; to alleviate depression

Caution: Avoid exposing skin to sunlight after using this oil until after bathing or showering to remove it.

Peppermint   13

Mentha piperta

Characteristics: one of the most useful essential oils. It is stimulating, refreshing, cooling, and restorative and uplifts the mind and body.

Uses: relaxes the muscles of the digestive system and stimulates bile flow; relieves gas, colic, and indigestion; refreshes tired head and feet. Inhale briefly from bottle or apply one drop on a tissue and inhale to revive during travel. Blend with rosemary and juniper to make a stimulating morning bath.

Caution: Can cause a burning sensation and irritate skin if too much is used or it is not diluted well. Can neutralize homeopathic medicines.

Eucalyptus

Eucalyptus globulus

Characteristics: energizing and stimulating; cleanses and purifies

Uses: helps relieve respiratory congestion, colds, fevers, and pain. Kills airborne bacteria.

Caution: Should not be used if pregnant or on pregnant clients or by people who have epilepsy. Can neutralize homeopathic medicines.

Tea Tree   28

Melaleuca alternifolia, M. linariifolia, M. uncintata

Characteristics: powerful antiseptic, antifungal, and antiviral agent

Uses: to reduce acne, cold sores, warts, and burns; cleansing agent for the skin; can be used as a vapor to kill airborne germs; helps combat foot odor and athlete's foot

Caution: May be used full strength as a first aid application. However, it is best to do a patch test on extremely sensitive skin. Limit usage to problem area if using undiluted.

40, 34, 21, 15

PROFILES OF FOUNDATIONAL OILS CONTINUED

Geranium

Pelargonium graveolens

Characteristics: both uplifting and calming
Uses: soothes certain skin conditions; helps relieve PMS, cramps, menstrual and menopausal issues; tension, anxiety, and depression; is an immunostimulant. Can be used as an aromatic insect repellant.
Caution: Should not be used if pregnant or on pregnant clients; should not be used on persons with a history of estrogen-dependent cancer.

Lavender

Lavendula augustifolia, L. officinalis, L. vera

Characteristics: the most versatile and valuable essential oil; helpful in many ways for the mind and body. Safe to use on children. Blends easily with many other oils.
Uses: helps heal wounds, cuts, burns; relieves headaches; acts as a local anesthetic to relieve pain from sunburn, asthma, and throat infections; relieves irritability and sleeplessness; is an immunostimulant. Can be used as an aromatic insect repellant.
Caution: Avoid high doses during pregnancy; can cause uterine contractions.

Chamomile (Roman Chamomile)

Chamaemelum nobile

Characteristics: relaxing; safe to use on children
Uses: to relieve pain; increase mental clarity; decrease anxiety, nervous tension, depression, anger, and irritability; soothe sunburn, earaches, toothaches, and headaches.
Caution: Can neutralize homeopathic medicines.

Cypress   *34*

Cupressus sempervirens

Characteristics: distilled from the twigs, needles, and cones of the cypress tree. Has a spicy, smoky, pungent, pinelike scent.
Uses: antispasmodic; warming; diuretic; helps relieve edema, asthma, hot flashes; assists in balancing hormonal levels; helps relieve pain from varicose veins and hemorrhoids; decreases the appearance of thread veins; supports weight reduction
Caution: Should not be used if pregnant or on pregnant clients; should not be used on persons with a history of estrogen-dependent cancer.

Marjoram

Origanum Marjorana, Majorana hortensis

Characteristics: calming, relaxing, and sedating
Uses: relieves pain, insomnia, headaches, constipation, and colds; increases circulation; helps regulate menstrual cycle; helps relieve anxiety; makes an excellent after-sports rub because of its pain-relieving ability
Caution: Should not be used if pregnant or on pregnant clients; should not be used on persons with a history of estrogen-dependent cancer.

Rosemary

Rosemarinus officinalis, R. coronarium

Characteristics: revives, warms, stimulates, and restores
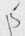
Uses: refreshes tired muscles and feet; increases mental concentration; perfect in pre- and postsports rubs to maintain suppleness; helps combat water retention; combats fatigue; clears a stuffy atmosphere.
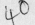
Caution: Should not be used by or on people who are pregnant, by or on people who have epilepsy, or by people who have untreated high blood pressure. Can neutralize homeopathic medicines.

(Buckle, 2007; Price and Price, 2007; Rose, 1999; Shutes and Weaver, 2008; Tisserand, 1985; Worwood, 1999)

ADDITIONAL ESSENTIAL OILS

On the following pages are some additional essential oils to consider. They are useful for a variety of conditions and can be easily added to the practitioner's collection.

WAYS TO USE ESSENTIAL OILS IN A SPA OR PRIVATE PRACTICE

Diffusers

Aromatherapy diffusers come in many sizes, shapes, and styles. The basic diffuser is a ceramic pot with a small bowl to hold water and essential oils (four to six drops), *21* heated by a small candle (see ▶Figures 8.4 a and b on page 280). The warmth of the candle releases the properties in the essential oils. Another type of aromatherapy diffuser uses the warmth of hot water indirectly. A plate is placed over a pot filled with hot water, and four to six drops of essential oil are placed on the plate. As the plate warms, the essential oil evaporates and diffuses into the air (see Figure 8.4 c on page 280). There are also electric diffusers, some with fans, some made of glass (see ▶Figures 8.5 a and b on page 280). These diffusers disinfect and scent the atmosphere by releasing droplets of essential oil as a cool mist.

TO GET YOU STARTED

For relaxation
4 drops Roman chamomile
4 drops lavender or rose or rose absolute

For insomnia
4 drops Roman chamomile
2 drops lavender
2 drops marjoram

To help with grieving
4 drops Roman chamomile
3 drops bergamot
3 drops marjoram

To relieve sore muscles
Try adding the following blend to a massage oil or massage crème (recipes under the section "Scented Oils and Crèmes")
1 drop peppermint
2 drops Roman chamomile
1 drop rosemary
1 drop juniper
3 drops lavender

Clarity temple massage
Use this massage blend to facilitate creative work, clear your mind, and enhance concentration.
    To 1 tablespoon of carrier oil, add
3 drops clary sage
3 drops bergamot or sweet orange

Aroma mist
Use this mist for everything from scenting a room to freshening a client's feet.
2 oz spray bottle
5–6 drops essential oil per ounce
2 oz of purified water or mineral water

Fill bottle halfway with water, add essential oils and shake. Fill bottle to the top and shake again.
    Place one or two drops of the mixture on your fingertips and gently massage your temples. Close your eyes as the warm, sweet aroma of the blend penetrates; envision the creative work before you and proceed.

PROFILES OF ADDITIONAL FOUNDATIONAL OILS

Grapefruit   30 .

Citrus x paradisi
Characteristics: from the peel of the common grapefruit. It has a fresh, sweet, bitter, citrus aroma and is both cleansing and uplifting.
Uses: digestive and lymphatic stimulant; detoxification; helps relieve muscle pain and fatigue; antidepressant; antiseptic; antiviral; astringent. Used to scent citrus perfumes, soaps, creams, and lotions
Caution: Avoid exposing skin to sunlight after using this oil until after bathing or showering to remove it.

Orange, Mandarin

Citrus reticulata
Characteristics: from the peel of the orange. Intense, sweet, fresh scent, similar to tangerine but with neroli-like floral aromas. Cheery and uplifting; blends well with other citrus oils and spice oils such as cinnamon and clove.
Uses: aids digestion; helps relieve hiccups and anxiety; assists liver functions in the elderly. Mandarin essential oil is also commonly used in soaps, cosmetics, perfumes, and men's colognes.
Caution: Avoid exposing skin to sunlight after using this oil until after bathing or showering to remove it.

Neroli (Orange Blossom)

Citrus aurantium
Characteristics: from the blossom of bitter orange; fresh, floral, sweet, and distinctive
Uses: antibacterial; anti-inflammatory; antiseptic; astringent; helps relieve depression; aids digestion; stimulates circulation.
Caution: No known cautions—oil is considered nontoxic and nonsensitizing.

Birch   30

Betula lenta
Characteristics: sweet, sharp scent. Shares similar chemistry, properties, and uses with wintergreen and white birch oil.
Uses: relieves muscular and arthritic pain; is a diuretic; stimulates circulation; soothes skin irritations and psoriasis; softens the skin. It is an effective addition to massage lubricants for sore muscles, sprains, and painful joints because of its anti-inflammatory and antispasmodic properties.
Caution: Because of its potentially toxic effects, this essential oil should be used with caution and should always be diluted. Because it has a sweet, candylike scent, it should be stored safely away from children.

PROFILES OF FOUNDATIONAL OILS CONTINUED

Clary Sage 30

Salvia sclarea

Characteristics: spicy, haylike, bittersweet aroma that is long lasting. It combines well with coriander, cardamom, citrus oils, sandalwood, cedarwood, geranium, and lavandin (a cross between English lavender and spike lavender).

Uses: helps relieve muscle and nervous tension, pain, menstrual cramps, PMS and menopausal problems, such as hot flashes; relaxation and stress relief; encourages dreaming, visualization, and a sense of clarity and balance.

Caution: Those with estrogen-related disorders should avoid long-term use.

Avoid if using alcohol because it can exaggerate the effects and induce a narcotic effect.

Juniper Berry

Juniperus communis

Characteristics: distilled from the dried ripe berry of the juniper tree. It has a fresh, warm, balsamic, woody pine needle odor. Used with citrus oils in room sprays and in masculine perfumes, aftershaves, and spicy colognes. Blends well with clary sage, sandalwood, bergamot, geranium, rosemary, chamomile, and eucalyptus.

Uses: helps relieve arthritic and rheumatic pain; enhances meditative practices because it is considered purifying and clearing; diuretic; detoxification; supports weight loss.

Caution: Should not be used if pregnant or on pregnant clients since it stimulates uterine contractions.

Wintergreen

Gaultheria procumbens

Characteristics: intense, sweet, woody aroma; contains methyl salicylate, giving it analgesic properties. Dried wintergreen leaf and stem are currently in the British Herbal Pharmacopoeia as a treatment for rheumatoid arthritis. Blends well with oregano, peppermint, thyme, and ylang-ylang.

Uses: anti-inflammatory; helps relieve arthritic and other joint and muscular pain, and pain from sciatica, neuralgia, and myalgia. It is an effective addition to massage lubricants.

Caution: Because of its potentially toxic effects, this essential oil should be used with caution and always be diluted. Because it has a sweet, minty, candylike scent, it should be stored safely away from children.

Rose

Rose damascena or centifolia

Characteristics: strongly floral and sweet. Gives a feeling of joy, well-being, happiness, and peace; known as the "oil of love."

Uses: soothes the skin; eases grief; encourages contentment; dissipates guilt; detoxifies the liver; opens the heart; helps relieve depression, menstrual tension, and menopausal symptoms; eases the effects of a hangover.

Caution: No known cautions—oil is considered nontoxic and nonsensitizing.

Frankincense

Boswellia carterii

Characteristics: spicy, balsamic, green-lemon–like, and peppery. It modifies the sweetness of citrus oils such as orange and bergamot. It is also the base for incense-type perfumes and is used in Asian, floral, spicy, and masculine fragrances.

Uses: enhances meditative practices, visualization, and mental clarity; is an antiseptic, anti-inflammatory, and antifungal; helps heal skin infections; good for wound care.

Caution: No known cautions—oil is considered nontoxic and nonsensitizing.

Myrrh

Commiphora myrrha

Characteristics: warm, rich, spicy balsamic aroma. Blends well with lavender, palmarosa, sandalwood, frankincense, rosewood, tea tree, and thyme.

Uses: enhances meditative practices, centering, and visualizing; antiseptic; antifungal. It is an effective addition to massage lubricants for sore muscles, sprains, and painful joints because of its anti-inflammatory and antispasmodic properties.

Caution: Should not be used if pregnant or on pregnant clients; can possibly be toxic in high concentrations.

Sandalwood

Santalum album

Characteristics: rich sweet, woody aroma, a warm balsamic scent that improves with age. Blends well with most essential oils, especially rose, lavender, neroli, and bergamot.

Uses: induces calm and relaxation of the body, mind, and spirit; cleansing; astringent; soothes the skin; often added to massage and facial lubricants, bath oils, aftershaves, lotions, and crèmes.

Caution: No known cautions—oil is considered nontoxic and nonsensitizing.

(Buckle, 2007; Price and Price, 2007; Rose, 1999; Shutes and Weaver, 2008; Tisserand, 1985)

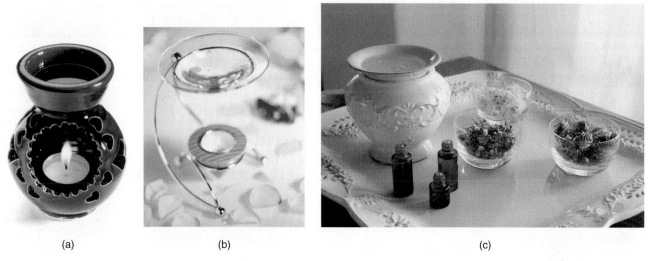

(a)   (b)   (c)

▶ **Figure 8.4** Aromatherapy diffusers come in different sizes, shapes, and styles. A pot of hot water and a plate can make an effective diffuser. *(Photos (a) courtesy of Jules Selmes © Dorling Kindersley and (b) Mauritius, GMBH/Phototake NYC)*

Light Bulb Rings

Light bulb rings sit on top of light bulbs (see ▶Figure 8.6). When the light is turned on, the warmth of the bulb diffuses the essential oils into the room.

Aromastone 35

Aromastones are made of porcelain or ceramic and plug into electrical outlets (see ▶Figure 8.7). Essential oil is poured directly onto the heated porcelain or ceramic surface; no water is needed.

Scented Candles

Candles come in all different sizes, shapes, and scents. They can be made of paraffin, soywax, or beeswax. High-quality candles that burn cleanly and are scented with pure essential oils are the best to use.

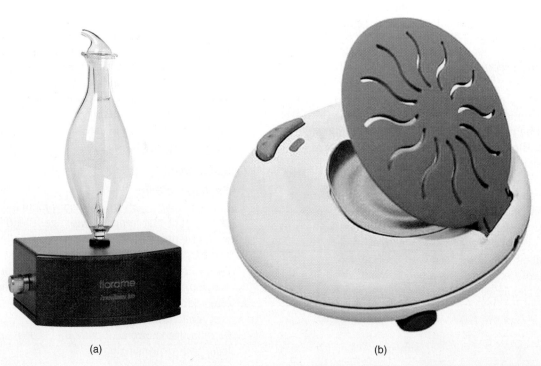

(a)   (b)

▶ **Figure 8.5** Electric diffusers come in many styles and shapes. *(Photos (a) courtesy of © Florame Aromatherapy and (b) Serenity Health)*

20
42
44

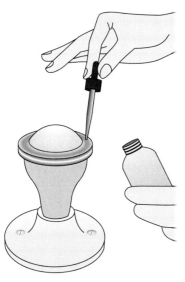

▶ **Figure 8.6** Another type of diffuser is a light bulb ring, which sits on top of a light bulb, using the bulb's heat to diffuse the essential oil into the room.

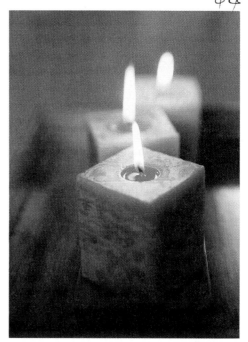

(Getty Images, Inc.)

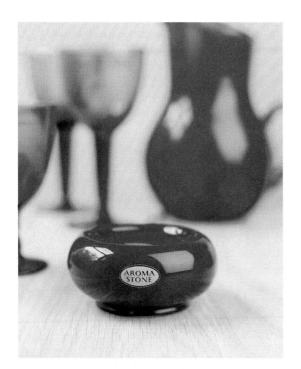

▶ **Figure 8.7** Porcelain or ceramic aromastones plug directly into electrical outlets to diffuse essential oils into a room. *(Image courtesy of Dezac Group Ltd.)*

Scented Massage Oils, Lotions, and Crèmes

To prepare one application, dilute ten to twelve drops of essential oil with one ounce of either a carrier oil or an unscented lotion. If preparing a four- or eight-ounce bottle of oil or lotion, the addition of a few drops of jojoba oil, vitamin E oil, or wheat germ oil will act as a preservative.

Liniments

Liniments are liquid preparations that cause a soothing, cooling, warming, or analgesic action when applied to the skin. The therapeutic action of a liniment application is to increase blood flow to the area and to stimulate the receptors that feel heat and cold. The sensation of hot or cold distracts the brain from the original pain, reducing the perception of pain and offering temporary relief. An example of a heating liniment is one that uses capsicum; an example of a cooling liniment is one that uses menthol or mint.

Some recipes of liniments follow. These are recipes that have been handed down through generations and have been found to be effective. NOTE: Liniments should not be used over areas of the skin that have wounds, infection, or a rash.

TO GET YOU STARTED

Aromatherapy massage oil
2 oz bottle
20–24 drops essential oil (10–12 drops per oz)
Unscented massage oil of choice

Fill bottle halfway with oil; add essential oils and shake. Fill bottle to the top with massage oil and shake again. Oil can be kept for up to six months.

Aromatherapy massage lotion
2 oz bottle
20–24 drops essential oil (10–12 drops per oz)
Unscented massage lotion of choice

Fill bottle halfway with lotion; add essential oils and shake. Fill bottle to the top with massage lotion and shake again. Lotion can be kept for up to six months.

Aromatherapy massage crème
4 oz jar
40–48 drops essential oil (10–12 per oz)
4 oz unscented massage crème of choice

Fill jar halfway with unscented crème, add essential oils, and mix well. Fill jar to top with crème and mix again. Crème can be kept for up to six months.

Rose and Lavender Crème
4 oz jojoba oil
3 oz distilled water
½ oz beeswax
20 drops rose absolute
15 drops lavender

Using a double boiler, slowly melt the beeswax in the jojoba oil. Add the distilled water in a thin stream while vigorously beating the mixture with a wire whisk. Remove from heat and continue whisking the oil while adding the essential oils drop by drop. Crème can be kept for up to 6 months.

Simple Inhalation and Facial Sauna Treatments Using Essential Oils

Simple inhalation treatments are excellent for relieving head congestion and sinus infections. Boil one quart of water, and while it is still boiling, pour it into a large bowl. Add five to eight drops of the desired essential oil and stir. Cover head with a towel and lean over the water (▶Figures 8.8 a and b). Keep eyes closed and breathe deeply through the nose for 5 to 15 minutes, depending on one's level of comfort. Rinse face with cool water and gently blot skin dry.

Essential oils can also be used in steam cabinets; just add five to eight drops to the water.

TO GET YOU STARTED

All-Purpose Liniment
2 oz tincture of capsicum (red pepper)
2 oz extract of lobelia
1/8 oz each of rosemary, wormwood, and spearmint oil

Combine and shake well. Massage into the skin over areas of pain, especially for pain from arthritis, sprains, bruises, neuralgia (general nerve pain), and stiff joints.

Liniment for Muscle Pain
1 oz oil of camphor
4 oz almond or sesame oil
(or combination of 2 oz each)

Combine and shake well. Massage into the skin over areas of general muscular pain.

Arthritis Rub
1 pint rubbing alcohol
1 oz olive oil
1 oz witch hazel
1 oz peppermint spirits*
1 oz oil of wintergreen*
1 oz oil of pine*
25 menthol crystals*
*These are usually available at local pharmacies.

Combine and shake well. Massage into the skin over areas of pain, especially for pain from arthritis.

Warming Liniment
1 tbsp cayenne powder
1 pint apple cider vinegar

Combine ingredients in a small pot. Bring to a slow boil, and boil for 10 minutes. Bottle while hot. Liniment can be used while warm or at room temperature. Massage into the skin over areas of tightness and pain. Do not use over areas of inflammation.

Wintergreen Liniment
30 aspirin (methyl salicylate*)
2 tbsp oil of wintergreen
1 pint rubbing alcohol
*People with aspirin sensitivity should not use this liniment.

Crush aspirin and dissolve in rubbing alcohol. Add oil of wintergreen. Shake well. Massage into the skin over areas of muscle tension and pain.

Hot and Cold Compresses

The hot and cold compresses discussed in Chapter 4 can be enhanced by adding four to five drops of desired essential oil to the compress water.

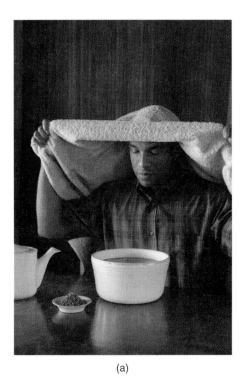
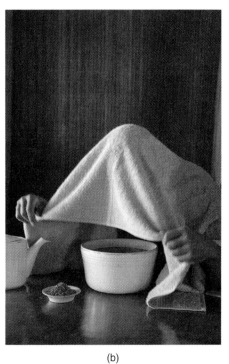

(a)   (b)

▶ **Figure 8.8** Simple inhalation treatments are excellent for relieving head congestion and sinus infections.

TO GET YOU STARTED

To relieve congestion
3–5 drops eucalyptus

To relieve nervous tension and anxiety
1 drop vanilla essential oil
1 drop tangerine essential oil

For insomnia
5 drops lavender, chamomile, jasmine, or bergamot essential oil
OR
3 drops lavender
1 drop bergamot

To relieve headache
5 drops lavender essential oil

To energize
2 drops rosemary
2 drops bergamot
OR
1 drop peppermint
2–3 drops bergamot

To refresh and rehydrate the skin
3 drops Roman chamomile
3 drops lavender

Manual Exfoliations Using Natural Substances

The manual exfoliations using natural substances discussed in Chapter 5 and the salt glow discussed in Chapter 6 can be enhanced by adding two to three drops of the desired essential oil to the manual exfoliation mixture.

Aromatic Baths

Adding essential oils to a bath is another way to get the benefits of essential oils through absorption and inhalation. It is best to dilute four to six drops of essential oil in one teaspoon of carrier oil and then add the mixture to the bath. (It is easier for the essential oil to disperse in the water if it is in a carrier oil.) If peppermint is being used, no more than three drops should be added; more than that may irritate sensitive skin.

USING HERBS IN SPA AND HYDROTHERAPY TREATMENTS

Herbs are invaluable additions to spa and hydrotherapy treatments. There are many from which to choose, and, as with essential oils, the sheer number of them may be daunting for practitioners just learning how to use them.

TO GET YOU STARTED

To help release anger
3 drops chamomile
3 drops ylang-ylang
3 drops marjoram

To help release sadness
4 drops chamomile
3 drops bergamot
3 drops marjoram

For relaxation
4 drops chamomile or neroli
4 drops lavender or rose or rose absolute

To energize
3 drops rosemary
2 drops lemon
2 drops frankincense

For insomnia
4 drops chamomile
2 drops lavender
2 drops neroli
2 drops marjoram

For stress reduction
3 drops orange, sweet
2 drops lavender
2 drops clary sage
1 drop ylang-ylang

To help soften the skin
4 drops lavender
2 drops ylang-ylang
2 drops geranium

To help relieve sore muscles
1 drop peppermint
2 drops Roman chamomile
1 drop rosemary
1 drop juniper
3 drops lavender

Aromatic bath to help relieve depression
1/2 cup honey (or almond, canola, or safflower oil)
3 drops lavender essential oil
3 drops ylang-ylang essential oil
2 drops basil essential oil
2 drops geranium essential oil
1 drop grapefruit essential oil

Combine and add to bath water. Soak for at least 20 minutes. Rest and keep body warm after bath.

Aroma Bath Soak
2 cups baking soda
5–10 drops essential oil

Mix well and keep in a pint jar. Let sit for 1 week, shaking daily, to allow the essential oil to permeate the baking soda. Add entire jar to bath and soak. Jar of bath soak can be kept for up to 6 months.

Aromatic bath salts
2 cups salt (Epsom, sea salt, Dead sea salt, desert mineral salt)
½ cup baking soda
40–48 drops essential oil
Organic vegetable food coloring (optional)
Dried herbs (optional; herbs are discussed in the next section of this chapter)
Pint jar

Pour salt and baking powder into a bowl and mix well with fingers. Add essential oil and mix well. Pour into the pint jar. If you are using the vegetable food coloring and want more than one color, separate salt mixture into one or two other bowls. Add coloring and mix well. Pour layers of different colors into a pint jar. Aromatic bath salts can be kept up to 6 months.

When bathing, use at least 1 cup of the mixture per bath, or the whole jar can be used for maximum benefit.

Jars of bath salts make excellent gifts. For example, decorate the jar of salts with raffia and a colorful label.

▶Table 8.3 shows common herbs and other plants that have many uses. As practitioners become more comfortable working with herbs, they may discover that they want to work with a greater variety of them. Or they may discover that using just these is enough for the treatments they perform. Practitioners may also discover useful plants that are indigenous to their geographical areas. For example, in the Southwest, poultices can be made from prickly pear pads (after the needles are removed, of course). In the Northeast, chickweed can be used for body wraps. Hayflower grows abundantly in Germany, and spas there have long incorporated it into treatments. Hayflower treatments are now becoming popular in the United States.

Purchasing and Storing Herbs and Plants

Some herbs can be purchased in grocery stores, but the selection may be limited. Organic and natural food stores may be better places to find a variety of herbs, and the quality may be better. There are also many internet sources.

Herbs can be purchased either fresh or dried. If fresh plants are desired, only purchase as much as will be used for specific treatments to ensure they do not spoil before

TABLE 8.3

Common Herbs for Use in Spa and Hydrotherapy Treatments

Stress-Relief and Relaxation 23	Energizing and Balancing	Detoxification 22
Lavender	Chamomile	Juniper
Chamomile	Clary sage	Ginger
Clary Sage	Rosemary	Grapefruit zest
Jasmine	Geranium	Eucalyptus
Marjoram	Lemongrass	Clove
Linden flowers	Orange zest	Lemon balm
Hops	Ylang ylang	Hayflower 22
Valerian		Oatstraw
Passionflower		Fennel
		Nettle

(Ody, 2002; Ody, 1993)

the next use. Plants can also be dried by gathering them in small bundles, tying them together with string, and hanging them upside down. Hanging them this way makes it easier to pull leaves off stems.

When the herbs are fully dried, they can be stored in glass jars with tight lids. Even dried plants do not last more than a couple of months before they lose their potency. If a continual supply of high-quality, fresh plants is desired, planting an herb garden may be the solution (Biggs, McVicar and Flowerdew, 2006; Ody, 2002; Dobelis, 1986).

Herbal Infusions

Infusions are one of the easiest methods to prepare herbs for use in spa and hydrotherapy treatments. The infusion water can then be used in simple inhalations and facial saunas, herbal wraps, baths, poultices, and compresses.

Herbal Baths

Herbal infusions can be added to baths; simply add the infused water to warm bath water. The bath should then be soaked in for at least 20 minutes.

CLINICAL ALERT !

Practitioners and clients can be allergic to any and all herbs and other plants. It is important for the practitioner to find out from clients any allergies they may have, and note them on an intake form so there is written documentation. Practitioners allergic to any or all herbs or other plants should never use them on clients even if requested to do so, either by clients or employers.

People can develop allergies throughout their lives; therefore, every time a client arrives for a treatment, the practitioner should do a quick allergy update. Before any treatment is performed, the herb or plant should be applied to a small area on the client's skin and the practitioner's skin, usually the forearm, to see if there is an allergic reaction.

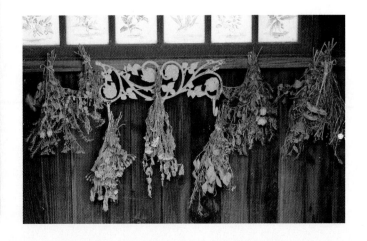

TREATMENT 8.1

Equipment and Supplies

- large muslin drawstring bag (approximately 10″ × 12″) or cheesecloth square (at least 20″ × 20″) tied with a string
- 1–2 cups of dried herbs; double the amount if the herbs are fresh
- large pot or an electric roaster
- 1–4 quarts of water (1 quart of water for baths and inhalations; up to 4 quarts for herbal wraps, in which sheets will be placed to soak, and compresses, in which towels are placed to soak)

Procedure

1. Place herbs in the large muslin drawstring bag or cheesecloth square with a string, and fasten securely (▶Figures 8.9 a and b).

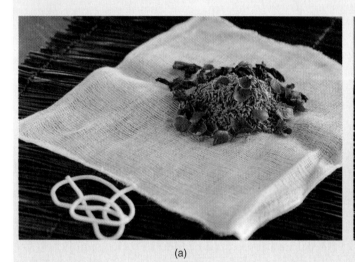

(a)

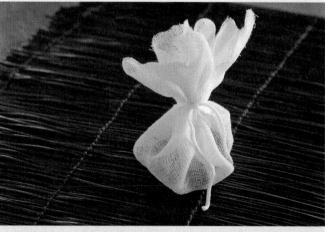

(b)

▶ **Figure 8.9**

2. Bring the quart of water to a rolling boil. Turn off heat and add herbs.
3. Allow the herbs to steep for a minimum of 15 to 30 minutes or longer; the longer the infusion steeps, the stronger it will be.
4. An option is to add herbs directly to the hot water, just like making tea with loose tea leaves (▶Figure 8.10).

Hygiene

Discard the used herbs. Launder the muslin drawstring bag or cheesecloth square with hot water and detergent after each use. Wash the pot or roaster with warm, soapy water and rinse after each use.

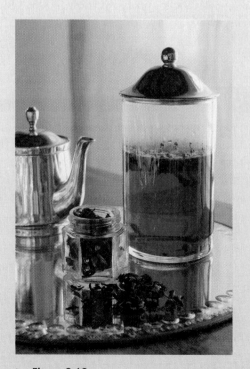

▶ **Figure 8.10**

TREATMENT 8.1 CONTINUED

Herbal Wrap

The herbal wrap is probably the most popular and best-known herbal spa treatment. It is a full-body moist heat treatment, using multiple towels or muslin sheets soaked in an herbal infusion. The herbal wrap treatment can easily be incorporated into a 60-minute treatment; the wrap itself typically takes 20 to 30 minutes. It can be an individual treatment or preceded by an exfoliation and followed by complementary therapy. For best results, warm the client's body first with a warm foot bath or a hot, nonalcoholic beverage such as tea. Using dark-colored sheets and/or towels is recommended; practitioners should be aware that placing cloth sheets into the herbal infusion may cause them to become stained.

Rationale

An herbal·body wrap can be done for any or all of the following physiological effects:

- Tonifier: strengthens vitality and the immune system
- Vasodilator: increases local blood flow
- Analgesic: relieves pain
- Detoxifier: elimination of toxins
- Emollient: soothing to the skin
- Sedative: induces a state of deep relaxation
- Thermodynamic: sends deep, penetrating heat into muscles and joints

Indications

- tight joints (from noninflammatory conditions)
- muscle spasms, tightness, or strain
- need to soften and smooth the skin
- need to balance skin's pH
- need for relaxation
- need for detoxification
- need for skin cleansing

Contraindications

- heart conditions
- untreated hypertension
- numbness or loss of sensation
- neuropathy
- vascular disorders
- burns
- flare-up stages of autoimmune disorders such as lupus, rheumatoid arthritis, and multiple sclerosis (there is generally a great deal of pain with flare-up stages; the heat from the herbal wrap would only be more painful and debilitating)
- any disorders with accompanying vascular issues or neuropathy, such as diabetes
- inflammation
- intolerance to heat
- high body temperature (fever)
- broken or irritated skin
- skin conditions made worse by heat and moisture
- pregnancy
- claustrophobia

Equipment and Supplies

- large muslin drawstring bag (approximately 10″ × 12″) or cheesecloth square (at least 20″ × 20″) tied with a string
- 1–2 cups of dried herbs; double the amount if the herbs are fresh
- large pot or an electric roaster filled with at least at least 1 quart of water

- exfoliation tools or ingredients for a scrub
- washcloth
- small bowl
- cool water
- five cloth sheets; muslin works best (one fitted and four flat). If performing an exfoliation prior to the body wrap, six cloth sheets will be needed (two beach towels, approximately 35″ × 70″, can be used instead of two sheets).
- one large towel, approximately 30″ × 60″
- insulating sheet (rubber, plastic, Mylar, etc.)
- wool blanket

Preparation

1. Prepare the herbal infusion
2. Layer the table in the following order (see ▶Figure 8.11):
   - Fitted sheet to protect table
   - Large towel placed horizontally across the head of the table, leaving enough room for the head
   - Wool blanket placed horizontally across the table, on top of the towel, leaving enough room for the head to rest on the towel
   - Flat sheet placed horizontally on top of the wool blanket
   - Insulating sheet on top of the cloth sheet
   - 1 flat sheet placed horizontally on top of the insulating sheet (extend the cloth sheet at least 1 inch beyond the wool blanket and insulating sheet at the head of the table so it can be folded over the wool blanket once the client is wrapped. This helps protect the client from being in contact with the wool, which may be itchy.
   - If performing an exfoliation, place two flat sheets horizontally on top of the insulating sheet.

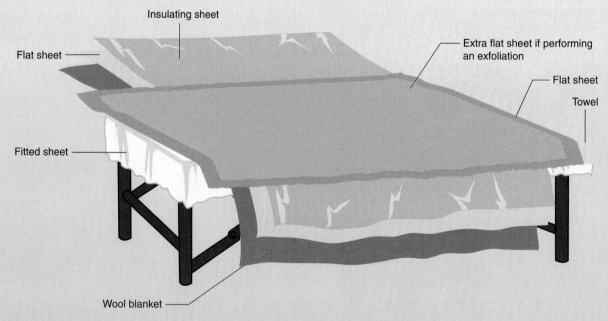

▶ **Figure 8.11**

3. Fold two cloth sheets in half lengthwise, then in half lengthwise again. Fold each sheet in half width-wise, and then roll each sheet up (see ▶Figure 8.12). If using beach towels, fold each one in half length-wise, and then roll each one up. Place both sheets (or towels) in the herbal infusion and allow them to become thoroughly saturated.

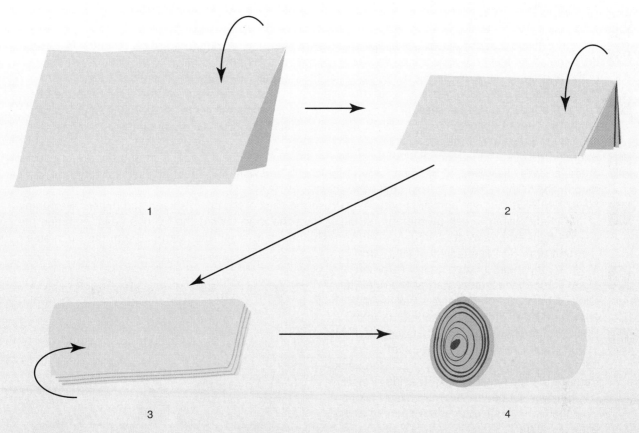

1   2   3   4

▶ **Figure 8.12**

4. Fill the small bowl with cool water and place the washcloth in it. Position it within easy reach.

Procedure

A pre–body wrap exfoliation can be performed. The quick-prep dry-brushing procedure from Chapter 5 is described here, but any of the exfoliation treatments in Chapter 5 can be performed.

1. Standing at the foot of the table, undrape the client's left leg and gluteal region. Working toward the client's heart, start brushing at the feet, move up the leg, and include the gluteals. Redrape the client's left leg. Move to the client's right leg. Undrape and brush the foot, leg, and gluteal region the same as for the left leg. Redrape the client's right leg.

CLINICAL ALERT !

Check with the client about pressure and adjust as necessary.

2. Move to the client's left arm and undrape it. Brush the palm of the client's hand and fingers. Beginning at the client's wrist, brush up the arm, stroking from the wrist toward the client's heart. Redrape the client's left arm. Move to the client's right arm. Undrape and brush the hand and arm the same as for the left arm. Redrape the client's right arm.

TREATMENT 8.1 CONTINUED

3. Move to the head of the table and undrape the back. Starting at the neck and shoulders, brush down to the client's mid-back. Move to the right side of the table. Reaching across the client's back, brush the client's left lumbar to mid-back area, using angling, upward strokes toward the client's heart. Move to the left side of the table. Brush the client's right lumbar to mid-back area the same as for the left side. Redrape the back.

4. Help the client turn over.

5. Standing at the foot of the table, undrape the client's right leg. Working toward the client's heart, start brushing at the feet and move up the leg. Redrape the client's right leg. Move to the client's left leg. Undrape and brush the foot and leg the same as for the right leg. Redrape the client's left leg.

6. Move to the client's abdomen and drape the large towel across the client's chest area. Have the client hold it firmly as you pull the sheet inferiorly until the client's abdomen is undraped. Using smaller strokes, brush the client's abdomen in a clockwise direction. Finish the abdomen by brushing up each side and coming to the center of the abdomen.

7. Redrape the client's abdomen by pulling the sheet up over the client's abdomen and the draping towel on the client's chest area. Move to one side of the client, and while the client holds the sheet firmly, gently pull the draping towel out from under the sheet.

8. Move to the client's right arm and undrape it. Brush the back of the client's hand and fingers. Beginning at the client's wrist, brush up the arm, stroking from the wrist toward the client's heart. Redrape the client's right arm. Move to the client's left arm. Undrape and brush the hand and arm the same as for the right arm. Redrape the client's left arm.

9. Move to the head of the table. To brush the client's upper chest area, start at the right clavicle and brush downward three times; then brush downward three times from the left clavicle.

10. If an exfoliation was performed, assist the client off the table, making sure the client stays securely draped with a sheet opening at the back. Remove the top sheet and set it aside. If an exfoliation was not performed, make sure the client is draped with a sheet or towel opening at the back (▶Figure 8.13).

11. Take the one cloth sheet out of the herbal infusion and thoroughly wring it out. To prevent heat loss from the sheet, quickly unroll it and unfold it widthwise; then lay it horizontally along the massage table. It should be even with the edge of the wool blanket at the head of the table, and depending on the length of the sheet, it may hang off the foot of the table. Unfold the sheet lengthwise once so that it is the width of the massage table (it should still be folded in half lengthwise) (see ▶Figure 8.14). If towels are being used, unroll and unfold one and lay it lengthwise on the massage table.

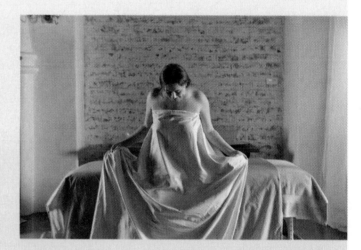

▶ **Figure 8.13**

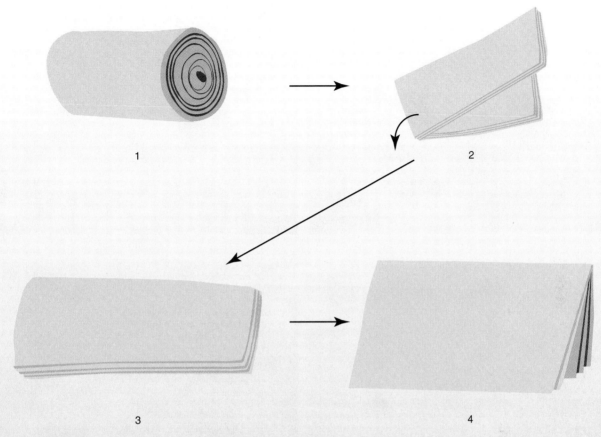

1

2

3

4

▶ **Figure 8.14**

12. Help the client quickly lie supine on top of the wet sheet, spreading the sheet or towel drape out on both sides of the client so that the client is lying directly on the wet sheet.

13. Remove second sheet (or towel) from the herbal infusion and wring out thoroughly, unrolling and unfolding the same as in step 2, and place it on top of client (removing the drape from underneath). To retain the heat in the wet sheets, begin at the feet. If the wet sheets are hanging off the foot of the table, fold up over the client's legs, covering the feet. Wrap the rest of the client's body one layer at a time. The wrap should be snug, but not tight. The client's arms can be at the sides of the body or crossed over the chest. For best results, the client's arms should be inside the wrap. However, if the client is more comfortable or feeling slightly claustrophobic, the arms can be left outside the wrap (▶ Figures 8.15 a, b, c, and d).

TREATMENT 8.1 CONTINUED

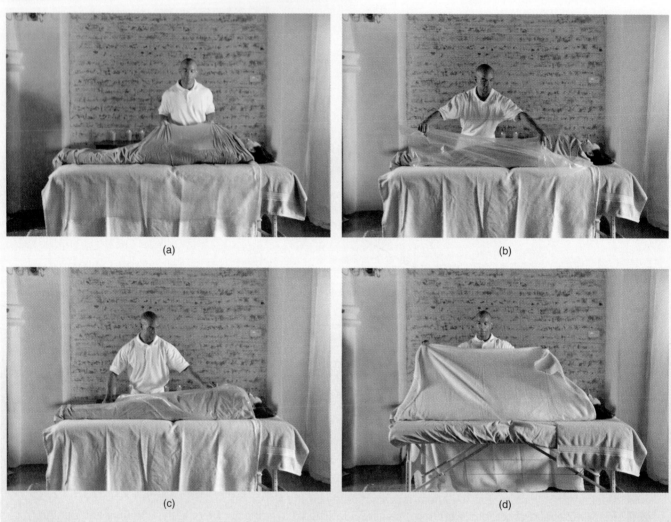

(a)

(b)

(c)

(d)

▶ **Figure 8.15**

14. Secure the towel at the head of the table around the client's neck and shoulders (▶ Figures 8.16 a and b).

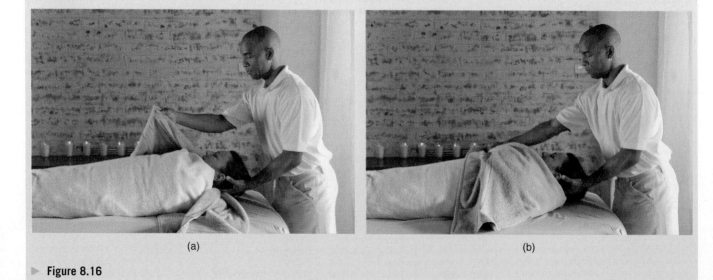

(a)

(b)

▶ **Figure 8.16**

Each layer of the wrap should be tucked snugly under the client's body (▶Figure 8.17).

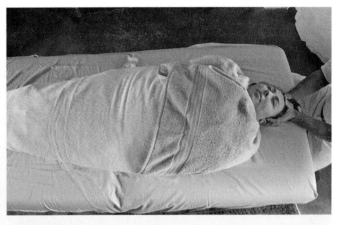

▶ **Figure 8.17**

15. Make sure the client is comfortable, using bolsters, pillows, or other props as needed. An extra blanket can be added for more warmth. The client should remain wrapped for 20 to 30 minutes. During this time, a scalp and facial massage can be given or the client's feet can be unwrapped for a foot massage. Another option is to sit quietly at the head or foot of the table (▶Figure 8.18). When the client begins to feel hot, a cool, moist washcloth can be placed on the forehead and a cool drink of water can be offered.

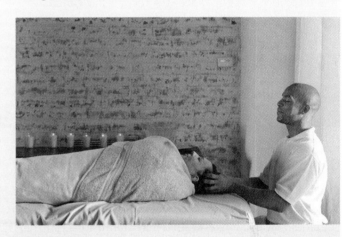

▶ **Figure 8.18**

CLINICAL ALERT !

It is important to stay near the client; some clients may become claustrophobic or overheated and need to have the wrappings removed as soon as they start feeling uncomfortable.

16. When the time is up, unwrap the client quickly. Cover the client with the original sheet drape or large towel as layers are removed. The air will feel chilly so it is important to redrape the client as quickly as possible.

After the Treatment
Encourage the client to rest and drink plenty of water after treatment. The client's skin may show a slight flush since being wrapped for the treatment increases body warmth and improves circulation.

Hygiene
Any leftover infusion water should be discarded after each client. The sheets, towels, and washcloth should be laundered with hot water and detergent after each use. The insulating sheet should be sprayed with alcohol or other disinfectant and allowed to dry after each use and before folding and storing. It can also be washed with soap and water, but it should still be sprayed with disinfectant after washing. If brushes were used for the exfoliation, wash them in warm, soapy water and rinse. After rinsing, place them in rubbing alcohol for at least 20 minutes; then let them air dry. The tools can also be washed in a dishwasher. Store them in an airtight container. If the exfoliation was done using a natural substance, any leftover exfoliation mixture should be immediately discarded. All bowls should be washed in warm, soapy water and rinsed between each use.

TO GET YOU STARTED

For relief from muscle pain
4 tbsp dried lavender
2 tbsp bay leaves
4 tbsp dried marjoram
4 tbsp dried rosemary

To induce sleep
4 tbsp dried chamomile
2 tbsp dried passionflower
1 tbsp dried valerian
4 tbsp dried lemon balm

To promote circulation
1 tbsp dried lemon peel (or 1 lemon, quartered)
3 tbsp dried rosemary
2 tbsp dried juniper
2 tbsp dried ginger powder (or 4 tbsp freshly grated ginger root)

For general relaxation
4 tbsp dried lavender
2 tbsp dried chamomile
2 drops clary sage essential oil
2 drops marjoram essential oil

To uplift the spirit
4 tbsp dried lavender
2 tbsp dried lemon or orange zest
2 drops neroli essential oil
1 drop mandarin orange essential oil
1 drop grapefruit oil

For headache relief
2 tbsp dried peppermint
4 tbsp dried lemon balm
3 tbsp dried ginger powder (or 4 tbsp freshly grated ginger)
4 tbsp dried lavender

To prevent a cold
3 tbsp dried ginger powder (or 4 tbsp freshly grated ginger)
4 tbsp dried rosemary
3 tbsp dried eucalyptus
4 tbsp dried lavender

Compresses

Before applying a cold or hot compress (Chapter 4), the towels can be soaked in an herbal infusion. (Practitioners should be aware, however, that herbal infusions can stain the towels.) Any of the infusions described under herbal wraps, facial saunas, and herbal baths can be adapted for use with compresses.

Poultices

Poultices are treatments applied to a specific area of the body. They are soft, moist masses of substance that are applied either directly or encased in a clean cloth such as flannel, cheesecloth, or muslin. The poultice is then covered and left for a period of time. Today's body wraps evolved from the use of poultices. The procedures are the same: a substance is applied to the body and then covered by cloth. In fact, a body wrap can be thought of as a poultice applied to the entire body. For more information on herbal poultices, see Appendix 1.

TREATMENT 8.2

Simple Inhalation and Facial Sauna Treatments Using Herbs

Rationale

A simple inhalation or facial sauna treatment can be done for any or all of the following physiological effects:

- Decongestant: clears mucus from respiratory passageways
- Vasodilator: increases local blood flow
- Analgesic: relieves pain
- Detoxifier: elimination of toxins
- Emollient: soothing to the skin
- Sedative: induces a state of deep relaxation

Indications

- congestion from respiratory infections, sinus infections, colds, flu, and bronchitis
- pain relief from sore throat and laryngitis
- need to soften the skin on the face
- need for relaxation

Equipment and Supplies

- large muslin drawstring bag (approximately 10″ × 12″) or cheesecloth square (at least 20″ × 20″) tied with a string
- 1–2 cups of dried herbs; double the amount if the herbs are fresh
- large pot or an electric roaster
- 1 quart of water
- washcloth
- small bowl (for cool water)

Contraindications

- numbness or loss of sensation in the face
- burns
- inflammation
- high body temperature (fever)
- broken or irritated skin
- skin conditions made worse by heat and moisture
- intolerance to heat

Preparation

1. Place herbs in the large muslin drawstring bag or cheesecloth square with a string, and fasten securely (▶Figures 8.19 a and b).

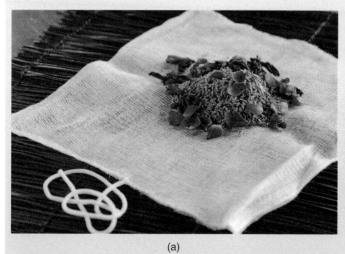

(a)

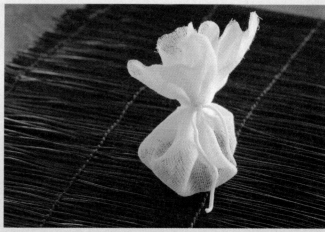

(b)

▶ **Figure 8.19**

2. Bring the quart of water to a rolling boil. Turn off heat.
3. Put the bag of herbs in the hot water and allow them to steep for a few minutes.
4. Fill the small bowl with cool water and place the washcloth in it.

TREATMENT 8.2 CONTINUED

Procedure

1. Tent head with the towel and stand or sit over the pot (▶Figures 8.20 a and b).

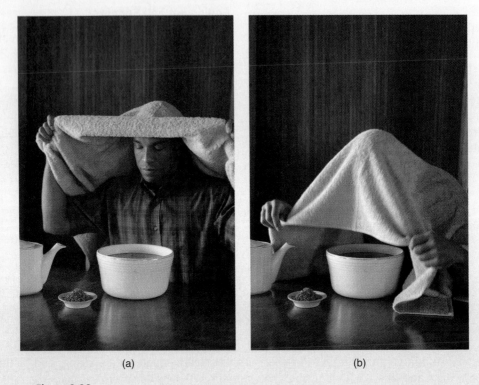

(a)   (b)

▶ **Figure 8.20**

2. Breathe slowly and deeply; inhale vapor for 5 to 10 minutes at a time. Wipe face with cool, moist wash-cloth as needed.

After the Treatment
Drink plenty of water.

Hygiene
Discard the used herbs. Launder the muslin drawstring bag or cheesecloth square and towel with hot water and detergent after each use. Wash the pot or roaster with warm, soapy water and rinse after each use.

TO GET YOU STARTED

Here are some simple inhalations you can try.

For insomnia
1 cup dried lavender, chamomile, or jasmine flowers

To relieve headache
1 cup dried lavender flowers

Here are some facial saunas you can try.

Hydrating facial toner
1 quart water
3 chamomile tea bags (or ½ cup dried chamomile flowers in muslin drawstring bag or wrapped in cheesecloth)
1 tbsp fennel seeds

Bring the water to a rolling boil. Add the herbs and turn off the heat. Stir and let it sit for 5 to 10 minutes. Place the pot on a table and tent head with the towel. Stand or sit over the pot and steam your face for 5 to 15 minutes. Rinse face with cool water and gently blot dry. You can save the tea infusion; put it in a spray bottle and chill it to use later for a facial toner.

Herbal deep pore cleanser
1 quart water
1 cup herbs
juice and peel of ½ lemon

Bring the water to a rolling boil. Add the herbs and lemon, and turn off the heat. Stir and let it sit for 5 to 10 minutes. Place the pot on a table and tent head with the towel. Stand or sit over the pot and steam your face for 5 to 15 minutes. Rinse face with cool water and gently blot dry.

Rose petal steam
1 quart water
1 cup rose petals

Bring the water to a rolling boil. Add the rose petals and turn off the heat. Stir and let it sit for 5 to 10 minutes. Place the pot on a table and tent head with the towel. Stand or sit over the pot and steam your face for 5 to 15 minutes. Rinse face with cool water and gently blot dry. You can save the rose infusion; put it in a spray bottle and chill it to use later for a facial toner.

Herbal skin detoxifier
2 quarts water
½ cup dried lavender flowers (antiseptic, antidepressant, stress relieving, and calming properties)
½ cup dried juniper berries (detoxifying properties)
½ cup dried chamomile flowers (soothing and calming properties)
½ cup dried calendula flowers (healing and softening properties)
1 drop patchouli essential oil (especially good for dry or mature skin; moisturizer, regenerator, and fungicide)
2 drops tea tree essential oil (antiseptic, antifungal, and good for all types of skin)
3 drops geranium essential oil (good for cellular regeneration, balancing, and rejuvenating)

Combine the dry herbs and put them in a muslin drawstring bag or wrap in cheesecloth. (You could also simply add dry herbs directly to hot water.) Bring the water to a rolling boil. Add the herbs and turn off the heat. Add the essential oils. Stir and let sit for 5 to 10 minutes. Place the pot on a table and tent head with the towel. Stand or sit over the pot and steam your face for 5 to 15 minutes. Rinse face with cool water and gently blot dry.

TO GET YOU STARTED

For relaxation
½ cup dried rose petals
½ cup dried lavender

General relaxation
4 tbsp dried lavender
2 tbsp dried chamomile
2 drops clary sage essential oil
1 drop ylang-ylang essential oil

For relief of muscle pain
4 tbsp dried lavender
2 tbsp bay leaves
4 tbsp dried marjoram
4 tbsp dried rosemary

To induce sleep
4 tbsp dried chamomile
2 tbsp dried passionflower
1 tbsp dried valerian
4 tbsp lemon balm (melissa)

To promote circulation
1 tbsp dried lemon peel (or 1 lemon, quartered)
3 tbsp dried rosemary
2 tbsp dried juniper
2 tbsp dried ginger powdered (or 4 tbsp fresh grated ginger root)

TO GET YOU STARTED CONTINUED

To relieve symptoms of premenstrual syndrome
½ cup dried orange peel (or ½ fresh orange, sliced)
3 tbsp dried jasmine flowers
3 tbsp dried sandalwood chips

To soothe the skin
4 tbsp dried calendula
3 tbsp dried comfrey
2 tbsp dried sandalwood chips

To relieve headache
2 tbsp dried peppermint
4 tbsp dried lemon balm (melissa)
3 tbsp dried ginger powder (or 4 tbsp fresh grated ginger root)
4 tbsp dried lavender

To prevent a cold
3 tbsp dried ginger powder (or 4 tbsp fresh grated ginger root)
4 tbsp dried rosemary
3 tbsp dried eucalyptus
4 tbsp dried lavender

To uplift the spirit
4 tbsp dried lavender
2 tbsp dried lemon or orange zest
2 drops neroli essential oil
1 drop mandarin orange essential oil
1 drop lemon essential oil

TO GET YOU STARTED

The following are other herbal treatments to try.

Aroma Clay Mask
2 tbsp clay of choice
1 tbsp soy powder
8–10 drops essential oil
Dried herbs of choice
Water
Small, nonmetal bowl
Washcloth

Mix ingredients together in a clean jar or reclosable plastic sandwich bag; then pour the mixture into a small bowl. Add enough water to make a thick paste and apply to face. When completely dried, rinse face thoroughly with warm water, and use a warm, moist washcloth to remove the mask. Splash face with cold water and gently blot dry.

Cucumber Mask
½ cucumber
1 egg white
1 tbsp lemon juice
1 tsp mint
Small bowl
Washcloth

Place all ingredients in a blender and puree. Pour the mixture into a small bowl and refrigerate for 10 minutes.

Apply to face and leave on for 15 minutes. Rinse face with hot and then cool water. Use a moist washcloth to remove the mask. Gently blot the skin dry.

Almond Face and Body Scrub
⅔ cup ground almonds
⅓ cup ground or fine oatmeal
½ tsp dried herbs of choice
Yogurt, milk, buttermilk, or floral water, enough to make a paste
5 drops essential oil, optional
Washcloth

Combine dry ingredients in a blender or food processor and process until they are reduced to a coarse meal. Keep this "exfoliation base" in a glass jar in the refrigerator until needed.

For a facial scrub: use about one teaspoon and mix with enough yogurt, milk, or floral water to make a paste. Apply to face, avoiding eyes, and allow to dry. Rinse with hot and then cool water. Use a moist washcloth to remove residue. Gently blot the skin dry.

For a body scrub: use ½ cup and mix with enough yogurt, milk, or floral water to make a paste. Apply to the body and exfoliate using small circular strokes. Leave on until dry. Rinse with hot and then cool water. Use a moist washcloth to remove residue. Gently blot the skin dry.

Summary

Although *aromatherapy* has become an umbrella term for just about anything that is pleasantly scented, it is an actual art and science. Humans have used plants for their healing properties, as well as for food, since prehistory. The ancient Aztecs, Native Americans, Greeks, Romans, Chinese, and ancient Egyptians all used aromatic oils and made their own herbal remedies. The term *aromatherapy* was coined in the early 1900s by French chemist Rene-Maurice Gattefosse. French physician Dr. Jean Valnet, French biochemist Marguerite Maury, Micheline Arcier, and Robert Tisserand all furthered the study of aromatherapy and helped make it as well known as it is today.

Essential oils are the volatile oils that aromatic plants, trees, and grasses produce. About 200 different essential oils have been extracted for use in aromatherapy, and they have myriad effects on the body, such as rejuvenation, relaxation, and stimulation.

There are ten recommended foundational essential oils that practitioners can purchase to create a "starter set." These are bergamot, chamomile, cypress, eucalyptus, geranium, lavender, marjoram, peppermint, rosemary, and tea tree. There are many ways to use essential oils in a spa or massage and bodywork practice, including in diffusers, light bulb rings, aromastones, scented candles, scented oils and lotions, steam inhalation treatments, hot and cold compresses, poultices, salt glows, and aromatic baths.

Herbs can also be useful adjuncts to spa and hydrotherapy treatments. Some basic herbs to use include chamomile, clary sage, clove, eucalyptus, geranium, ginger, grapefruit, hops, jasmine, juniper, lavender, lemon balm, lemongrass, linden flowers, marjoram, orange, rosemary, valerian, and ylang-ylang. Herbs can be prepared using an infusion. The infusion can be used for inhalation treatments and facials or added to bath water for immersion or partial baths. For a hot or cold compress treatment or herbal sheet wrap, the towels and sheets can be soaked in the infusion.

Activities

1. What is your favorite essential oil? What do you like about it?

   _____

   _____

   _____

   _____

2. Make flash cards of essential oils with their properties, benefits, indications, and contraindications.

3. Make an aroma mist using peppermint. Use it while on a plane flight, road trip, or just in a depleting situation. How did you feel immediately afterward? 24 hours later? 48 hours later?

   _____

   _____

   _____

   _____

4. Make an aroma mist using lavender. Use it when you need to feel calm. How did you feel immediately afterward? 24 hours later? 48 hours later?

   _____

   _____

   _____

   _____

5. Place a couple of drops of an essential oil of choice on a cotton ball and place it in the air conditioning vent of your car. How do you feel when you smell the essential oil while driving? 24 hours later? 48 hours later?

   _____

   _____

   _____

6. Place a couple of drops of eucalyptus essential oil on a cotton ball, and with a client's permission, place it under the edge of a face cradle cover. Does the eucalyptus help combat the congestion clients may experience when resting the face in the face cradle?

_____

_____

7. Take a rosemary bath in the morning. Does it help you start your day more energized?

_____

_____

8. Take other aromatic or herbal baths. How did you feel immediately afterward? 24 hours later? 48 hours later?

_____

_____

_____

_____

_____

9. Make a massage oil, lotion, or crème, and with their permission, use it on clients. Did they like it? Why or why not? Did you like it? What benefits did the clients experience from it?

_____

_____

_____

_____

_____

10. Try a facial using essential oils or herbs or both. How did you feel immediately afterward? 24 hours later? 48 hours later?

_____

_____

_____

11. Try an inhalation treatment using essential oils or herbs or both. How did you feel immediately afterward? 24 hours later? 48 hours later?

_____

_____

_____

_____

_____

12. Receive a compress treatment using essential oils or herbs or both. How did you feel immediately afterward? 24 hours later? 48 hours later?

_____

_____

_____

_____

13. Receive an herbal body wrap treatment. Describe which type of wrap you received. What did you like about it? What did you not like about it? What would you have done differently? How did you feel 24 hours after the treatment? 48 hours after the treatment?

_____

_____

_____

_____

_____

14. Make your own herbal resource file. Go to a natural foods market or nursery and see which herbs are available. Smell them, take pictures of them, and write down where you can find each herb. Make a list of each herb's properties, benefits, indications, and contraindications.

_____

_____

_____

_____

_____

Study Questions

1. The term for the therapeutic use of plants is
    a. aromatherapy
    b. phytotherapy
    c. infusion
    d. distillation

2. Who became interested in studying essential oils when his burned hand was healed by a vat of lavender essential oil?
    a. Ibn Sina
    b. Dr. Jean Valnet
    c. Robert Tisserand
    d. Rene-Maurice Gattefosse

3. Vaporizing easily at low temperatures is the definition of
    a. compress
    b. detoxification
    c. volatile
    d. extraction

4. Which of the following oils would be safe to use on a pregnant client?
    a. Cypress
    b. Bergamot
    c. Geranium
    d. Eucalyptus

5. Which of the following herbs is used for detoxification?
    a. Clove
    b. Lemon balm
    c. Clary sage
    d. Lavender

6. Which of the following herbs would be used for energizing and balancing?
    a. Lavender
    b. Ylang-ylang
    c. Valerian
    d. Fennel

7. What is the minimum amount of time herbs should be allowed to steep while making an infusion?
    a. 5 minutes
    b. 15 minutes
    c. 20 minutes
    d. 25 minutes

8. Essential oils are used for the purposes of
    a. increasing pain sensations
    b. increasing anxiety and insomnia
    c. stimulating the immune system
    d. stimulating bacterial growth

9. Which of the following is a base note essential oil?
    a. Peppermint
    b. Coriander
    c. Lemongrass
    d. Frankincense

10. To make a 3% dilution, how many drops of essential oil should be added to one ounce of carrier oil?
    a. 5–6
    b. 10–12
    c. 15–18
    d. 25–30

Case Samples

A. Jordan Nelson is a thirty-three-year-old mother of two-year-old twins. She is a stay-at-home mom whose husband is working eighty hours a week starting up his own carpet-cleaning business. Once a month, Jordan can afford the time and money to get away for a relaxing treatment. She has decided to try aromatherapy. A friend of hers recommended Amrit Gupta, a shiatsu practitioner whose practice also includes aromatherapy and herbal treatments.

1. Which aromatherapy/herbal treatments would be best for Jordan to receive?
2. What are the rationale, equipment and supplies, indications, contraindications, preparation, after-treatment care, and hygiene for these treatments?
3. Which questions should Amrit ask Jordan to determine which treatment would be most beneficial?

B. Martin Grant is coming down with a cold. He is having trouble breathing because he has a lot of nasal and sinus congestion.

1. What aromatherapy or herbal treatment could he do at home to help relieve the congestion?
2. What are the rationale, equipment and supplies, indications, contraindications, preparation, after-treatment care, and hygiene for these treatments?

C. Jaime Marquez competes in triathlons. To get ready for his next event, he has been training 4 hours a day, 6 days a week for the past 2 months, and he has been experiencing quite a bit of generalized muscle pain.

1. Which aromatherapy or herbal treatments would help reduce his discomfort?
2. What are the rationale, equipment and supplies, indications, contraindications, preparation, after-treatment care, and hygiene for these treatments?

Poultices

Poultices are treatments applied to a specific area of the body. They are soft, moist masses of substance that are applied either directly to the body or encased in a clean cloth such as flannel, cheesecloth, or muslin and then covered and left for a period of time. Today's body wraps evolved from the use of poultices. The procedures are the same: a substance is applied to the body and then covered by cloth. In fact, a wrap can be thought of as a poultice applied to the entire body (Barron, 2003).

Poultices have been used in various cultures throughout history. The ancient Romans, Chinese, Indians, and Native Americans discovered the usefulness of applying various substances onto areas of the body for healing purposes, such as to soothe inflamed areas; stimulate circulation; warm and relax muscles; and draw out toxins, infection (pus), or foreign particles (Williams, 2007).

The word *poultice* comes from the Latin *pultes,* meaning "porridge" because, historically, certain poultices were made from bread or other cereals (www.Infoplease.com, 2008; Merriam-Webster Dictionary, 2004). However, mud, clay, seaweed, and fresh or dried plant materials have all been used for poultices. Old-fashioned mustard and onion plasters are, in fact, poultices.

Poultices can be applied in spas and massage and bodywork offices and at home. They are relatively simple to perform, and the supplies are readily available; many commercial poultices are also on the market. Poultices can be hot or cold, depending on the therapeutic need. Generally, cold poultices are used to withdraw heat from an inflamed or congested area, and hot poultices are used to relax spasms, reduce pain, and draw out infection or insect venom. Some poultices can be used either hot or cold, and some can be applied at room temperature and still be effective (Barron, 2003; Nikola, 1997).

What follows is a basic poultice procedure; specific types of poultices and their effects on the body are described next. The equipment and supplies for poultices can be purchased at local stores, except for certain items such as mud, peat, clay, sea mud, and seaweed, which need to be purchased through a spa treatment supply store.

Mud, Peat, Clay, Sea Mud, or Seaweed Poultice

The mud, peat, or clay can be warmed or used at room temperature; either way, each is effective. The many benefits of mud, peat, or clay poultices include:

- increased blood and lymphatic flow in the area
- pain relief from tight joints and muscle spasms, tightness, or strain
- relaxation and stress relief
- deep, penetrating heat sent into muscles and joints
- balanced pH of the skin
- loosening old scar tissue
- detoxification
- cleansed skin
- soothed skin, especially for eczema and psoriasis
- strengthened vitality and immune system
- pain relief from osteoarthritis and a noninflammatory state of rheumatoid arthritis
- pain relief from old injuries or broken bones

ADDITIONAL POULTICE RECIPES

Clay and Essential Oil
Add twelve drops of a desired essential oil to each teaspoon of clay. See Chapter 8 for the therapeutic benefits, indications, and contraindications of various essential oils.

Clay and Apple Cider Vinegar
This can be used to soothe inflamed skin, bruises, sprains, and acne and can draw out toxins, infections, and insect venom. Mix ¼ cup clay powder with enough organic apple cider vinegar to make a thick paste. Apply the paste directly to the skin and allow it to dry completely before removing it.

TREATMENT

Equipment and Supplies

- Poultice substance (this makes enough for one poultice; if successive poultices are desired, then double or triple the amount)
  ¼ cup mud; peat; or clay, mud, peat, or clay powder mixed with water into a thick paste, or ¼ cup mud or peat gel
  OR
  ¼ cup sea mud powder mixed with water or ¼ cup seaweed mud, gel, or crème
  OR
  1–2 cups of dried herbs (double the amount if using fresh)
  ¼ cup flour, cornmeal, or flaxseed oil
- soft cloth (flannel, cheesecloth, or muslin), approximately 18″ × 30,″ if enclosing the poultice substance in cloth before applying to the skin. (This is for one poultice; if successive poultices are desired, then two or three cloths will be needed.)
- small, nonmetal bowl; nonmetal because most poultice substances react chemically with metal, which will cause the properties of the poultice substance to change. Likewise, poultice substances should not be stored in metal containers.
- If the poultice substance is to be warmed before use, a small crock pot or small electric warmer is necessary. If using a small electric warmer, another bowl will be needed. (Poultice substances should never be warmed by microwaving; this destroys their therapeutic properties.)
- hydrogen peroxide and cotton balls (to clean the skin before and after applying the poultice)
- plastic wrap
- dry towel, approximately 18″ × 30″
- warm, moist towel, approximately 18″ × 30″ (to wipe residue after the poultice is removed); a towel cabi or crock pot can also be used to keep the towel warm and moist.
- hydrocollator pad, heating pad, warmed gel pack, or hot water bottle to place over the poultice if using heat

Preparation

1. If making an herb poultice:
   - Dried herbs—moisten then mix with moistened flour, cornmeal, or flaxseed oil into a thick paste; this makes the herbs more adhesive
   - Fresh herbs—bruise or crush the medicinal parts of the plant (the leaves, stems, buds, or flowers, depending on the herb used) into a paste; add water if necessary
2. To warm the poultice substance using a crock pot, place the substance in one small bowl, then put the bowl in a small crock pot with one inch of hot water. If using a small electric warmer, place the substance in one small dish then put that dish inside another dish that has about one inch of water in it, and place both bowls on the warmer (see ▶ Figure A1.1).
3. If using a crock pot or towel cabi to warm the towel for substance removal at the end of the treatment, turn it on. Moisten the towel and put it in the crock pot or cabi. If using the basin of warm water and towel, place the basin in a convenient place to fill it with warm water toward the end of the treatment.

Procedure

1. Using the hydrogen peroxide and cotton balls, clean the skin in the area where the poultice will be applied.
2. If enclosing the poultice substance in cloth, spread the mixture onto half of the cloth and then fold the cloth over. If applying the mixture directly onto the skin, spread it evenly over the area of discomfort.

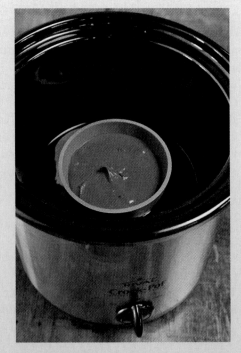

▶ **Figure A1.1**

TREATMENT CONTINUED

3. Cover the poultice mixture with plastic wrap, and then the dry towel for insulation (▶Figure A1.2).

4. A hydrocollator pack, heated gel pack, heating pad, or hot water bottle can be placed on top of the poultice to increase the heating effect.

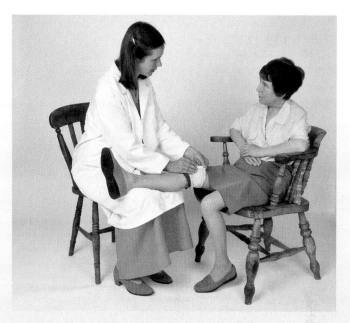

▶ **Figure A1.2** *(Andy Crawford © Dorling Kindersley)*

CLINICAL ALERT

To prevent burning, remove the pack immediately if the temperature is uncomfortable.

---

5. Leave the poultice on for 30 to 60 minutes while resting comfortably. If the poultice is applied to a client, the practitioner can give the client complementary massage on the scalp, face, feet, or other area. Another option is to just sit quietly with the client. It is important to stay near the client; if the poultice becomes too hot or uncomfortable, it needs to be removed immediately.

6. After lifting off the small towel and plastic wrap, remove the poultice residue from the skin with the moist warm towel or rinse the area under warm water.

7. If desired, another poultice may be applied to the area.

8. After the last poultice is removed and the area where it was applied is wiped off, clean the area with hydrogen peroxide and cotton balls.

After the Treatment

The skin may show a slight flush since some poultice substances improve circulation and retain heat, which allows increased blood to flow to the surface of the skin. Massage the area afterward if warranted and appropriate, such as if the poultice was applied to loosen tight muscles. Be sure to drink plenty of water afterward (or encourage the client to do so).

Hygiene

Any leftover poultice substance should be discarded after each use. The small bowl should be washed in warm, soapy water and rinsed after each use. The towel cabi should be washed out daily and sprayed with disinfectant. Used towels should never be placed back in it. Any towels or the piece of flannel should be laundered with hot water and detergent after each use. If a hydrocollator pad was used, place it back into the hydrocollator. At an average temperature of 160°F, the hydrocollator water is hot enough to sterilize the pad. If a heating pad or gel pack was used, wash the cover after each use. If a hot water bottle was used, it should be wiped down with a disinfectant after each use. If a crock pot was used, it should be washed in warm, soapy water, rinsed, and sprayed with disinfectant after each use.

Some conditions, however, warrant caution in using a mud, peat, or clay poultice. It should not be used on or by people who have:

- ► heart conditions
- ► vascular disease
- ► numbness or loss of sensation in area
- ► a high body temperature (fever)
- ► inflammation

- ► broken or irritated skin
- ► an intolerance to heat
- ► become pregnant

Herbal Poultice

Chapter 8 discusses various herbs and plants, including their therapeutic benefits and indications and contraindications for use. Any of them can be used to make poultices.

MORE POULTICE RECIPES

Cold Poultices

These are applied without the use of heat.

Aloe vera

Excellent for relieving inflammation, sunburn, or infection. Remove a leaf from an aloe vera plant (aloe vera pulp or gel can also be used). Carefully slice it in half and apply directly to the area of inflammation, sunburn, or infection. Place gauze or cheesecloth over the area and secure it. Reapply as often as desired.

Cayenne

Increases local circulation; beneficial for reducing inflammation, swelling, chest congestion; relaxes tense muscles. Cayenne is an irritant so it should be placed between two pieces of cloth, not directly on the skin.

Chamomile

Soothing and healing for all skin conditions; especially beneficial for mild eye ailments.

Chaparral (Creosote), Dandelion, and Yellow Dock

Can be used to treat acne, eczema, itchy or dry skin, psoriasis, and rashes. The greatest benefit is obtained by using a combination of all three, but they can be used individually (chaparral works best individually).

Charcoal

Alone or combined with lobelia to treat insect bites, bee stings, and other minor wounds.

Coffee

Traditional Chinese remedy for insect bites. Mix ground coffee with citronella, pennyroyal, or eucalyptus herbs or essential oils; sesame, safflower, or oregano oil can be added.

Comfrey

Beneficial for mild wound care and infection. The ancient name for comfrey was knitbone, a reminder of its traditional use in healing fractures. The herb contains allantoin, which encourages bone, cartilage, and muscle cells to grow. Make a paste of the powdered root and water and apply to wounds. Once broken bones have been set by a health care professional, a poultice puree can be made from the leaves and applied to the skin over broken bones to assist in the healing process.

Elderberry

Relieves pain associated with hemorrhoids.

Fenugreek, flaxseed, and slippery elm

Can be combined to treat inflammation. Slippery elm can also be used alone to help heal minor wounds.

Goldenseal

A traditional healing herb of the Native Americans. Taken internally for indigestion and as an appetite stimulant. As a poultice, it relieves inflammation and reduces chest congestion and abdominal cramping from premenstrual syndrome.

Nopal (Prickly Pear Cactus)

The pulp of the prickly pear cactus pad can be used to relieve aching muscles and joints, help heal minor wounds and burns, and reduce inflammation. Burn or cut off the prickly spines, and slice the pad open. Place the inside of the pad directly onto the skin. The inner surface of the split pads can be used to take the venom out of insect and scorpion stings.

Onion

Good for chest congestion, boils, and sores that refuse to heal. Finely chop one onion and place it between two pieces of cloth to apply; do not place the onion directly on the skin because it is an irritant.

Raw Potato

Can assist in healing conjunctivitis. Grate one raw white potato and then wrap it in gauze or a soft cloth and apply to the eye.

Mustard Plaster

Relieves chest congestion from colds, flu, and bronchitis.
¼ cup dry mustard powder
1 egg white

Make a paste from the mustard powder and egg white. Spread it on a soft cloth, paper towel, or coffee filter; apply the cloth, towel, or filter to the chest. Never apply this poultice directly to skin because the dry mustard can be irritating. Reapply as often as desired.

MORE POULTICE RECIPES CONTINUED

Bread and Milk
Draws out infection
1 slice white bread
¼ cup milk

Break the bread into small pieces and moisten with milk. Either apply to the area directly and cover with a clean cloth, or wrap the mixture in gauze or soft cloth and apply. Reapply as often as needed.

Poultices That Can Be Either Hot or Cold

Cabbage
Soothes skin disorders such as shingles and eczema; helps draw out infection.
Cabbage leaves, either cooked or raw
If making a hot poultice, blanch the leaves. Either apply them to the area directly and cover with a clean cloth or wrap them in gauze or soft cloth and apply. Reapply as often as needed.
If making a cold poultice, chop the leaves to make a pulp. Either apply to the area directly and cover with a clean cloth or wrap the mixture in gauze or soft cloth and apply. Reapply as often as needed.

Garlic
Garlic is an antiseptic as well as being antiviral and antifungal; draws out infection; relieves chest congestion and inflammation.
Garlic—either grated or crushed, raw or cooked; enough to cover the area where it will be applied.
If applying directly to the skin, first apply a layer of olive oil to prevent irritation. Cover with a clean cloth. Another option is to wrap the garlic in gauze or soft cloth and apply. Reapply as often as needed.

Carrot
Draws out infection; helps heal cysts, boils, cold sores, and impetigo.
2–3 large carrots
1–2 tbsp vegetable oil

If making a hot poultice, boil carrots until soft and then mash them to a pulp. Mix with enough vegetable oil to make a thick paste. Either apply the mixture to the area directly and cover with a clean cloth or wrap the mixture in gauze or soft cloth and apply. Reapply as often as needed.

If making a cold poultice, grate the carrots raw. Mix with enough vegetable oil to make a thick paste. Either apply to the area directly and cover with a clean cloth or wrap the mixture in gauze or soft cloth and apply. Reapply as often as needed.

Linseed
Reduces pain and swelling, especially from arthritis.
Ground linseed
⅛ cup lime juice
Boiling water

Mix four parts ground linseed with ten parts boiling water.
Make a paste with the linseed mixture and lime juice to help heal a minor burn.

Hot Poultices

Ginger and Onion
Relieves chest congestion from colds, flu, and bronchitis
1 large onion, chopped
¼ cup grated, unpeeled ginger root

Cook the onion and ginger with a little water until they are soft. Mash them together and spread the mixture on a soft cloth, paper towel, or coffee filter; then apply the cloth, towel, or filter to the chest. Never apply this poultice directly to skin because the ginger and onions are irritants.

Comfrey Wintergreen
Relieves pain and inflammation from old sprains and strains; heals, soothes, and reduces bruising; helps heal cuts, insect bites, and stings.
1 oz dried comfrey
1 oz dried wintergreen
1 pint distilled water

Bring water to a boil, reduce heat and add dried herbs. Simmer gently for 5 minutes. Remove from heat and drain off water, reserving herbs to use in poultice.

Mullein
Helps reduce inflamed hemorrhoids; relieves chest congestion from colds, flu, and bronchitis; relieves pain from tonsillitis, sore throat, and laryngitis.
Mix four parts mullein with one part water and one part hot apple cider vinegar.

Spa treatments based on Ayurvedic principles have grown in popularity over the past decade. *Ayurveda* is a Sanskrit word that means "science of life"—*ayus* meaning "life" or "living" and *veda* meaning "knowledge" or "science" (Douillard, 2004). A traditional medical system from India, Ayurveda is a holistic approach to life and health that encompasses nutrition, meditation, yoga, essential oils, medicinal herbs, positive thinking, breathing, and exercise. The Ayurvedic system dates back at least 5,000 years and is one of the oldest medical systems in the world (Miller and Miller, 1995).

The origin of current Ayurvedic spa treatments can be traced to Dr. Deepak Chopra, who is the grandson of a traditional Ayurvedic medicine practitioner. Dr. Chopra was trained in Western science and medicine, specializing in internal medicine and endocrinology. In the 1980s, after meeting Dr. Vaidya Triguna, an Ayurvedic physician from India, Dr. Chopra became a leader in the transcendental meditation movement and then broadened out into researching mind-body healing and treatments. He cofounded the Chopra Center in 1996, a clinic for health and healing based on meditation, Ayurveda, and yoga (Chopra, 2005a, 2005b).

Brief History of Ayurveda

Ayurveda is a complex medical system encompassing knowledge based on natural rhythms and life cycles. Ayurvedic theory states that health results from harmony within oneself, which is harmony among the purpose for being, thoughts, feelings, and physical actions. Temperature, light, herbs, foods, minerals, exercise, and engaging the mind and emotions through meditation are the means by which health, or balance and harmony in the body, can be achieved. Emphasis is placed on prevention of ill-health.

In India, holy men called *rishis* developed Ayurveda, which grew and changed as it was handed down through oral tradition until it incorporated surgery, herbal medicine, medicinal effects of minerals and metals, exercise, physiology, human anatomy, and psychology. Ayurveda spread to other civilizations and influenced traditional medicine in Tibet, China, Persia, Egypt, Greece, Rome, and Indonesia.

The traditional healing methods of Ayurveda were outlawed during British rule of India (1858–1947). Because rural areas of the country were not as well controlled as urban areas by the British, Ayurveda continued to be practiced there and thus came to be known as folk medicine for almost 100 years. With India's independence in 1947, Ayurveda started to reemerge and gradually gained equal footing with Western medicine. Seventy percent of India's population is treated Ayurvedically (Miller and Miller, 1995).

Ayurvedic Principles

Ayurveda encompasses a huge body of knowledge, and comprehensive programs of study teach it. What follows are the basic principles of Ayurveda.

The theory behind Ayurveda is that all matter in the universe is made up of five elements or building blocks, and these elements are reflected in the human body. These elements are:

▶ **earth:** the solid state of matter; earth represents the physical structures of the body
▶ **water:** fluid movement and change, just like rivers that are always flowing; water represents blood, lymph, and other fluids of the body that are constantly moving
▶ **fire:** the power to transform solids to liquids, to gas, and back again; fire represents the body's energy, such as the energy needed to contract muscles or send nerve impulses, or the conservation of energy, which is shown by the conversion of excess food to fat
▶ **air:** gaseous form of matter, which is mobile and dynamic; air represents the oxygen the body needs to live
▶ **ether:** the space in which everything happens, from the space in the universe to the space inside one cell; ether represents the spaces or distances between structures of the body, such as the space between organs, the space inside hollow organs, and the space inside cells

The five elements combine in pairs to form three dynamic forces called *doshas*. *Dosha* means "that which changes" because doshas are constantly interacting with one another or moving in dynamic balance. The three primary doshas are:

- **Vata:** combination of ether and air; means "that which moves things"; main function is that of propulsion and movement (Ninivaggi, 2008); controls all movement in the mind and body—nerve impulses, thoughts, air in and out of the lungs, blood and lymph flow, food moving through the digestive tract, and waste elimination from the body (Miller and Miller, 1995)
- **Pitta:** combination of fire and water; means "the principle of transformation"; main function is transformation, also heat production and digestion (Ninivaggi, 2008); controls enzymes that digest food, hormones that regulate metabolism, and transformation of nerve impulses into thoughts (Miller and Miller, 1995)
- **Kapha:** combination of water and earth; means "that which is solid and grounded"; main function is providing cohesion, binding, and containment (Ninivaggi, 2008); controls structure and lubrication, such as the cells that make up the organs and the fluids that nourish and protect them (Atreya, 1999; Miller and Miller, 1995)

Vata, Pitta, and Kapha are constantly changing and balancing one another. It is this interaction or dynamism that is the source of life.

Physical features, stamina, temperament, way of thinking, methods of communication, and even dreams determine the dosha of which a person is part. Individual doshas, such as whether the person is a Vata, Pitta, or Kapha, or a combination, can be discovered by completing a thorough constitutional analysis ("constitution" refers to a person's physical, mental, and emotional makeup). The analysis consists of a list of questions about, for example, physical frame, body weight, skin color and type, hair color and texture, eye color and size, lip color and size, teeth color and size, nail appearance, overall strength, physical activities, appetite, emotional temperament, memory, speech, quality of sleep, elimination of wastes, and the overall types of imbalances to which the person is prone (Miller and Miller, 1995).

Vata Types

Attributes: light, erratic, sinuous, thin, cold, dry, excitable, creative and spiritually oriented

Characteristics: physically thin with prominent joints and long limbs; dark skin that tans easily; prone to dry skin, chapped lips, and headaches; sleep is light or disturbed; flexible thinker; does many projects at once

Benefit from: treatments that slow them down and encourage stillness and peacefulness

Pitta Types

Attributes: hot, moist, radiant, intense, focused, oily, passionate, confident

Characteristics: medium, athletic build; fair skin that burns easily; prone to oily skin, cold sores, and stomach aches; sleep is moderate with active dreams; competitive; organized thinker

Benefit from: treatments that are relaxing, cooling, and soothing

Kapha Types

Attributes: solid, heavy, slow, dense, smooth, round, methodical, articulate, easy going, and faithful

Characteristics: large frame and heavy build; skin tans evenly; prone to obesity and sinus congestion; need motivation to stay healthy; sleep is sound and deep; calm and patient. (Douillard, 2004)

Benefit from: regimented treatments that are structured and invigorating (Douillard, 2004; Tirtha, 2007).

Prana is another Ayurvedic concept. Basically prana is the life force or energy of the body (it is comparable to Qi in traditional Chinese medicine), and its vehicle is the breath. Prana gives and maintains life and unifies the person. Prana travels throughout the body and can be accessed at *marmas*, which are energetic points located near the surface of the body (Ninivaggi, 2008). There are about 100 marmas, and they are concentrated at the junctions of muscles and tendons, in the joints, and along blood vessels.

Some Ayurvedic schools of thought believe that marmas are too delicate to be addressed directly through massage, whereas other Ayurvedic practices include massage on these points. However, since the points are considered sacred, the massage needs to be done in a very specific manner (Douillard, 2004).

Chakras are centers of prana. They are located along the spinal column in the areas of certain glands and nerve plexuses (*plexus* means "braid" or "network"). Chakras are the link between the prana of the universe and the prana of the individual. Chakra translates as "wheel," and Chakras are indeed wheels of energy that govern the various physical organs as well as emotions. ▶Table A2.1 describes the seven chakras of the body (Douillard, 2004, Ninivaggi, 2008) and ▶Figure A2.1 shows their locations.

Treatments

Many Ayurvedic-based methods address imbalances in the body. For example, yoga is designed to open chakras and bring out the positive qualities associated with the individual chakras. Other types of exercise, colors, sounds, foods, and massage with specific types of oils and with the use of aromatherapy can be used to bring about har-

TABLE A2.1

The Seven Chakras of the Body

Number	English name	Indian name	Associated color	Governing element	Location	Function
1	Root chakra	*Muladhara*	Red	Earth	Perineum (anal area)	Main foundation or support of chakras above it
2	Sacral chakra	*Svadhisthana*	Orange	Water	Genital region	Controls reproduction, adrenal glands, and prostate
3	Solar plexus chakra	*Manipura*	Yellow	Fire	Navel areas	Controls the connection of the person to the universe
4	Heart chakra	*Anahata*	Green	Air	Near the heart	Controls the sacred heart or the connection to pure consciousness
5	Throat chakra	*Vishuddha*	Blue	Ether	At the throat	Regulates the connection between mind and body
6	Brow chakra	*Ajna*	Indigo	The mind (not governed by an element)	Between the eyebrows	Also called the "third eye"; connected to the meditative process, insight, and development of higher consciousness
7	Crown chakra	*Sahasrara*	Silver, gold, white, violet	Not governed by an element	Beyond the top of the head	Not exactly a chakra; activates all the brain centers; associated with the highest refinement of consciousness and the connection of individual prana with universal prana

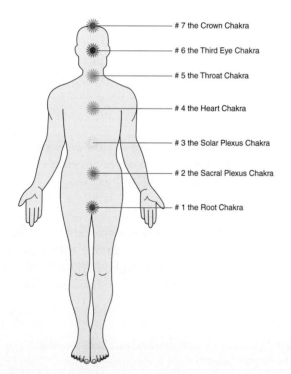

7 the Crown Chakra
6 the Third Eye Chakra
5 the Throat Chakra
4 the Heart Chakra
3 the Solar Plexus Chakra
2 the Sacral Plexus Chakra
1 the Root Chakra

▶ **Figure A2.1** There are seven chakras, or centers of energy, within the body, and each governs various organs and emotions based on its location. Image courtesy Rev. Larissa Dahroug, Reiki M/T, Clear & Balanced Energy Work.

mony in a person, both in terms of chakras and in terms of Vata, Kapha, and Pitta.

In a plant:

▶ Vata is concentrated in the flowers, fruits, and leaves
▶ Kapha is concentrated in the roots
▶ Pitta is found in the plant's essential oils, resins, and sap

Plants have varying concentrations of Vata, Pitta, and Kapha, therefore specific plants and parts of those plants can be used in Ayurvedic massage and aromatherapy to alter the body's proportions of Vata, Pitta, and Kapha and bring about balance (Miller and Miller, 1995). ▶Table A2.2 shows the carrier oils, essential oils, and dry powders that can be used for each of the doshas.

Popular Ayurvedic Treatments in the American Spa

Abhyanga Massage

Abhyanga massage is a firm, flowing full-body massage with one or two practitioners massaging the client at the same time. Warmed herbal oils that are selected according to the client's dosha are used, and the treatment typically lasts 45 to 60 minutes, after which a

TABLE A2.2

Carrier Oils, Essential Oils, and Dry Powders for each of the Doshas

Dosha	Carrier Oils	Essential Oils	Dry Powders
Vata	Sweet almond	Lavender	Fenugreek seed
	Avocado	Juniper	Garbanzo
	Castor	Sage	Oat
	Olive	Geranium	Lentil
	Sesame	Patchouli	Triphala
	Wheat germ	Cedarwood	
	Bala	Tulsi	
	Amla	Myrrh	
Pitta	Sweet almond	Lavender	Barley
	Calendula	Sandalwood	Fenugreek seed
	Coconut	Marjoram	Sweet garbanzo
	Safflower	Cedar	Rice
	Sunflower	Gardenia	Triphala
	Pumpkin	Seed	Jasmine
	Rice	Bran	Saffrom
			Vetivert
Kapha	Sweet almond	Sage	Blue corn
	Jojoba	Peppermint	Millet
	Olive	Rosemary	Fenugreek seed
	Sesame	Eucalyptus	Corn
	Corn	Lavender	Vitamin A
	Mustard	Basil	Garbanzo
	Safflower	Camphor	

steam or sauna is recommended. Abhyanga decreases stress and anxiety, nourishes the body, helps improve sleep, improves skin texture, and promotes overall physical health.

Shirodara

In Shirodara, an herbal oil or infusion with medicated milk or buttermilk is poured in a steady stream on the client's forehead for 20 to 50 minutes, followed by a gentle scalp massage and possibly a facial or a head and neck massage. With the goal of balancing the doshas, this treatment focuses on relaxing the nervous system and balancing the prana around the head. It improves the function of the five senses and helps with insomnia, stress, anxiety, depression, hair loss, and fatigue (see ▶Figure A2.2).

Bindi Exfoliation and Massage

Bindi means "point of origin"—the point from which everything begins and ends. This treatment uses ancient recipes of herbal-infused oils and dry powders for exfoliation body masks, and massage may be performed afterward. The goal is detoxification and deep cleansing of the body, and the skin is left soft, smooth, and nourished. The combination of herbs and oils strengthens the immune system and eliminates feelings of anxiety and stress.

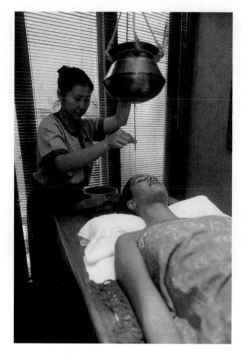

▶ **Figure A2.2** In Shirodara, an herbal oil or infusion with medicated milk or buttermilk is poured in a steady stream on the client's forehead for 20 to 50 minutes, followed by a gentle scalp massage and possibly a facial or head and neck massage.
(Jochen Tack/Das Fotoarchiv/Peter Arnold, Inc.)

TREATMENT

Equipment and Supplies

- massage table
- large funnel with a regulating tap
- large bowl to catch the oil
- small table on which to set bowl
- 4 cups warmed sesame oil

Procedure

The client lies on the massage table with the head tilted slightly off the head of the table. A large bowl (to catch the oil) is positioned on a small table or stool under the client's head. The funnel is filled with the warm sesame oil and positioned over the middle of the person's forehead (over the third eye). The temperature of the oil is tested by the practitioner to make sure it is comfortably warm for the client. The tap is adjusted so that the oil runs slowly over the client's forehead, through the hair, and into the bowl while the scalp, face, head, or neck are massaged. The person is encouraged to rest or move slowly after the treatment.

TREATMENT CONTINUED

Tridosha Ayurvedic Exfoliation

1 cup besan (chickpea flour)
1 tsp cardamon
1 tsp fennel
1 tsp nutmeg
½ tsp cinnamon
½ tsp tumeric
½ tsp ginger powder
8 tbsp crushed rice
1 tbsp rose water (more may be used if needed)
10–12 drops sandalwood essential oil
2 tsp sesame oil

Mix all ingredients together to make a thick paste. Massage paste over entire body. Rinse off in shower and gently blot the skin dry.

Milk and Honey Body Polish

2 cups grated cucumber
¾ cup warmed honey
½ cup heavy cream

Slowly add one teaspoon of cream at a time to the warmed honey. When completely combined, massage the mixture over the entire body; then apply the grated cucumber (the cucumber tightens the skin) over the mixture. Leave on for 10 to 15 minutes. Rinse completely and gently blot the skin dry.

Exfoliating and Restorative Recipes from Bali

Balinese Boreh

4 tsp sandalwood oil
2 tsp whole cloves
2 tsp ginger powder
1 tsp cinnamon
1 tsp coriander seeds
1–2 tsp brown rice powder
1 tsp tumeric
1 tsp nutmeg
1–2 tbsp rose water or sesame oil
1 cup yogurt or 1 cup grated carrot

Mix all ingredients together to make a thick paste. Massage paste over entire body to exfoliate. Apply the grated carrot or yogurt over the paste and leave on for 10 to 15 minutes. Rinse completely and gently blot the skin dry.

*Javanese Lulur**

2 tbsp sesame oil
2 tbsp brown rice powder
1 tsp tumeric
1 tsp sandalwood oil
2 drops jasmine essential oil
a splash of floral or distilled water, enough to make a paste
2 cups natural plain yogurt

Coat the body with a thin coat of sesame oil. Mix the remaining ingredients together into a thick paste. Massage paste over entire body to exfoliate. Allow to dry; then apply the yogurt (which restores skin's natural pH). Leave on for 10 to 15 minutes. Rinse completely and gently blot the skin dry.

*The Javanese Lulur treatment is used for cleansing the bride before marriage and to prepare a woman for childbirth.

Resources

EQUIPMENT AND SUPPLIES

General Equipment and Supplies

Banyan Botanicals (Ayurveda products)
6705 Eagle Rock Ave. NE
Albuquerque, NM 87113
Phone: (800) 953-6424 (toll free)
(541) 488-9525
Email: info@banyanbotanicals.com
www.banyanbotanicals.com

By the Planet (Ayurveda products)
c/o Your Body Naturally
P.O. Box 1008
Silver Lake, WI 53170
Phone: (800) 742-5841 (toll free)
Fax: (800) 905-6887 (toll free)
Email: BythePlanet@YourBodyNaturally.com
www.bytheplanet.com

Health-Enhancement-Accessories-Training
Spa Kur Development, Inc.
P.O. Box 1177
Calistoga, CA 94515
Phone: (707) 942-6633
Fax: (707) 942-0734
www.h-e-a-t.com

Innovative Spa Technologies
607 W. Broadway Ave., Suite 133
Fairfield, IA 52556
Phone: (888) 942-5428 (toll free)
(641) 469-5299
www.innovativespa.com

Massage Warehouse and Spa Essentials
360 Veterans Parkway, Suite 115
Bolingbrook, IL 60440-4607
Phone: (800) 910-9955 (toll free)
Fax: (630) 771-7500
www.massagewarehouse.com

New Life Systems
2853 Hedberg Dr.
Minnetonka, MN 55305
Phone: (800) 852-3082 (toll free)
Fax: (888) 717-7701 (toll free)
Email: webmaster@newlifesystems.com
www.newlifesystems.com

Pure Essential, Inc.
P.O. Box 33044
1299 Oxford St. East
London, Ontario N5Y 5L4
Canada
Phone: (519) 488-1432
Fax: (519) 433-7970
Email: info@pureessentialoils.com
www.essential-oil.org

The Sauna Warehouse
6 Orchard, Suite 201
Lake Forest, CA 92630
Phone: (800) 906-2242 (toll free)
(949) 609-2202
Email: sales@saunas.com
www.saunas.com

SpaElegance
1350 Old Pond Rd.
Second Floor
Bridgeville, PA 15017
Phone: (877) 200-7727 (toll free)
Fax: (412) 220-7750
www.spaelegance.com

SpaEquip
Phone: (877) 778-1685 (toll free)
Fax: (310) 544-4210
Email: assist@spaequip.com
www.spaequip.com

The Spa Specialist
12910 N. Zuni St.
Westminister, CO 80234
Phone: (888) 478-2224 (toll free)
(303) 920-1495
www.spaspecialist.com

Steam Embrace, Inc.
3251 Corte Malpaso, #502-3
Camarillo, CA 93010
Phone: (800) 231-7832 (toll free)
(805) 384-5454
Fax: (805) 384-5458
Email: steam@steamembrace.com
www.steamembrace.com

Steamy Wonder
Natural Health Technologies, Inc.
P.O. Box 2222
Fairfield, IA 52556
Phone: (800) 417-6789 (toll free)
Fax: (641) 472-5117
Email: info@steamywonder.com
www.steamywonder.com

Thermophore
Battle Creek Equipment Co.
307 West Jackson Street
Battle Creek, MI 49015
Phone: (877) 565-8833 (toll free)
www.thermophore.com

TouchAmerica
P.O. Box 1304
Hillsborough, NC 27278
Phone: (800) 678-6824 (toll free)
Fax: (919) 732-1173
Email: info@touchamerica.com
www.touchamerica.com

Universal Companies, Inc.
18260 Oak Park Dr.
Abingdon, VA 24210
Phone: (800) 558-5571 (toll free)
Fax: (800) 237-7199 (toll free)
Email: info@universalcompanies.com
www.universalcompanies.com

Water Werks
10740 Lyndale Ave., South, Suite 12W
Minneapolis, MN 55420
Phone: (800) 884-7343 (toll free)
Fax: (952) 887-9054
Email: info@vichyshower.com
www.vichyshower.com

Muds, Peats, Clays, Salts, Seaweed

Ahava Essential Dead Sea Treatment
www.ahava.com

Eyton's Earth
www.eytonsearth.org

Moor Spa Inc.
7-13680 Bridgeport Rd.
Richmond, BC V6V 1V3
Canada
Phone: (800) 666-7987 (toll free)
(604) 279-5561
Fax: (604) 279-5541
Email: sherry@moorspa.com
www.moorspa.com

Nature's Body Beautiful
626 Scheel
Kyle, TX 78640
Phone: (800) 915-2529 (toll free)
(512) 804-5909
Email: Info@NaturesBodyBeautiful.com
www.naturesbodybeautiful.com

Pascalite, Inc.
329 Lawson
P.O. Box 104
Worland, WY 82401
Phone: (307) 347-3872
Fax: (307) 347-2346
Email: pascalite@rtconnect.net

Premier USA
Dead Sea products
3336 Montreal Station
Atlanta, GA 30084
Phone: (866) 594-7546 (toll free)
Fax: (770) 730-8249
www.premierdeadsea.com

Redmond RealSalt
Redmond Trading Company, L.C.
475 W. 910 South
Heber City, UT 84032
Phone: (800) 367-7258 (toll free)
Email: mail@realsalt.com
www.realsalt.com

San Francisco Bath Salt Company
30997 Huntwood Ave., Suite 102
Hayward, CA 94544
Phone: (800) 480-4540 (toll free)
Fax: (510) 477-9621
Email: customerservice@sfbc.com
www.sfbc.com

Torf Spa LLC
184 Joy Rd.
Middlebury, CT 06762
Phone: (877) 811-1008 (toll free)
Fax: (866) 606-4718 (toll free)
Email: info@torfspa.com
www.torfspa.com

Well, Naturally Ltd.
12706-114A Ave.
Surrey, BC V3V 3P4
Canada
Phone: (604) 580-3468
Fax: (604) 580-9548
www.wellnaturally.com

Bottles and Packaging

SKS Bottle and Packaging, Inc.
2600 7th Ave., Bldg. 60 West
Watervliet, NY 12189
Phone: (518) 880-6980
Fax: (518) 880-6990
www.sks-bottle.com

Specialty Bottle LLC
5200 4th Ave., S.
Seattle, WA 98108
Phone: (206) 340-0459
Fax: (206) 903-0785
Email: service@specialtybottle.com
www.specialtybottle.com

Bags and Bows
500 Main St.
Groton, MA 01471
Phone: (800) 225-8155 (toll free)
Fax: (800) 225-8455 (toll free)
www.bagsandbowsonline.com

Packaging Specialties
515 S. Michigan
Seattle, WA 98108
Phone: (206) 762-0540
Fax: (206) 762-4413
www.ps-stores.com

Herbs

Mountain Rose Herbs
P.O. Box 50220
Eugene, OR 97405
Phone: (800) 879-3337 (toll free)
Fax: (510) 217-4012
www.mountainroseherbs.com

Blessed Herbs
109 Barre Plains Rd.
Oakham, MA 01068
Phone: (800) 489-4372 (toll free)
(508) 882-3839
Fax: (508) 882-3755
Email: info@blessedherbs.com
www.blessedherbs.com

Organic Essential Oils

Enfleurage
321 Bleeker St.
New York, NY 10014
Phone: (888) 387-0300 (toll free)
(212) 691-1610
Fax: (212) 337-0842
Email: jasmine@enfleurage.com
www.enfleurage.com

Essential Aura Aromatherapy
1935 Doran Rd.
Cobble Hill, BC V0R 1L0
Canada
Phone: (250) 733-2035
Fax: (250) 733-2036
Email: info@essentialaura.com
www.essentialaura.com
www.organicfair.com

Fragrant Earth International Limited
Unit 21 The Beckery
Glastonbury, Somerset BA6 9NX
United Kingdom
Phone: +44 (0) 1458 831 216
Fax: +44 (0) 1458 831 361
www.fragrantearth.com

Florihana
Les Grand Pres
06460 Caussols
France
Phone: +33 (0) 493 09 06 09
Fax: +33 (0) 493 09 86 85
Email: info@florihana.com
www.florihana.com

Omega Nutrition
6515 Aldrich Rd.
Bellingham, WA 98226
Phone: (360) 384-1238
Fax: (360) 384-0700
Email: info@meganutrition.com
www.omeganutrition.com

Original Swiss Aromatics
P.O. Box 6842
San Rafael, CA 94903
Phone: (415) 459-3998
Fax: (415) 479-0614
Email: osa_pia@yahoo.com
www.originalswissaromatics.com

Oshadhi Ltd.
Oshadhi House
Unit 6, Sycamore Close
Cambridge, Cambridgeshire CB18PG
United Kingdom
Phone: +44 (0) 1223 242 242
Fax: +44 (0) 8701 224 638
Email: info@oshadhi.co.ul
www.oshadhi.co.uk

Universal Companies, Inc.
18260 Oak Park Dr.
Abingdon, VA 24210
Phone: (800) 558-5571 (toll free)
Fax: (800) 237-7199 (toll free)
Email: info@universalcompanies.com
www.universalcompanies.com

Organic Vegetable Oils

Florihana
Les Grand Pres
06460 Caussols
France
Phone: +33 (0) 493 09 06 09
Fax: +33 (0) 493 09 86 85
Email: info@florihana.com
www.florihana.com

Oshadhi Ltd.
Oshadhi House
Unit 6, Sycamore Close
Cambridge, Cambridgeshire CB18PG
United Kingdom
Phone: +44 (0) 1223 242 242
Fax: +44 (0) 8701 224 638
Email: info@oshadhi.co.ul
www.oshadhi.co.uk

Universal Companies, Inc.
18260 Oak Park Dr.
Abingdon, VA 24210
Phone: (800) 558-5571 (toll free)
Fax: (800) 237-7199 (toll free)
Email: info@universalcompanies.com
www.universalcompanies.com

SPA LOCATION SEARCH SITES

SpaFinder
www.spafinder.com

Spagazers.com
www.thespasdirectory.com

SpaLifeOnline.com
www.spalifeonline.com

Spas.about.com
www.spas.about.com

BUSINESS AND MARKETING

Natural Touch Marketing
P.O. Box 1038
Olympia, WA 98507-1038
Phone: (800) 754-9790 (toll free)
(360) 754-9799
Fax: (360) 705-3864
Email: info@naturaltouchmarketing.com
www.naturaltouchmarketing.com

Plus One Health Management
75 Maiden Lane, Suite 801
New York, NY 10038
Phone: (800) 518-9083 (toll free)
www.plusone.com

Sharper
110 Pacific Ave., Suite 850
San Francisco, CA 94111-1900
Phone: (800) 561-6677 (toll free)
Fax: (888) 251-4454 (toll free)
Email: info@e-sharper.com
www.e-sharper.com

Sohnen-Moe Associates, Inc.
3900 W. Costco Dr., Suite 168-367
Tucson, AZ 85741-2999
Phone: (800) 786-4774 (toll free)
Fax: (520) 743-3656
Email: sma.info@sohnen-moe.com
www.sohnen-moe.com

SpaTrade
Email: info@spatrade.com
www.spatrade.com

VistaPrint
Phone: (800) 961-2075 (toll free)
www.vistaprint.com

ASSOCIATIONS

American Massage Therapy Association
500 Davis St., Suite 900
Evanston, IL 60201-4695
Phone: (877) 905-2700 (toll free)
(847) 864-0123
Fax: (847) 864-1178
Email: info@amtamassage.org
www.amtamassage.org

Associated Bodywork and Massage Professionals
1721 Sugarbush Dr.
Evergreen, CO 80439
Phone: (800) 458-2267 (toll free)
(303) 674-8478
Fax: (800) 667-8260 (toll free)
Email: expectmore@abmp.com
www.abmp.com

Canadian Federation of Aromatherapists (CFA)
110 Thorndale Pl.
Waterloo, ON N2L 5Y8
Canada
Phone: (519) 746-1594
Fax: (519) 746-9493
Email: cfamanager@cfacanada.com
www.cfacanada.com

Council on Naturopathic Medical Education (CNME)
Executive Director
P.O. Box 178
Great Barrington, MA 01230
Phone: (413) 528-8877
Fax: (413) 528-8880
Email: staff@cnme.org
www.cnme.org

The Day Spa Association
520 23rd St.
Union City, NJ 07087
Phone: (201) 865-2065
Fax: (201) 865-3961
Email: info@dayspaassociation.com
www.dayspaassociation.com

National Association for Holistic Aromatherapy
3327 W. Indian Trail Rd., PMB 144
Spokane, WA 99208
Phone: (509) 325-3419
Fax: (509) 325-3479
Email: info@naha.org
www.naha.org

National Certification Board for Therapeutic Massage and Bodywork (NCBTMB)
1901 S. Meyers Rd., Suite 240
Oakbrook Terrace, IL 60181
Phone: (800) 296-0664 (toll free)
(630) 627-8000
Email: info@ncbtmb.org
www.ncbtmb.org

Worldwide Aquatic Bodywork Association
P.O. Box 1817
Middletown, CA 95464
Phone: (707) 928-5860
Fax: (707) 317-0052
Email: info@waba.edu
www.waba.edu

International SPA Association
2365 Harrodsburg Rd., Suite A325
Lexington, KY 40504
Phone: (888) 651-4772 (toll free)
Fax: (859) 226-4445
Email: ispa@ispastaff.com
www.experienceispa.com

TREATMENT CLINICS

Naturopathic

Bastyr Center for Natural Health
3670 Stone Way N.
Seattle, WA 98103
Phone: (206) 834-4100
Fax: (206) 834-4107
www.bastyrcenter.org

Boucher Naturopathic Medical Clinic
Boucher Centre
320-435 Columbia St.
New Westminister, BC V3L 5N8
Canada
Phone: (604) 540-2873
Fax: (604) 540-2879
Email: clinic@binm.org
www.binm.org/Teaching_Clinic.htm

The University of Bridgeport's Naturopathic Center
60 Lafayette Ave.
Warner Hall
Bridgeport, CT 06604
Phone: (203) 576-4349
Fax: (203) 576-4776
Email: sookraja@bridgeport.edu
www.bridgeport.edu/pages/4412.asp

Canadian College of Naturopathic Medicine
Robert Schad Naturopathic Clinic
1255 Sheppard Ave. East
Toronto, Ontario M2K 1E2
Canada
Phone: (416) 498-9763
www.ccnm.edu/?q=robert_schad_naturopathic_clinic

National College of Naturopathic Medicine
Natural Health Center—First Avenue
2220 SW First Ave.
Portland, OR 97201
Phone: (503) 552-1551
www.ncnm.edu/natural-health-center-clinics.php

Southwest Naturopathic Medical Center
8010 E. McDowell Rd. #111
Scottsdale, AZ 85257
Phone: (480) 970-0000
www.scnm.edu/medcenter/index.php

Ayurveda

Chopra Center
2013 Costa del Mar Rd.
Carlsbad, CA 92009
Phone: (888) 424-6772 (toll free)
(760) 494-1608
www.chopra.com

SCHOOLS AND PROGRAMS OF STUDY

Aromatherapy

The East West School for Herbal and Aromatic Studies
335 Amber Lane
Willow Spring, NC 27592
Phone: (919) 892-7230
Email: info@theida.com
www.theida.com

Essential Oil Resource Consultants
Au Village
83840 La Martre
Provence, France
Phone: +33 (0) 494 84 29 93
Fax: +33 (0) 632 39 58 43
Email: essentialorc@club-internet.fr
www.essentialorc.com

Pacific Institute of Aromatherapy
P.O. Box 6723
San Rafael, CA 94903
Phone: (415) 479-9120
Fax: (415) 479-0614
Email: osa_pia@yahoo.com
www.pacificinstituteofaromatherapy.com

Ayurveda

The Ayurvedic Institute
P.O. Box 23445
Albuquerque, NM 87192-1445
Phone: (505) 291-9698
Fax: (505) 294-7572
www.ayurveda.com

Hot and Cold Stone Therapy

LaStone Therapy
www.lastonetherapy.com

Naturopathic Education

Bastyr University
14500 Juanita Dr. NE
Kenmore, WA 98028-4966
Phone: (425) 823-1300
Fax: (425) 823-6222
www.bastyr.edu

Boucher Institute of Naturopathic Medicine
Boucher Center
300-435 Columbia St.
New Westminister, BC V3L 5N8
Phone: (604) 777-9981
Fax: (604) 777-9982
Email: info@binm.org
www.binm.org

**University of Bridgeport
College of Naturopathic Medicine**
126 Park Ave.
Bridgeport, CT 06604
Phone: (203) 576-4552
(800) 392-3582 (toll free)
www.bridgeport.edu

Canadian College of Naturopathic Medicine
1255 Sheppard Ave. East
Toronto, Ontario M2K 1E2
Canada
Phone: (416) 498-9763
www.ccnm.edu

National College of Naturopathic Medicine
049 SW Porter St.
Portland, OR 97201
Phone: (503) 552-1555
www.ncnm.edu

Southwest College of Naturopathic Physicians
2149 E. Broadway Rd.
Tempe, AZ 85282
Phone: (480) 858-9100
Fax: (480) 858-9116
Email: admissions@scnm.edu
www.scnm.edu

Watsu® and Aquatic Massage

Aquatic Massage
Phone: (707) 995-9090
Email: watsuem@inreach.com
www.aquaticmassage.com

Watsu®
P.O. Box 1817
Middletown, CA 95464
Phone: (707) 928-5860
Fax: (707) 317-0052
www.watsu.com/index.html

PUBLICATIONS

Aromascents Journal
1226 Killarney St.
Penticton, BC V2A 4R2
Canada
Phone: (250) 493-0363
Email: robyn@aromascentsjournal.ca
www.aromascentsjournal.ca

Spa Management Journal
P.O. Box 2699
Champlain, NY 12919-2699
Phone: (514) 274-0004
Fax: (450) 833-2444
Email: info@spamanagement.com
www.spamanagement.com

Spa Wire
An online news digest and resource portal for the spa, salon, and wellness industry.
www.spawire.com

The International Journal for Clinical Aromatherapy
Au Village
83840 La Martre
Provence, France
Phone: +33 (0) 494 84 29 93
Fax: +33 (0) 632 39 58 43
Email: editorijca@club-internet.fr
www.ijca.net

Massage Magazine
5150 Palm Valley Rd., Suite 103
Ponte Vedra Beach, FL 32082
Phone: (800) 533-4263 (toll free)
Fax: (904) 285-9944
Email: cstsrv@massagemag.com
www.massagemag.com

Massage Therapy Journal
500 Davis St., Suite 900
Evanston, IL 60201-4695
Phone: (877) 905-2700 (toll free)
Fax: (847) 864-1178
www.amtamassage.org/journal

Massage and Bodywork
1271 Sugarbush Dr.
Evergreen, CO 80439-9766
Phone: (800) 458-2267 (toll free)
Email: editor@abmp.com
www.massageandbodywork.com

Research

The Dead Sea Research Center
www.deadsea-health.org

PubMed
National Center for Biotechnology Information (U.S. National Library of Medicine and National Institutes of Health)
www.ncbi.nlm.nih.gov

Herb Research Foundation
4140 15th St.
Boulder, CO 80304
Phone: (303) 449-2265
Fax: (303) 449-7849
Email: customerservice@herbs.org
www.herbs.org

Appendix 4

Answers to Study Questions

CHAPTER 1

1. a
2. c
3. b
4. d
5. c
6. a
7. d
8. c
9. b
10. c
11. a
12. b
13. c
14. b
15. d
16. b

CHAPTER 2

1. c
2. c
3. b
4. a
5. d
6. c
7. d
8. d
9. a
10. c
11. b
12. c
13. d
14. a
15. b
16. c
17. c
18. c
19. b
20. d

CHAPTER 3

1. d
2. b
3. c
4. a
5. d
6. c
7. d
8. d
9. a
10. b

CHAPTER 4

1. a
2. d
3. b
4. c
5. d
6. c
7. c
8. b
9. a
10. c
11. b
12. b
13. a
14. c
15. d
16. b
17. d
18. d
19. b
20. c

CHAPTER 5

1. b
2. a
3. c
4. b
5. c
6. a
7. b
8. d
9. c
10. d

CHAPTER 6

1. b
2. d
3. a
4. c
5. d
6. b
7. a
8. d
9. b
10. c
11. a
12. c
13. b
14. c

CHAPTER 7

1. c
2. a
3. b
4. d
5. b
6. b
7. d
8. a
9. c
10. b

CHAPTER 8

1. b
2. d
3. c
4. b
5. a
6. b
7. b
8. c
9. d
10. c

Appendix 5

References

Abehsera, Michel (2001). *The Healing Power of Clay.* New York: Kensington Publishing Corp.

Abel, Ann (2005). "Masquerade." Retrieved 12 May 2008 from http://www.spafinder.com/Article/216-Masquerade.

Ashworth, William, and Charles E. Little (2001a) "Fuller's Earth." Retrieved 10 May 2008 from *Encyclopedia of Environmental Studies.* In *Science Online,* Facts On File, Inc.: http://www.fofweb.com/activelink2.asp?ItemID=WE40&SID=5&iPin=envrnstud1332&SingleRecord=True.

Ashworth, William, and Charles E. Little (2001b). "Soil." Retrieved 10 May 2008 from *Encyclopedia of Environmental Studies.* In *Science Online,* Facts On File, Inc.: http://www.fofweb.com/activelink2.asp?ItemID=WE40&SID=5&iPin=envrnstud2945&SingleRecord=True.

Atreya (1999). *Ayurvedic Healing for Women.* York Beach, ME: Samuel Weiser, Inc.

Ball, Aimee Lee (2008). "Spa Rx: Ocean Notion." Retrieved 12 May 2008 from http://www.spafinder.com/archive/article.jsp?id=257.

Barron, Patrick (2003). *Hydrotherapy Theory and Technique.* St. James City, FL: Pine Island Publishers, Inc.

Benjamin, Patricia J., and Frances M. Tappan (2005). *Tappan's Handbook of Healing Massage Techniques.* Upper Saddle River, NJ: Pearson Prentice Hall.

Biggs, Matthew, Jekka McVicar, and Bob Flowerdew (2006). *Vegetables, Herbs and Fruit, an Illustrated Encyclopedia.* Buffalo, NY: Firefly Books, Inc.

Bruggemann, W. (1982). *Kneipp Vademecum Pro Medico.* Wurzburg, Germany: Sebastian Kneipp Publications.

Buckle, Jane (2007). *Clinical Aromatherapy, Essential Oils in Practice.* New York: Churchill Livingstone.

Calistoga Spas (2008). "The Mud Baths." Retrieved 10 May 2008 from http://www.calistogaspas.com/mud-baths/.

Cargill (2007). "The History of Salt." Retrieved 10 May 2008 from http://www.cargillsalt.com/dc_salt_about_hist_salt.htm.

Charton, Barbara (2001). *The Facts on File Dictionary of Marine Science.* New York: Facts on File, Inc. (Checkmark Books)

Chopra, D. (April 23, 2005a). "Intelligent Design Without the Bible." Retrieved 11 May 2008 from http://www.huffingtonpost.com/deepak-chopra/intelligent-design-withou_b_6105.html.

Chopra, D. (August 24, 2005b). "Rescuing Intelligent Design—But from Whom?" Retrieved 11 May 2008 from http://www.huffingtonpost.com/deepak-chopra/rescuing-intelligent-desi_b_6164.html.

Colbert, Bruce J., Jeff Ankney, and Karen T. Lee (2007). *Anatomy and Physiology for Health Professions.* Upper Saddle River, NJ: Pearson Prentice Hall.

Crebbin-Bailey, Jane, John Harcup, and John Harrington (2005). *The Spa Book, Official Guide to Spa Therapy.* Stamford, CT: Habia Thomson.

Croutier, Alev Lytle (1992). *Taking the Waters.* New York: Abbeville Press, Inc.

Curtis, Rick (2002). "Outdoor Action Guide to Hypothermia and Cold Weather Injuries." Retrieved 15 May 2008 from http://www.cdc.gov/nasd/docs/d001201-d001300/d001216/d001216.html

de Vierville, Jonathon Paul (2000). "Taking the Waters, A Historical Look at Water Therapy and Spa Culture Over the Ages." In *Massage and Bodywork* (February/March 2000). Retrieved 15 May 2008 from http://www.massagetherapy.com/articles/index.php/article_id/323.

Diracdelta Science and Engineering Encyclopedia (2006). "Specific Heat Capacity." Retrieved 11 May 2008 from http://www.diracdelta.co.uk/science/source/s/p/specific%20heat%20capacity/source.html.

Dobelis, Inge N., Project Editor (1986). *Magic and Medicine of Plants.* Pleasantville, NY: Reader's Digest Association, Inc.

Douillard, John (2004). *The Encyclopedia of Ayurvedic Massage.* Berkeley, CA: North Atlantic Books.

Ellis, Richard (2000). *Encyclopedia of the Sea.* New York: Alfred A. Knopf.

Encyclopedia Britannica (2008a). "Borax." Retrieved 11 May 2008 from http://www.britannica.com/eb/article-9080702.

Encyclopedia Britannica (2008b). "Epsom and Ewell." Retrieved 11 May 2008 from http://www.britannica.com/eb/article-9032828.

Encyclopedia Britannica (2008c). "Fuller's Earth." Retrieved 10 May 2008 from http://www.britannica.com/eb/article-9035638/fullers-earth.

Encyclopedia Britannica (2008d). "Paraffin Wax ." Retrieved 11 May 2008 from http://www.britannica.com/eb/article-9058378.

Epsom Salt Industry Council (2008). "Health Benefits." Retrieved 11 May 2008 from http://www.epsomsalt-council.org/health_benefits.htm.

Eyton's Earth (2007a). "Bentonite: Public Research Project, an Educational Compilation of Related Commentaries and Articles: 1995 & 2006." Retrieved 10 May 2008 from http://www.eytonsearth.org/pascalite-calcium-bentonite.php.

Eyton's Earth (2007b). "Eyton's Earth—Introduction." Retrieved 10 May 2008 from http://www.eytonsearth.org/introduction-clays.php.

Food and Agricultural Organization of the United Nations (2001). "Lecture Notes on the Main Soils of the World." Reference Soil Groups, Set #1, Organic Soils, Histosols. Retrieved 10 May 2008 from http://www.fao.org/docrep/003/y1899e/y1899e04.htm#P0_0.

Fritz, Sandy (2008). *Fundamentals of Therapeutic Massage,* 4th ed. St. Louis, MO: Mosby Elsevier.

Fritz, Sandy, and James Grosenbach (2008). *Essential Sciences for Therapeutic Massage: Anatomy, Physiology, Biomechanics and Pathology.* St. Louis, MO: Mosby Elsevier.

Frohlich, Hans Horst (1997). *The Nature Gardens of Sebastian Kneipp.* New York: Sterling Publishing Co., Inc.

Glen Ivy Hot Springs Spa (2008). "Hot Springs Spa, History." Retrieved 10 May 2008 from http://www.glenivy.com/index.php/resort/C8/.

Infoplease.com (2008). "Poultice." Retrieved 13 May 2008 from http://dictionary.infoplease.com/poultice.

Jouan, Alain (2008). "Back to Thalassotherapy." Retrieved 12 May 2008 from http://www.spamanagement.com/education/thalaso/thalaso_nx.html.

Kellogg, John Harvey (1903). *Rational Hydrotherapy, Part 1 and 2.* Philadelphia: F.A. Davis Company.

Keville, Kathi, and Mindy Green (1995). *Aromatherapy, A Complete Guide to the Healing Art.* Berkeley, CA: The Crossing Press.

Kneipp, Sebastian (1956). *My Water-Cure.* Mokelumne Hill, CA: Health Research.

Knishinsky, Ran (1998). *The Clay Cure, Natural Healing from the Earth.* Rochester, VT: Healing Arts Press.

Latona, Valerie (March 2000). "Get Glowing." *Vegetarian Times,* 271, 88–92.

Lauste, L. W. (May 1974). "Dr. Richard Russell, 1687–1759." In *Journal of the Royal Society of Medicine.* Retrieved 12 May 2008 from http://www.pubmedcentral.nih.gov/pagerender.fcgi?artid=1645547&pageindex=1#page.

Lynch, Benjamin (April 12, 2000). "Patient Care: Effective Balneo Therapeutic Procedures at Home." Retrieved 10 May 2008 from http://www.spawire.com/Articles/TorfPeatLynch.htm.

Marie, Elaine (2008). "Aquatic Massage." Retrieved 14 May 2008 from http://www.aquaticmassage.com/coursedescriptions.html.

Martin, Ingrid (2007). *Aromatherapy for Massage Practitioners.* Philadelphia: Lippincott, Williams and Wilkins.

McConnell, David (2001). "The States of Water." Retrieved 14 May 2008 from *The Good Earth,* McGraw Hill Higher Education: http://www.mhhe.com/earthsci/geology/mcconnell/atm/wstates.htm.

Merriam-Webster Dictionary (2004). Springfield, MA: Merriam-Webster, Inc.

Miller, Todd (2008). "Preparing for Cold Weather Exercise." *NSCA Performance Training Journal,* 3, no.1. Retrieved 14 May 2008 from the National Strength and Conditioning Association: https://www.nsca-lift.org/Perform/articles/03016.pdf.

Miller, Light, and Bryan Miller (1995). *Ayurveda and Aromatherapy.* Twin Lakes, WI: Lotus Press.

Minton, Melinda (2008a). "Healing from the Sea." Retrieved 12 May 2008 from http://www.massagemag.com/spa/treatment/sea.php.

Minton, Melinda (2008b). "Mud: Dig It!" Retrieved 10 May 2008 from www.massagemag.com/spa/treatment/mud.php.

Mitchell J. K. (1993). *Fundamentals of Soil Behavior,* 2nd ed. New York: John Wiley and Sons, Inc.

Moor Spa (2008). "Moor properties." Retrieved 10 May 2008 from http://www.moorspa.com/moor_properties.html.

Mulvihill, Mary Lou, Mark Zelman, Paul Holdaway, Elaine Tompary, and Jill Raymond (2006). *Human Diseases, A Systemic Approach,* 6th ed. Upper Saddle River, NJ: Pearson Prentice Hall.

NAHA (2005a). "About Aromatherapy." Retrieved 15 May 2008 from http://www.naha.org/about_aromatherapy.htm.

NAHA (2005b). "Aromatherapy Regulation." Retrieved 15 May 2008 from http://www.naha.org/faq_regulation.htm#11.

Nelson, Mary, and Jane Scrivner (2004). *The Official LaStone™ Manual.* London, England: Piatkus Books Ltd.

Nikola, R. J. (1997). *Creatures of Water.* Salt Lake City, UT: Europa Therapeutic.

Ninivaggi, Frank John (2008). *Ayurveda, A Comprehensive Guide to Traditional Medicine for the West.* Westport, CT: Praeger.

Ody, Penelope (2002). *Essential Guide to Natural Home Remedies.* London, England: Kyle Cathie Limited.

Ody, Penelope (1993). *The Medicinal Herbal.* New York: Dorling Kindersley.

O'Rourke, Maureen (1995). *Hydrotherapy and Heliotherapy.* Miami, FL: Educating Hands, Inc.

Pernetta, John (1994). *Philip's Atlas of the Oceans*. New York: Sterling Publishing Co.

Price, Shirley, and Len Price (2007). *Aromatherapy for Health Professionals*, 3rd ed. Philadelphia: Churchill Livingstone Elsevier.

Proksch, Ehrhardt, Hans-Peter Nissen, Markus Bremgartner, and Colin Urquhart (February 2005). "Bathing in a Magnesium-Rich Dead Sea Salt Solution Improves Skin Barrier Function, Enhances Skin Hydration, and Reduces Inflammation in Atopic Dry Skin." *International Journal of Dermatology*, 44, no. 2, 151–157.

Pure Essential, Inc. (2007). "Essential Oils and Perfume Notes." Retrieved 15 May 2008 from http://www.essential-oil.org/essential_oils_notes.asp.

Rhines, Erin M. (2007). "Superior Customer Service." *Massage Magazine*, 132, 27–30.

Rose, Jeanne (1999). *375 Essential Oils and Hydrosols*. Berkeley, CA: Frog Ltd.

Roy, Robert L. (2004). *Sauna: A Complete Guide to the Construction, Use, and Benefits of the Finnish Bath*. White River Junction, VT: Chelsea Green Publishing Co.

Salt Institute (2008). "Rock Salt Mining." Retrieved 10 May 2008 from http://www.saltinstitute.org/14.html.

Salvo, Susan G., and Sandra K. Anderson (2004). *Pathology for Massage Therapists*. St. Louis, MO: Mosby Elsevier.

Santa Clarita Valley History (2008). "Borax: The Twenty Mule Team, An Enduring Symbol." Retrieved 11 May 2008 from http://www.scvhistory.com/scvhistory/borax-20muleteam.htm.

Shutes, Jane, and Christina Weaver (2008). *Aromatherapy for Bodyworkers*. Upper Saddle River, NJ: Pearson Prentice Hall.

Sinclair, Marybetts (2008). *Modern Hydrotherapy for the Massage Therapist*. Philadelphia: Lippincott, Williams and Wilkins.

Sohnen-Moe, Cherie (2008). *Business Mastery: A Guide for Creating a Fulfilling, Thriving Business and Keeping It Successful*, 4th ed. Tucson, AZ: Sohnen-Moe Associates.

SpaElegance.com (September 20, 2000). "Magical Mud of the Neydharting Moor." Retrieved 10 May 2008 from http://spaelegance.com/spavivantDetail.asp?CurrentPage=3&SpaVivantID=34&Type=6&Page=

Thrash, Agatha, and Calvin Thrash (1981). *Home Remedies*. Seale, AL: Thrash Publications.

Tirtha, Swami Sadashiva (2007). *The Ayurveda Encyclopedia*. Bayville, NY: Ayurveda Holistic Center Press.

Tisserand, Robert B. (1985). *The Art of Aromatherapy*. Essex, England: Saffron Walden, The C. W. Daniel Company Ltd.

Tisserand, Robert B., and Tony Balaz (1995). *Essential Oil Safety: A Guide for Health Care Professionals*. London, England: Churchill Livingstone.

Tortora, Gerard J., and Bryan Derrickson (2006). *Principles of Anatomy and Physiology*, 11th ed. Hoboken, NJ: John Wiley and Sons, Inc.

Torv Forsk, Swedish Peat Research Foundation, 2008. "Facts About Peat." Retrieved 10 May 2008 from http://www.torvforsk.se/torvfaktaeng.html.

Trieste, Diane (2003). "Spa-Management Opportunities for Massage Therapists." *Massage Magazine*, 102, 64–68.

Turkce Bilgi (2008). "Bathing Machine." Retrieved 12 May 2008 from http://english.turkcebilgi.com/Bathing_machine

U.S. Geological Survey (1999). "Environmental Characteristics of Clays and Clay Mineral Deposits." Retrieved 10 May 2008 from http://pubs.usgs.gov/info/clays/.

Valnet, Jean (1996). Edited by Robert Tisserand. *The Practice of Aromatherapy*. Essex, England: Saffron Walden, The C. W. Daniel Company Ltd.

Venclik, Carol (2007). "Talking to Clients About Spa Therapies." *Massage Magazine*, 130, 32–34.

WABA (Worldwide Aquatic Bodywork Association) (2008a). "Aquatic Bodywork." Retrieved 14 May 2008 from http://www.waba.edu/.

WABA (Worldwide Aquatic Bodywork Association) (2008b). "What Is Waterdance?" Retrieved 14 May 2008 from http://www.waba.edu/school/waterdance.htm.

Walton, John K. (2005). "The Seaside Resort: A British Cultural Export." Retrieved 12 May 2008 from http://www.history.ac.uk/ihr/Focus/Sea/articles/walton.html.

Werner, Ruth (2008). *A Massage Therapist's Guide to Pathology*, 4th ed. Philadelphia: Lippincott Williams and Wilkins.

Wiedner, Robin (2007). "Spas, the Marriage of Healing and Business." *Massage Therapy Journal*, 46, no. 1, 79–87.

Williams, Anne (2007). *Spa Bodywork, A Guide for Massage Therapists*. Philadelphia: Lippincott, Williams and Wilkins.

Williams, William David (November 1, 1999). "What Future for Saline Lakes?" Retrieved 10 May 2008 from http://www.encyclopedia.com/doc/1G1-19123452.html.

Williamson, John (August 1, 2003). "Dead Sea Under Threat." Retrieved 11 May 2008 from http://www.encyclopedia.com/beta/doc/1G1-106560239.html.

Worwood, Valerie Ann (1999). *The Fragrant Heavens*. Novato, CA: New World Library.

Glossary

Abhyanga Massage—Ayurvedic treatment; firm, flowing, full-body massage with one or two practitioners massaging the client at the same time. Warmed herbal oils that are selected according to the client's dosha are used, and the treatment typically lasts 45 to 60 minutes, after which a steam or sauna is recommended. Abhyanga decreases stress and anxiety, nourishes the body, helps improve sleep, improves skin texture, and promotes overall physical health.

Absolute—the most concentrated form of essential oil. Plant parts are placed in a volatile solvent, and as the solvent evaporates, it leaves behind a natural wax. The fluid that is then separated from the wax is the absolute.

Acid—a substance that dissociates into one or more hydrogen ions (H^+) and one or more anions when it is in water; a solution that has a pH of less than 7.

Acidosis—condition in which blood pH is below 7.35.

ADH (antidiuretic hormone)—hormone that stimulates water reabsorption from the kidneys back into the blood.

Adipose—fat.

Afferent (sensory) nerves—peripheral nerves that send nerve impulses into the CNS; nerves that detect sensations.

Affusion—the act of pouring water onto the body, usually through a hose.

Aldosterone—hormone that promotes sodium and water reabsorption from the kidneys into the blood.

Algae—groups of aquatic organisms that perform photosynthesis.

Alkali (base)—substance that dissociates into one or more hydroxide ions (OH^-) and one or more cations when it is in water; a solution that has a pH of more than 7.

Alkalosis—condition in which blood pH is higher than 7.45.

Allopathic, allopathy—relating to or being a system of medicine that combats disease by using remedies such as medications or surgery; also known as Western medicine.

Alphahydroxy acids (AHA)—mild acids found in commercial products and occurring naturally in certain fruits; used for chemical, enzyme, or dissolving exfoliation; loosen the keratin that holds skin cells together, allowing the cells to be easily sloughed off.

Analgesic—pain reliever.

Anaphylactic reaction—a severe allergic response that can include increased mucus production, hives, and impaired breathing (resulting from constricted airways); severe anaphylactic reactions may require medical attention.

Anecdotal—based on or consisting of reports or observations by nonscientists.

Anesthetic—substance or application that decreases or numbs sensations.

Anion—negatively charged ion; results when an atom gains electrons.

Antidiuretic hormone (ADH)—hormone that stimulates water reabsorption from the kidneys into the blood.

Antipyretic—substance or application that decreases fever.

Antiseptic—substance that kills microorganisms on living tissue.

Antispasmodic—substance or application that relieves muscle spasms.

Aquatic massage—derivative of Watsu that has the same principles and techniques but a shorter program of study.

Aristotle (384–322 BC)—Greek philosopher, student of Plato, and teacher of Alexander the Great; he wrote about physics, metaphysics, poetry, theater, music, logic, rhetoric, politics, government, ethics, biology, and zoology. One of the founders of Western philosophy and contributor to physical sciences; he opened the first Western university in Athens in 346 BC.

Aromatherapy—therapeutic use of the preparation of fragrant essential oils extracted from plants.

Aromatic—having a distinct, strong smell.

Asclepios—Greek god of healing and medicine; Roman spelling of his name is Aesculapius.

Atom—the basic unit of matter that retains the characteristics of the element.

Autoimmune disorders—any of a large group of disorders characterized by an alteration in the immune system so that the immune system is unable to distinguish body tissues from nonbody substances; the immune system attacks the body tissues, resulting in tissue damage, inflammation, and pain. Autoimmune disorders generally have periods of flare-up (in which the immune system attacks the tissues) and periods of remission (when the immune system stops attacking the tissues).

Autonomic nervous system (ANS)—division of the peripheral nervous system that controls the cardiac muscle of the heart, the muscle in organs, and glandular secretions.

Avascular—without blood vessels.

Avicenna (973–1037)—also known as Ibn Sina; Persian physician who practiced throughout Arabia. He based his practice on the teachings of Galen and did further research and experimentation in medicine. His chief work, *Canon Medicinae,* served as the most important textbook for physicians in Western society until the Renaissance.

Ayurveda—Sanskrit for "science of life"—*ayus* meaning "life or living" and *veda* meaning "knowledge or science". This is a traditional medical system from India that dates back at least 5,000 years and involves a holistic approach to life and health that encompasses nutrition, meditation, yoga, essential oils, medicinal herbs, positive thinking, breathing, and exercise.

Balnea—private or neighborhood Roman baths; used only cold water and were employed for cleansing after physical exercise.

Balneology—science of baths and bathing.

Banya—Russian hot vapor bath that evolved from portable sweat lodges used by nomadic tribes. It is a small wooden room or hut with benches that is heated by steam from water poured on hot stones for ritual and/or therapeutic sweating. The treatment ends with a cold plunge into icy water or snow.

Base (alkali)—substance that dissociates into one or more hydroxide ions (OH⁻) and one or more cations when it is in water; a solution that has a pH of more than 7.

Base notes—essential oil classification by the French perfume industry; notes refer to scent characteristics and the rate at which the oil evaporates; base notes are intense, heavy, long-lasting fragrances that evaporate slowly.

Bastyr, Dr. John (1912–1995)—"Father of Naturopathic Medicine"; modalities included hydrotherapy, homeopathy, botanical medicine, nutrition, and chiropractics. In 1956, he established the National College of Naturopathic Medicine in Seattle, WA.

Bentonite—clay named for the Benton Formation in eastern Wyoming; discovered around 1890. Closely resembling montmorillonite, this is a smectite that is usually found as green clay with a high pH. The quality of these clays varies according to the location of the deposit, and the mineral content varies quite a bit among sources.

Betahydroxy acids (BHA)—mild acids found in commercial products and occurring naturally in certain fruits; used for chemical, enzyme, or dissolving exfoliation; loosen the keratin that holds skin cells together, allowing the cells to be easily sloughed off.

Blitzguss (jet Blitz)—therapeutic cold shower treatment using a high-pressure stream of water directed at different parts of the body, focusing on muscular areas. This is stimulating and intense and is done for strengthening the body's vitality and immune response by decreasing superficial circulation, driving blood to the core of the body. The temperature and duration of the treatment vary depending on the goals of the treatment.

Bobet, Louison—French Tour-de-France cyclist who was injured in a car accident. He achieved great recovery results through the use of the seawater in Roscoff, France, and was so impressed that he helped bring the use of thalassotherapy into popular focus. In 1964, he opened the first contemporary establishment for seawater therapy.

Body brushing (dry brushing)—exfoliation using brushes or fiber tools.

Body polish—gentle form of exfoliation using softer granules such as those found in fine blue cornmeal or finely ground natural substances such as crushed almonds or grape seed meal.

Borax (sodium borate)—mineral mined near Death Valley, CA, as well as in Tibet and Italy. It is a mineral salt that is naturally fine grained and is frequently used in lotions and face crèmes; added to soaps, ointments, and eye solutions; can be added to a bath or used for a body polish to soften and soothe the skin.

Brine—water saturated with salt, such as seawater or water from a salt lake.

Brown seaweeds—brown pigment masks the green of the chlorophyll; most numerous of the seaweeds in moderate and polar climate regions and grow at depths of 50 to 75 feet. The two major groups of brown seaweeds used in spa treatments are the *Laminaria* species (commonly known as kelp) and the *Fucus* species (commonly known as wracks). Brown seaweeds are used for detoxification, revitalization (through increased local blood and lymph circulation), slimming, and skin tightening.

Buffer—substance or application that balances pH of skin.

Buoyancy—the power of a fluid to exert an upward force on a body placed in it.

Caldarium—the hot bath in a Roman bath; a large tub or small pool with very hot water.

Capital expenditures (expenses)—payment by a business for basic assets such as property, fixtures, or equipment, but not for day-to-day operations such as payroll, inventory, maintenance, and advertising.

Carrageen or carrageen moss *(Chondrus crispus*, Irish moss)—red seaweed that grows in shallow waters, especially around the British Isles; it is used in spa and hydrotherapy treatments for detoxification, revitalization (through increased local blood and lymph circulation), slimming, skin tightening, and moisturizing.

Carrageenan—product made from processing carrageen (Irish moss); used as a thickener in many foods.

Carrier oil—base oil in which essential oil must be diluted before applying to the body. These are typically plant-based oils used to dilute essential oils for use on the skin, as in massage. They can also serve to moisturize the skin and keep essential oils on the skin longer.

Cation—positively charged ion; results when an atom loses electrons.

Cauldron—large kettle or boiler.

Celsus (circa AD 175)—prominent Roman physician who incorporated baths as an integral part of his remedies.

Central nervous system (CNS)—brain and spinal cord.

Centrifugation—process that involves the use of centripetal force (force produced from extremely rapid spinning) for the separation of mixtures. In the case of essential oils, plants are spun very rapidly to separate the oils from the plant matter.

Chakras—in Ayurveda, translates as "wheel"; centers of prana; located along the spinal column in the areas of certain glands and nerve plexuses; the link between the prana of the universe and the prana of the individual.

Chemical bond—the force that holds together the atoms of a molecule or a compound.

Chemical (enzyme, dissolving) exfoliation—uses exfoliants that consist of chemicals or enzymes that work by dissolving dead skin cells; after application, the enzymes are washed or rubbed off.

Chondrus crispus **(Irish moss, carrageen, carrageen moss)**—red seaweed that grows in shallow waters, especially around the British Isles; it is used in spa and hydrotherapy treatments for detoxification, revitalization (through increased local blood and lymph circulation), slimming, skin tightening, and moisturizing.

Compress—soft cotton cloths soaked in hot or cold water and applied to the body.

Code of conduct—principles, values, standards, or rules of behavior that guide the decisions, procedures, and systems of an organization in a way that contributes to the welfare of its participants and respects the rights of those affected by the operations of the organization.

Cold plunge—a short, immersion in cold water or snow; the temperature for a cold plunge is usually much lower than that for a cold bath. Examples include the plunges taken by members of "polar bear clubs" into icy rivers and lakes or plunges into snow or icy water after being heated in a sauna, steam room, or sweat lodge.

Conduction—transfer of heat from objects in direct contact with each other; the transmission of nerve impulses.

Conduction system—specialized pathway that generates nerve impulses that travel through the heart and make its chambers contract in a synchronized manner.

Consensual (reflex) response—stimulation such as application of heat or cold to one area of the body resulting in a response in another area.

Contraindication—factor or body condition that prohibits the administration of a treatment; administration of the treatment would, in fact, make the factor or body condition worse.

Convection—transfer of heat due to the movements (currents) of air or water.

Core temperature—temperature deep in the body underneath the skin.

Counterirritant—locally applied agent that produces superficial inflammation in an attempt to relieve a deeper, adjacent inflammation.

Covalent bond—chemical bond formed when atoms share electrons.

Cranial nerves—peripheral nerves that communicate directly with the brain.

Cross-contamination—spread of pathogens from one person to another via substances.

Cryotherapy—therapeutic use of cold as in the application of ice to the body.

Day spa—spa location to which guests travel to spend a day or part of a day. There are many different types, and menus of services vary depending on the individual spa. Examples include hair and nail treatments, bodywork and spa therapies, esthetic treatments, yoga classes, and weight loss consultations.

Dead Sea mud—mineral-rich, highly saline mud that draws impurities and retains heat; used for a wide range of skin disorders such as psoriasis and eczema; especially beneficial for muscle pain and stiffness, arthritis, and other joint pain.

Dead Sea salts—harvested from the Dead Sea; contain magnesium and potassium that are used for their cleansing, detoxification, and restorative properties, especially for the skin and muscles.

Decongestant—substance or application that breaks up mucus.

Dehydration—condition in which there is an abnormal depletion of body fluids.

de la Bonnardiere, Joseph—French physician who had a practice in the sea-bathing resort in the town of Arcachon; coined the word *thalassotherapy* in 1865 as the term to encompass the treatments based on the healing benefits of the sea.

Derivation—process of using heat to draw blood and lymph from one part of the body to the other.

Dermis—layer of skin underneath the epidermis; composed of connective tissue (protein and adipose tissue); blood vessels, nerves, sudoriferous (sweat) glands, sebaceous glands, and hair follicles are all embedded in the dermis.

Desert mineral salts—gathered from deserts that are the remnants of prehistoric oceans; the most common desert mineral salt is borax; another example is Redmond salt.

Destination spa—locations to which guests travel for multiple-day stays. The focal point of the programs offered is to enhance health and well being. Individualized for each guest, these programs can assist in detoxifying, smoking cessation, increasing strength and flexibility, better nutrition, and incorporating stress-reduction techniques into each guest's life. Guests' progress is closely monitored by health care professionals. Complementary treatments and activities help guests integrate their body, mind, and spirit. Examples include bodywork and spa therapies, yoga, hiking, labyrinth walking, and meditation.

Detoxifier—substance or application that helps eliminate toxins from the body.

Diaphoresis—perspiration or sweating.

Disinfectant—substance applied to nonliving objects to destroy microorganisms.

Dissolving (chemical, enzyme) exfoliation—uses exfoliants that consist of chemicals or enzymes that work by dissolving dead skin cells; after application, the enzymes are washed or rubbed off.

Distillation—process in which a solution, consisting of water and a substance such as parts of a plant, is boiled. The resulting evaporation is cooled or condensed, forming a liquid, which is then captured. It contains the "essence" of the plant that was distilled.

Dosha—term meaning "that which changes." According to Ayurvedic principles, five elements combine in pairs to form three dynamic forces called *doshas* that are constantly interacting with one another or moving in dynamic balance. The three primary doshas are Vata, Pitta, and Kapha.

Dry brushing (body brushing)—exfoliation using brushes or fiber tools.

Dry room—treatment room with no specialized shower facilities.

Edema—abnormal accumulation of interstitial fluid.

Effectors—muscle tissue and glands that respond to the nerve impulses.

Efferent (motor) nerves—peripheral nerves that carry nerve impulses away from the CNS to effectors; send impulses out to muscle tissue to make it contract or relax and/or to glands to make them increase or decrease their secretions.

Electrolytes—ionic compounds that dissociate into cations and anions in a solution; electrolytes are so called because their solutions can conduct electricity.

Electron—small, negatively charged particles that travel in a large space around the nucleus of an atom.

Element—substance that cannot be split into a simpler substance by ordinary chemical means; elements are the building blocks of all matter, living and nonliving.

Emollient—substance that makes the skin soft and supple.

Emperor Augustus (63 BC–AD 14)—Roman emperor who was cured of illness by cold baths; played a role in increasing the popularity of bathing in Rome.

Emulsifier—chemical that breaks large drops of fat into smaller drops so they mix better in a solution.

Emulsion—a fluid that has particles suspended in it because the particles do not dissolve.

Enzyme (chemical, dissolving) exfoliation—uses exfoliants that consist of chemicals or enzymes that work by dissolving dead skin cells; after application, the enzymes are washed or rubbed off.

Epidermis—superficial aspect of the skin, forming the surface of the body; it has many layers of densely packed cells and is avascular.

Epsom salt—named for the mineral-rich waters of Epsom, England, where it was first discovered in 1618; contains magnesium sulfate and can be used internally or externally for bath soaks to relieve aches and pains.

Erythrocyte—red blood cell; carries oxygen to the cells and a small amount of carbon dioxide from the cells.

Essence—a substance derived through physical or chemical means that possesses the special qualities (as of a plant) in concentrated form.

Essential oils—volatile plant oils extracted from certain aromatic plants that have both physiological and psychological effects on the human body.

Esthetician—person who specializes in the study of skin care and the application of skin care products and services.

Evaporation—the conversion from liquid into vapor.

Exfoliant—substance or process that removes dead skin cells.

Exfoliation—the peeling and sloughing off of dead skin cells from the surface of the body; from the Latin *exfoliare*, meaning "to strip of leaves."

Extractor—substance or application that draws impurities from the skin.

Fahrenheit, Daniel Gabriel (1686–1736)—German physicist and maker of scientific instruments; invented the alcohol thermometer in 1709 and the mercury thermometer in 1714; developed the Fahrenheit temperature scale, which is still in use in the United States.

Flotation (sensory deprivation) tank or room—tank or small tiled room that is filled with body-temperature water (94 to 98°F) to a depth of approximately 10 inches. Enough Epsom salt is dissolved in the water to allow the body to float. The tank or room can be closed to all exposure to sound and light so the client can experience true sensory deprivation for a session that lasts 20 to 60 minutes.

Floyer, Sir John (1649–1734)—English physician who was a passionate advocate of hydrotherapy. In 1697, he wrote *An Enquiry into the Right Use and Abuses of Hot, Cold and Temperate Baths in England*, which was later released as *The History of Cold Bathing*.

Fluid balance—condition in which the various parts of the body have the amount of water and solutes (dissolved particles) they need to function properly.

Fluxion—increased blood flow into an area; brings more blood cells and nutrients to the area and transports cell debris and other wastes away from the area.

Fomentation—hot compress.

French Argiletz clay—mined in Argiletz, France. It comes in all five clay colors and is used quite often for face, hand, and body masks. Sometimes this clay is referred to as French clay, as in French green or French white. French Argiletz clay is an illite.

Friction (scrub)—manual exfoliation method using salts or coarser organic substances.

Frigid—intensely cold.

Frigidarium—the cold room in a Roman bath; included a cold pool.

Fucus (wracks)—a brown seaweed used in spa and hydrotherapy treatments for detoxification, revitalization (through increased local blood and lymph circulation), slimming, and skin tightening.

Fuller's earth—smectite clay that draws oils; used therapeutically in masks for oily skin and to treat acne.

Galen (circa AD 200)—prominent Roman physician who studied the human body extensively; incorporated baths as an integral part of his remedies.

Galileo (1564–1642)—Italian physicist, mathematician, astronomer, and philosopher; credited with the invention of the thermometer in 1592.

Gattefosse, Rene-Maurice (1881–1950)—French chemist and perfumer; researched the benefits of essential oils, especially their antimicrobial properties; wrote several scientific papers about essential oils; in 1937, he wrote *Aromatherapie: Les Huiles essentielles, hormons vegetales (Aromatherapy: The Essential Oils, Vegetable Hormones); coined the term *aromatherapy.*

General (systemic)—the entire body; for example, a systemic treatment is applied to the entire body, and a systemic contraindication means that the treatment should not be applied anywhere on the body.

Geothermal—treatments involving hot stones; comes from the Greek words *geo*, meaning "earth" and *thermal* meaning "heat."

Green seaweeds—found near shores in shallow waters; usually grow in threadlike filaments, sheets, or branching fronds. One of the most common green seaweeds used in spa treatments is sea lettuce *(Ulva lactuca),* which is used in spa and hydrotherapy treatments to relieve inflammation and muscle soreness.

Hahn, Dr. Johann Sigmund (1696–1773)—influenced by Sir John Floyer's book, *The History of Cold Bathing*, he is credited with instituting the principles of modern hydrotherapy in Germany.

Hammam—Turkish bath. Bathers first relax in a warm, dry room that causes the bathers to perspire profusely and then move on to an even hotter room to perspire even more. After that, they splash themselves with cold water and then wash themselves completely in a warm room before receiving a massage. The massage is followed by sitting in a cooling room and relaxing for a period of time.

Heat capacity—measure of the heat energy required to increase the temperature of an object by a certain temperature interval.

Heat cramps—muscle cramps that result from loss of fluid and electrolytes from the body; can be remedied by stopping the heat treatment and replacing the fluids and electrolytes.

Heat exhaustion—symptoms include cool, moist, clammy skin (resulting from profuse sweating), and muscle cramps, dizziness, vomiting, and fainting from the loss of fluid and electrolytes; the client's body needs to be cooled down immediately and the fluids and electrolytes replaced. Medical intervention may be necessary.

Heat stroke—occurs when relative humidity and heat are high, making it difficult for the body to lose heat. In extreme cases, body temperature may reach 110°F, resulting in possible brain damage (death occurs at if body temperature reaches 112 to 114°F); because the body will not get back into homeostasis by itself, the person needs to be immersed in cool water and given fluids and electrolytes by health care professionals.

Henry VIII (1491–1547)—English king who closed holy wells that had been pilgrimage sites. This eventually led to the encouragement of public baths and the popularity of spa towns such as Bath, Buxton, and Harrogate.

Herb—plant or plant part valued for its medicinal, savory, or aromatic qualities.

Hippocrates (circa 460–370 BC)—Greek physician known as the "Father of Modern Medicine"; prescribed water to treat physical and mental disorders and documented the phenomenon of using water at various temperatures to create a healing response.

Homeostasis—relative consistency in the body's internal environment.

Hot towel cabi—electric cabinet that stores rolled moist towels at a temperature of about 175°F; many have a built-in UV sanitizer that keeps the towels hygienic until they can be used.

Hubbard tank—specially constructed full-immersion tank. It is equipped with a hoist for lifting and supporting patients who are injured or immobile. It has support bars for doing water exercise and jets for hydrotherapy massage. Therapists assist patients with stretching and joint mobilization exercises and gentle range of motion.

Hydration—condition in which the body has enough fluids.

Hydrocollator—an electronic stainless steel tank filled with water that is 160 to 165°F. Holds pads made of canvas and filled with heat-absorbing clay. Once heated, the pads are applied to the body and the heat penetrates to loosen tight muscles.

Hydrosol—the watery by-products from the distillation of plant products.

Hydrostatic pressure—when water is contained, the pressure or force it exerts against all sides of the container and against anything that is in the water.

Hydrotherapy—the use of water in the treatment of various mental and physical disorders; from the Greek *hydro* meaning "water" and *therapies* meaning "treatment," one of Kneipp's five fundamental principles described in *Meine Wasser Kur (My Water Cure).*

Hydrotherapy (hydro) tub—a large tub used for hydro massage. It is specially designed with jets and an underwater pressure hose that can be directed to areas of tension on the client's body.

Hygeia—Greek goddess of health and sanitation; daughter of Asclepios. Her name is the origin of the word *hygiene.*

Hygiene—conditions or cleanliness practices that are conducive to health.

Hyperemia—reddening of the skin caused by an increased blood flow to the area.

Hypertension—high blood pressure.

Hypocaust—system to heat Roman baths; pillars raised the floor off the ground and spaces were left inside the walls where hot air from the furnace could circulate.

Hypodermis (subcutaneous layer, superficial fascia)—layer underneath the dermis that is not part of the skin; anchors the skin to underlying structures such as muscles and bones.

Hypotension—low blood pressure.

Hypothalamus—controls many physiological functions and plays a major role in the regulation of homeostasis. It is responsible for, among other things, controlling the autonomic nervous system and regulating emotional and behavioral patterns.

Hypothermia—lowered core body temperature.

Ibn Sina (973–1037)—also known as Avicenna; Persian physician who practiced throughout Arabia. He based his practice on the teachings of Galen and did further research and experimentation in medicine. His chief work, *Canon Medicinae*, served as the most important textbook for physicians in Western society until the Renaissance.

Illite—a nonexpanding clay; it does not swell when in contact with water; an example of illite clay is French green.

Immersion bath—bath in which the person is submerged up to the neck.

Indication—a factor or body condition that would be relieved by the application of a particular treatment; a reason to perform a treatment.

Infusion—involves steeping plants, much like a tea, in hot water. Boiling water is poured over parts of a fragrant plant—leaves, flowers, or berries. The plants are then left to stand for 15 to 30 minutes, or longer for a stronger infusion. An oil infusion involves placing plant parts in oil and leaving them to stand for weeks. The herb or botanical is removed from the oil or water through straining, and the remaining oil or water then is used.

Ion—a positively or negatively charged atom; results from either gaining electrons, making it negatively charged (anion), or losing electrons, making it positively charged (cation).

Ionic bond—chemical bond formed between the attraction of a cation and an anion.

Irish moss (*Chondrus crispus*, carrageen, carrageen moss)—red seaweed that grows in shallow waters, especially around the British Isles; it is used in spa and hydrotherapy treatments for detoxification, revitalization (through increased local blood and lymph circulation), slimming, skin tightening, and moisturizing.

Interstitial fluid—fluid that surrounds body cells.

Jacuzzi® (whirlpool)—tub with high-pressure jets that circulate heated water. The temperature of the water is 100 to 108°F, and a session usually lasts 20 to 30 minutes.

Jet Blitz (Blitzguss)—therapeutic cold shower treatment using a high-pressure stream of water directed at different parts of the body, focusing on muscular areas. This is stimulating and intense and is done for strengthening the body's vitality and immune response by decreasing superficial circulation, driving blood to the core of the body. The temperature and duration of the treatment vary depending on the goals of the treatment.

Kaolinate—clay that has a low capacity to swell when in contact with water; commercial names for it are kaolin, China white, and China clay.

Kapha—in Ayurveda, means "that which is solid and grounded"; combination of water and earth; main function is providing cohesion, binding, and containment; controls structure and lubrication, such as the cells that make up the organs and the fluids that nourish and protect them. Kapha attributes are solid, heavy, slow, dense, smooth, round, methodical, articulate, easy going, and faithful. Kapha body types are physically large frames and heavy builds.

Kellogg, John Harvey (1852–1943)—medical superintendent of the Health Reform Institute, which became the Battle Creek Sanitarium; coined the term *sanitarium*; developed the "Battle Creek Idea" that good health and fitness were the result of good diet, exercise, correct posture, fresh air, and proper rest.

Kelp (*Laminaria*)—brown seaweed used in spa and hydrotherapy treatments for detoxification, revitalization (through increased local blood and lymph circulation), slimming, and skin tightening.

Keratin—protein, produced by keratinocytes, which makes skin waterproof.

Kinesiotherapy—movement, exercise, and massage; one of Kneipp's five fundamental principles described in *Meine Wasser Kur (My Water Cure)*.

Kneipp, Father Sebastian (1821–1897)—known as the "Father of Hydrotherapy," he wrote *Meine Wasser Kur (My Water Cure)*, published in 1866, which describes his course of water treatments. His approach to healing was holistic, encouraging "the balance between work and leisure, stress, and relaxation; and the harmony between the mental, emotional, physical, social, and ecological planes."

Labrum—waist-high fountain in the caldarium in a Roman bath; contained cool water to splash on the head and neck.

Laminaria (kelp)—brown seaweed used in spa and hydrotherapy treatments for detoxification, revitalization (through increased local blood and lymph circulation), slimming, and skin tightening.

Leukocyte—white blood cell; functions in protecting the body from disease.

Lichen (white algae)—combination of a fungus and an organism, usually a type of green algae, that produces food for the lichen from sunlight. Spirulina and white algae treatments are used in spa treatments for detoxification, revitalization (through increased local blood and lymph circulation), slimming, skin tightening, and moisturizing.

Limbic system—located within the higher brain, or cerebrum; sometimes referred to as the "emotional brain" because it has major role in a variety of emotions—pleasure, affection, passivity, fear, sorrow, sexual feelings, and anger. It is also involved in memory and olfaction.

Liniments—liquid preparations that cause a soothing, cooling, warming, or analgesic action when applied to the skin.

Lithothamnium—a type of red algae that leaves behind a calcified skeleton when it dies; it can be ground and used as a natural exfoliation substance.

Local (zonal, regional)—specific part of the body; for example, a local treatment is applied to one area of the body; a local contraindication means that a treatment should not be applied to that region but can be applied elsewhere on the body; a local response is one that occurs only in the area of the application.

Lust, Benedict (1872–1945)—combined the Kneipp cure with other modalities he had learned from many other European physicians who focused on natural cures; formed the foundation of naturopathic medicine as it is known today.

Lymphocyte—specialized type of white blood cell.

Manual exfoliation—physical process of applying friction with abrasives; manual exfoliants include dry brushes, mitts, loofahs, abrasive cloths, and abrasive natural substances such as salt, sugar, cornmeal, and coffee. These substances are typically mixed with water, oils, or crèmes before being rubbed over the surface of the skin.

Marma—in Ayurveda, energetic points located near the surface of the body.

Maury, Marguerite (1895–1968)—Austrian biochemist who lived in France; explored the psychological and physiological benefits from applying essential oils to the skin. She is credited with popularizing the topical application of essential oils and, of special interest to bodyworkers, incorporating the use of essential oils into massage therapy. Her work emphasized that using massage therapy and aromatherapy together created more benefit for the client than if each treatment were applied separately. This helped move aromatherapy into the realm of complementary therapies.

Medical spa (medspa)—The focus is on integrating the mind-body-spirit connection with medical procedures. Full-time, licensed health care professionals such as physicians, nurses, and nurse practitioners manage and oversee the programs and facilities. Guests are given thorough medical examinations and their health histories are discussed. Individualized treatment plans are designed for them and their progress is closely monitored. Some medical spas are for day use only; some have on-site accommodations for multiple-day stays.

Metabolic rate—the overall rate at which the chemical reactions of the body use energy.

Metabolism—all the chemical reactions of the body.

Microorganism—any life form that is microscopic; sometimes used instead of the term *pathogen*.

Middle notes—essential oil classification by the French perfume industry; notes refer to scent characteristics and the rate at which the oil evaporates; middle notes are warm, soft fragrances that unfold gradually. They are the balancing and harmonizing scents.

Mineral—inorganic element that occurs naturally in the Earth's crust.

Mineral spring spa—has as its basis a source of mineral or hot spring water; the waters are used for their healing properties. Some of these spas use seawater in addition to or instead of mineral springs. Generally, there are pools for guests to enjoy, and some mineral spring spas also offer bodywork and spa therapies. Spa may be for day use only, although certain ones have accommodations for multiple-day stays.

Molecule—the resulting combination when two or more atoms share electrons.

Montmorillonite—clay discovered in Montmorillon, France, in 1847. Found in many locations worldwide, it is a green clay and a smectite.

Moor mud—a type of peat also known as "black mud" because of its appearance. It is the mineral-rich sedimentation that is deposited at the bottom of lakes and rivers fed by both hot and cool springs.

Moor peat pack—organic moor peat sealed between layers of a permeable material and plastic. The permeable layer allows almost direct contact between the skin and the peat, while preventing the peat from sticking to the skin, and the plastic traps heat or cold and keeps it from leaving the body. These are sometimes called "foment pads."

Motor (efferent) nerves—peripheral nerves that carry nerve impulses away from the CNS to effectors; send impulses out to muscle tissue to make it contract or relax and/or to glands to make them increase or decrease their secretions.

Neuropathy—any disorder involving nerves.

Neutron—neutral particle found within the nucleus of an atom.

Nucleus—the dense center of an atom; found inside most body cells and contains the cell's genetic material (DNA).

Nutrition—the act or process of nourishing or being nourished; nutrition (a well-balanced diet) is one of Kneipp's five fundamental principles described in *Meine Wasser Kur* (*My Water Cure*).

O-furo—a Japanese family's deep-soaking tub.

Oil (sebaceous) gland—gland in the dermis of the skin that secretes oil (sebum).

Olfaction—sense of smell.

Olfaction bulbs—components of the limbic system; nervous tissue that plays a role in the brain's interpretation and differentiation of all the diverse aromas detected by the human nose; send nerve impulses along the olfactory tract.

Olfactory epithelium—specialized tissue with thousands of receptors for sense of smell located in the superior part of the nasal cavity. These receptors are the endings of nerve fibers that carry impulses for the sense of smell into the olfactory bulbs.

Olfactory tract—receives nerve impulses from olfaction bulbs; extends into parts of the brain that identify odors and that distinguish different odors; also extends into the part of the brain where conscious awareness of smell begins, as well as into the limbic system and hypothalamus. It is this connection to the limbic system and hypothalamus that accounts for emotional and memory-based responses to aromas.

Onsen—Japanese term for natural, mineral-rich hot springs.

Osmosis—movement of water from an area of higher concentration of solutes to an area of lower concentration of solutes.

Overhead—ongoing operating costs of running a business.

Parafango—mixture of dehydrated volcanic mud and paraffin, with talcum and magnesium oxide added; also provides the slow release of healing warmth.

Paraffin—waxy by-product from the processing of petroleum, wood, coal, or shale. Discovered to be a good insulator, it is used in spa and hydrotherapy treatments to increase heat penetration into the body.

Paraffin unit—an electronic appliance that safely melts paraffin and keeps it at the temperature required for application to the body (125 to 130°F).

Parasympathetic branch—division of the autonomic nervous system that is responsible for maintenance of the body's daily functions; also known as "rest and digest."

Partial bath—bath performed on body parts that need specific attention.

Pascalite—unearthed in Wyoming by French Canadian fur trapper Emile Pascale in 1830. It is a white clay that closely resembles montmorillonite and bentonite but is a nonswelling clay or illite.

Pathogen—disease-causing organism such as a bacterium, virus, or fungus.

Peat—organic soil that contains minerals, organic material, water, and trapped air. Because of their therapeutic properties, peats are used to help relieve aching muscles and joints and pain from muscle injuries and noninflammatory stages of arthritis and to soothe skin disorders.

Peloids (pelos)—fine grains making up muds, clays, and peat. They are highly absorbent and possess unique heat-retention abilities.

Pelotherapy—therapeutic use of muds, clays, peat, earth salts, paraffin, and stones; *pelo-* is Greek for "mud."

Percussion (jet) shower—shower in which a special high-pressure shower head called a Scotch douche produces a highly pressured stream of water of varying temperature (beginning at 94°F and increasing from there) that is directed at muscular areas of the body.

Peripheral nervous system (PNS)—all the nervous tissue outside the central nervous system.

pH—reflection of the acidity and alkalinity of solutions.

pH scale—scale that shows the acidity and alkalinity of solutions; 7 represents a neutral solution; lower numbers indicate increasing acidity and higher numbers indicate increasing alkalinity; each unit of measurement represents a tenfold change in acidity or alkalinity.

Phytotherapy—therapeutic use of plants; phytotherapy (natural herbal remedies, teas, oils, and juices) is one of Kneipp's five fundamental principles described in *Meine Wasser Kur (My Water Cure)*.

Pitta—In Ayurveda, means "the principle of transformation"; combination of fire and water; main function is transformation, also heat production and digestion; controls enzymes that digest food, hormones that regulate metabolism, transformation of nerve impulses into thoughts. Pitta attributes are hot, moist, radiant, intense, focused, oily, passionate, and confident. Pitta body types are physically medium, athletic builds.

Plasma—the liquid portion of blood.

Prana—Ayurvedic concept; life force or energy of the body (it is comparable to Qi in traditional Chinese medicine); its vehicle is the breath. Prana gives and maintains life and unifies the person. It travels throughout the body and can be accessed at *marmas*, which are energetic points located near the surface of the body.

Preissnitz, Vincent (1799–1851)—Austrian practitioner who is one of the people credited with bringing ancient hydrotherapy techniques to prominence today; designed the Priessnitz cure—a regimen of wrapping the body with wet sheets, cold baths, fresh air, healthy diet, and physical exercise. He also carefully organized and documented his treatments and was instrumental in bringing the world's attention to hydrotherapy.

Proton—positively charged particle found within the nucleus of an atom.

Pumice—volcanic rock.

Quinton, Rene—French marine biologist who wrote *L'Eau de Mer, Milleu Organique (Sea Water, Organic Medium)* in 1906; based on his studies of human blood plasma and lymph, Quinton discovered that seawater is chemically identical to both.

Radiation—transfer of heat in the form of infrared rays from warmer to cooler objects without contact.

Receptor—specialized nerve tissue that receives a stimulation or sensation and converts it to nerve impulses.

Redmond Salt—desert mineral salt initially discovered near Redmond, Utah. Redmond salt contains more than 50 trace minerals, which give it a slight pink color. It is certified kosher and comes in many grain sizes that can be used internally or externally for salt baths and exfoliations.

Red seaweeds—delicate and fernlike; many grow at great depths, down to 879 feet; their red pigment allows them to absorb the small amount of blue and violet light that penetrates to this level and use this light to produce oxygen. *Chondrus crispus* grows in more shallow waters, especially around the British Isles and is called Irish moss, carrageen, or carrageen moss. It is used in spa and hydrotherapy treatments for detoxification, revitalization (through increased local blood and lymph circulation), slimming, skin tightening, and moisturizing. *Lithothamnium,* another type of red algae, leaves behind a calcified skeleton when it dies that can be ground and used as a natural exfoliation substance.

Reflex (consensual) response—stimulation such as application of heat or cold to one area resulting in a response in another area of the body.

Regional (local, zonal)—specific part of the body; for example, a regional treatment is applied to one area of the body, and a regional contraindication means that a treatment should not be applied to that region but can be applied elsewhere on the body.

Regulative therapy—mental, emotional, and spiritual balance in one's life; one of Kneipp's five fundamental principles described in *Meine Wasser Kur (My Water Cure).*

Rehydration—process of replacing fluids to counteract dehydration.

Resort/hotel spa—spa in a setting such as hotels and cruise ships offering guests a menu of choices for relaxation, stress relief, and beauty enhancement.

Restorative—a substance or process that refreshes and renews the body.

Retrostasis—the act of pushing blood or lymph away from an area of the body by applying cold.

Revulsive—prolonged application of heat followed by a brief application of cold.

Russell, Dr. Richard (1687–1759)—English physician who published his *Dissertation on the Use of Sea Water* in 1752; it encouraged people to visit the seaside to improve their health, ushering in an era of seawater cures.

Ryokan—traditional Japanese inn.

St. Thomas Aquinas (1225–1274)—scholar, member of the Dominican order, and influential Christian philosopher. His study and interpretations of the works of Aristotle countered the Catholic Church's tendency to reject Greek philosophy and led, eventually, to a new acceptance of Aristotle's philosophies, including the virtues of cleanliness.

Sanitation—practices that ensure good health and cleanliness.

Sauna—Finnish hot vapor bath that evolved from portable sweat lodges used by nomadic tribes. It is a small wooden room or hut with benches that is heated by steam from water poured on hot stones for ritual and/or therapeutic sweating. The treatment ends with a cold plunge into icy water or snow.

Savusauna—smoke sauna that has a large wood-burning heater with 200- to 300-pound rocks and no stove pipe; the smoke is allowed to remain in the sauna while the sauna is heating up to the desired temperature. The smoke is released through a small vent before the sauna is used.

Scotch douche—special shower head that produces a highly pressured stream of water of varying temperature (beginning at 94°F and increasing from there).

Scrub (friction)—manual exfoliation method using salts or coarser organic substances.

Sea lettuce (*Ulva lactuca*)—common green seaweed used in spa and hydrotherapy treatments to relieve inflammation and muscle soreness.

Sea mud—collected from beaches at low tide and mixed with seawater. Like all sea products, it is used for its analgesic, warming, and sedative properties, as well as for detoxification. Sea mud can be used by itself or mixed with clays or paraffin.

Sea salt—formed by the natural evaporation of ocean water; harvested when seawater is left to dry in the sun. Sea salt can be used for salt scrubs, baths, and inhalation treatments.

Seaweed—an umbrella term for any marine plant or algae; it has chlorophyll, which allows it to produce oxygen as plants do, but it does not have true roots, stems, or leaves. Seaweed is actually algae, which are groups of aquatic organisms that perform photosynthesis.

Sebaceous (oil) gland—gland in the dermis of the skin that secretes oil (sebum).

Sedative—substance or application that calms muscles and nerves and can induce a state of relaxation.

Segment—each section of the spinal cord from which a pair of spinal nerves arises.

Sensory deprivation (flotation) tank or room—tank or small tiled room that is filled with body-temperature water (94 to 98°F) to a depth of approximately 10 inches. Enough Epsom salt is dissolved in the water to allow the body to float. The tank or room can be closed to all exposure to sound and light so the client can experience true sensory deprivation for a session that lasts 20 to 60 minutes.

Sensory (afferent) nerves—peripheral nerves that send nerve impulses into the CNS; nerves detect sensations.

Sento—Japanese public bath.

Shell temperature—temperature at the body's surface, or on the skin.

Shirodara—Ayurvedic treatment; herbal oil or infusion with medicated milk or buttermilk is poured in a steady stream on the client's forehead for 20 to 50 minutes, followed by a gentle scalp massage and possibly facial or head and neck massage. With the goal of balancing the doshas, this treatment focuses on relaxing the nervous system and balancing the prana around the head. It improves the function of the five senses and helps with insomnia, stress, anxiety, depression, hair loss, and fatigue.

Sitz bath—shallow, hip, or half bath (*sitz* means "sit" in German); partial bath that addresses the lower back, abdomen, pelvis, and lower extremities. Specially designed tubs are often found in hospitals and physical rehabilitation centers. In these facilities, a sitz bath is used most commonly after childbirth or to encourage postsurgical healing.

Smectite—clays that absorb water and swell considerably; examples of smectite clays are bentonites and Fuller's earth.

Solute—a dissolved substance.

Solution—the combination of a dissolved substance and the liquid in which the substance is dissolved.

Solvent—a liquid that dissolves another substance.

Somatic nervous system (SNS)—division of the peripheral nervous system that controls skeletal muscles and voluntary movements.

Spa—a mineral spring; a resort with mineral springs; a venue providing facilities devoted to health, fitness, weight loss, beauty, and relaxation; can also stand for *sanitas per agua* or *salud per agua*—health or healing via water.

Spa experience—subjective perception of a visit to a spa. Factors include health and wellness services, atmosphere, communication, staff professionalism, communication, and treatment-performance skills of practitioners.

Spinal nerves—peripheral nerves that communicate directly with the spinal cord.

Spirulina—a type of blue-green algae.

Standard (universal) precautions—protocols established by the Centers for Disease Control and Prevention (CDC) to reduce the chance of spreading contagious diseases within health care settings. These protocols are designed to protect both the patient and health care provider.

Stimulant—substance or application that excites the muscles and nerves and can invigorate the body.

Strigil—curved metal instrument Romans used to scrape off body dirt and oil.

Subcutaneous layer (hypodermis, superficial fascia)—layer underneath the dermis that is not part of the skin; anchors the skin to underlying structures such as muscles and bones.

Sudoriferous (sweat) gland—gland in the dermis of the skin that secretes perspiration (sweat).

Superficial fascia (hypodermis, subcutaneous layer)—layer underneath the dermis that is not part of the skin; anchors the skin to underlying structures such as muscles and bones.

Sweat (sudoriferous) gland—gland in the dermis of the skin that secretes perspiration (sweat).

Sweat lodge—Native American huts, lodges, caverns, or other small buildings that are heated by steam from water poured on hot stones for ritual and/or therapeutic sweating.

Sydenham, Dr. Thomas (1624–1689)—challenged common medical practices, especially that of blood letting. He did not believe in an authoritarian medical system; instead, he based his practice and teaching on independent reasoning. He

is considered one of the most important revivers of the views of Hippocrates, and he regularly used ancient applications, such as the use of water, to treat common ailments.

Sympathetic branch—division of the autonomic nervous system that overrides the parasympathetic branch during emergencies and exercise; also known as "fight or flight."

Systemic (general)—the entire body; for example, a systemic treatment is applied to the entire body; a systemic contraindication means that the treatment should not be applied anywhere on the body; a systemic response occurs within the entire body.

Taking the waters—term for traveling to mineral spring spas and spending time bathing in the water.

Temezcalli—sweat lodges in ancient Mexico; in the Aztec language of Nahuatl, *teme* meant "to bathe," and *calli* was the word for "house."

Tepid—moderately warm or lukewarm.

Tepidarium—the warm room in a Roman bath; had heated walls and floors, sometimes without a pool of water.

Thalassotherapy—use of the sea and sea products to maintain health and wellness; includes sea air, sea mud, sea salt, and seawater.

Thermae—public Roman baths.

Thermophore pad—electric heating pad covered in a fleece blend. The cover draws humidity from the air and retains it. When the pad is turned on, the heat forces moisture out of the cover and onto the body.

Thermoregulation—regulation of body temperature.

Thrombocyte—platelet; functions in clotting blood.

Tisserand, Robert—(b. November 11, 1948) well-known English aromatherapist and massage therapist who wrote the first edition of *The Art of Aromatherapy* in 1977. This work helped draw attention to aromatherapy in current culture. Tisserand works closely with doctors and herbalists and tracks all published scientific research relevant to essential oils. He lectures around the world and is the author of several more books on aromatherapy.

Tonic—treatments, such as those involving cold, that result in increased muscle tone.

Tonifier—substance or application that stimulates, invigorates, and strengthens vitality and the immune system.

Tonify—stimulate, invigorate, and strengthen vitality and the immune system.

Top notes—essential oil classification by the French perfume industry; notes refer to scent characteristics and the rate at which the oil evaporates; top notes have light, fresh, and uplifting qualities; since they evaporate quickly, their scents are usually not long lasting.

Turkish bath—common term for a *hammam*. Bathers first relax in a warm, dry room that causes them to perspire profusely and then move on to an even hotter room to perspire even more. After that, they splash themselves with cold water and then wash themselves completely in a warm room before receiving a massage. The massage is followed by sitting in a cooling room and relaxing for a period of time.

Ulva lactuca **(sea lettuce)**—common green seaweed used in spa and hydrotherapy treatments to relieve inflammation and muscle soreness.

Universal (standard) precautions—protocols established by the Centers for Disease Control and Prevention (CDC) to reduce the chance of spreading contagious diseases within health care settings. These protocols are designed to protect both the patient and health care provider.

Valnet, Dr. Jean (1920–1995)—French physician who further developed Gattefosse's findings; experimented with essential oils and, during World War II, used them as antiseptics in the treatment of wounded soldiers.

Vascular diseases—any of a number of diseases affecting blood vessels. Examples include Raynaud's disease, in which blood vessels in fingers and toes vasoconstrict abnormally in response to cold or emotional stress, or Buerger's disease (thromboangiitis obliterans), in which small and medium-sized arteries, usually in a foot or leg, become inflamed and subject to forming clots.

Vascular gymnastics (vasogymnastics)—pumping action of blood into and out of an area of the body.

Vasoconstriction—decrease in the diameter of a blood vessel resulting in less blood flowing through the vessel.

Vasoconstrictor—substance or process that decreases the diameter of a blood vessel.

Vasodilation—increase in the diameter of a blood vessel resulting in more blood flowing through the vessel.

Vasodilator—substance or process that decreases the diameter of a blood vessel.

Vasogymnastics (vascular gymnastics)—pumping action of blood into and out of an area of the body.

Vata—in Ayurveda, means "that which moves things"; the combination of ether and air; main function is that of propulsion and movement; controls all movement in the mind and body—nerve impulses, thoughts, air in and out of the lungs, blood and lymph flow, food moving through digestive tract, and waste elimination from the body. Vata attributes are light, erratic, sinuous, thin, cold, dry, excitable, creative, and spiritually oriented. Vata body types are physically thin with prominent joints and long limbs.

Vichy shower—shower with multiple nozzles that hang above the client. The practitioner controls the temperature, pressure, and amount of water used to rinse off the client.

Volatile—able to vaporize easily at low temperatures.

Water Dance (Wassertanzen®)—a form of underwater aquatic bodywork similar to Watsu except that both practitioner and client are completely underwater while the practitioner takes the client through a series of gentle gyrations and stretches.

Water intoxication—state in which excessive body water causes cells to swell dangerously because of lost body water and Na^+ being replaced by drinking plain water; characterized by convulsions, coma, and, possibly, death.

Watsu®—treatment performed in a pool of water at body temperature (98°F). The practitioner performs a series of stretches and pressure-point massage on the client to strengthen muscles and increase flexibility.

Wesley, John (1703–1791)—founder of the Methodist Church; recognized the correlation between bathing and health and coined the phrase, "Cleanliness is next to Godliness." In 1747, he wrote *Primitive Physick*, which asserted that cold baths could cure certain afflictions. This book brought social awareness to cold bathing and was a profound influence on the popularization of hydrotherapy.

Wet room—treatment room with a specialized water supply, such as showers, and floor drainage so that substances can be removed from clients' bodies; may also contain hydrotherapy tubs.

Wet table—treatment table with a drain so that substances can be removed from clients' bodies; may have an attached or separate water supply such as a Vichy shower.

Whirlpool (Jacuzzi)®—tub with high-pressure jets that circulate heated water. The temperature of the water is 100 to 108°F, and a session usually lasts 20 to 30 minutes.

White algae (lichen)—combination of a fungus and an organism, usually a type of green algae, that produces food for the lichen from sunlight. Spirulina and white algae treatments are used in spa treatments for detoxification, revitalization (through increased local blood and lymph circulation), slimming, skin tightening, and moisturizing.

White, Ellen G. (1827–1915)—one of the founders of Seventh Day Adventism and noted health reformer; focused on the importance and benefits of nature's remedies: pure water, clean air, sunshine, healthy diet, and exercise. Ellen and her husband James opened the Health Reform Institute in Battle Creek, MI, where hydrotherapy was practiced.

Wracks (*Fucus*)—a brown seaweed used in spa and hydrotherapy treatments for detoxification, revitalization (through increased local blood and lymph circulation), slimming, and skin tightening.

Zonal (local, regional)—specific part of the body; for example, a zonal treatment is applied to one area of the body, and a zonal contraindication means that a treatment should not be applied to that area but can be applied elsewhere on the body.

Index

Page numbers with f indicate figures; those with t indicate tables.